SOCIAL WORK with
HIV & AIDS

Also available from Lyceum Books, Inc.

Advisory Editor: Thomas M. Meenaghan, New York University

A Case-Based Guide

SOCIAL WORK with HIV & AIDS

DIANA ROWAN
and Contributors

LYCEUM
BOOKS, INC.

Chicago, IL 60637

© Lyceum Books, Inc., 2013

Published by
  LYCEUM BOOKS, INC.
  5758 S. Blackstone Ave.
  Chicago, Illinois 60637
  773-643-1903 (Fax)
  773-643-1902 (Phone)
  lyceum@lyceumbooks.com
  http://www.lyceumbooks.com

6 5 4 3 2 1   13 14 15 16

ISBN 978-1-933478-81-4

Cover photo by Diana Rowan. On left is Lamont Holley (chapter contributor) and on right is Kevin Edwards (chapter contributor).

Artwork for part openers by Richard Hull.

Printed in the United States of America.

Library of Congress Cataloging-in-Publication Data

Rowan, Diana.
  Social work with HIV & AIDS : a case-based guide / by Diana Rowan and Contributors.
    p. cm.
  ISBN 978-1-933478-81-4 (pbk. : alk. paper)
  1. AIDS (Disease)—Social aspects—United States. 2. HIV-positive persons—Services for—United States. 3. AIDS (Disease)—Patients—Services for—United States. 4. Social service—United States. 5. Social case work—United States. I. Title.
  RA643.83.R69 2013
  362.19697¢9200973—dc23

                                                          2012010909

When spiderwebs unite, they can tie up a lion.

—**Ethiopian proverb**

Contents

Boxes, Figures, and Tables

Figures

Tables

Foreword

I am deeply honored to have been invited to write the foreword for this important book on social work HIV (human immunodeficiency virus) and AIDS (acquired immune deficiency syndrome) practice. My work in this field has spanned more than twenty-five years, most of it related to my role as founder and ongoing chair of Boston College's Annual National Conference on HIV and AIDS Social Work. This conference is now in its twenty-fourth year of operation. During these years I have witnessed many ups and downs that have impacted our field of practice. My good friend and colleague, Alan Rice, provides expert reflections on many of these issues and events in Chapter 2.

From a Death Sentence to a Chronic Disease

Diana Rowan, the book's primary author, makes it clear from the outset that this book will primarily outline the current landscape of HIV and AIDS social work practice in this country. However, the book presents an excellent documentation of our history as well, and provides many helpful observations related to our future. Of special interest to me throughout the book are the many case examples, questions for reflection, and exercises that support the book's use in the classroom. However, this volume is not only useful in the classroom: the contributors have succeeded in developing a book that can be equally useful for our colleagues in the field who need a ready informational resource that can be referenced time and again in their daily HIV and AIDS social work practice activities. While every chapter presents unique topics for the reader, I noticed some observations, questions, and concerns that appear time and again in many of the chapters. Some of these include the following:

- We are at a crossroads in care and treatment.

- Leadership in our field needs to be strengthened.

- Most of us need to do more with less.

- There is a high degree of burnout among us.

- We have a difficult time recruiting and retaining social workers for our field of practice.

- Many -isms remain in our society that perpetuate disparities in health-care access and service delivery for those most in need.

- HIV and AIDS is still with us . . . and there are 50,000 new infections in the United States annually.

- We now have a National AIDS Strategy, but what does this really mean?

- We now have an Affordable Care Act, but what does this really mean?

- We see changes in Ryan White funding in ways that adversely impact psychosocial services to service consumers.

- How will health-care policy change after the 2012 elections?

- We have a newly formed professional association—Professional Association of Social Workers in HIV and AIDS (PASWHA). How can it be most helpful to those of us on the ground?

- We see a greater medicalization of care and treatment. What will this mean for social work?

- Do we wish to remain specialized in our work? Or do we wish to form new alliances with other health-care professional groups that will benefit us all?

Observations like these appear in many chapters. I think that the book's contributors have in an important way become truth-tellers for our field of practice. I suggest that these truth-tellers point us in an important new direction. This direction involves the need for transformational change on many fronts. This kind of change can only begin to happen if leaders emerge from within our ranks . . . and if those leaders can jumpstart a critical process of change.

We need many new transformational leaders who can inspire, motivate, and influence needed change. I would like to recommend that there be convened in the very near future a national leadership summit meeting composed of the contributors to this book, who are all leaders in their own right, in collaboration with leadership from our professional association (PASWHA) and with the leadership from Boston College's Annual National Conference on HIV and AIDS Social Work. The task of such a summit meeting would be for participants to craft a realistic, measurable, and achievable strategic action plan that can significantly enhance, improve, and advocate for our field of practice over the next critical decade in the areas of concern described earlier. The contributors to this important book have not only provided us with valuable content regarding our practice landscape, but also have (perhaps unwittingly) identified this as a true leadership moment in our field's history that needs to be grasped now. For this we are all grateful. Let's not miss the opportunity to take hold of this leadership moment and do what we can do to achieve real transformational change. This book can provide us a roadmap in this quest for such change. Let's get to work!

Vincent J. Lynch
Boston College Graduate School of Social Work
Chestnut Hill, Massachusetts
January 2012

Preface

I am the great granddaughter of four Polish immigrants who arrived in Buffalo, New York, via Ellis Island and the Erie Canal. My parents brought us up to follow the unwritten but much spoken rule of, "Don't talk to people outside of the family about politics, religion, sex, money, or nationality." These topics were off limits because they were potentially controversial and could bring up conflict, which was not something we entered into publically. The concept of nationality was my parents' version of racial stereotypes. The Polish community in Buffalo tried to keep its distance from the Italians, the Germans, and the other higher-ranking ethnic groups. I accepted these rules and played by the book until I pursued a professional social work education. All of a sudden, I was asked not only to think about politics, religions other than my own, sex, and discrimination on the basis of race or ethnicity, but also to champion conversations on these topics. I had some distance to go. However, my social work education prepared me with the knowledge, values, and skills necessary to serve marginalized populations. Yet when I began working with people living with HIV and AIDS, I realized that my current tool bag carried me only so far; social work with HIV and AIDS is so very complex.

More than fifteen years later, I am convinced that there is no more challenging group to work with. People living with HIV or AIDS need financial help, housing assistance, and referrals to a complex system of medical care. They need drugs, transportation, and advocacy in the workplace, and they need mental health support for issues related to fear, anger, grief, shame, loneliness, and pain. They have relational issues with family, friends, partners, lovers, and God; and they have problems with stigma and isolation, with discrimination, gender identity, and sexual orientation. They face changes in body image and self-esteem, and the challenge of planning for the future. Often they have co-occurring conditions, like substance abuse, other sexually transmitted diseases, and domestic violence. And, on top of all of that are issues of religion, sex, politics, and race or ethnicity. The work is complex.

Early on, I and other new social work practitioners getting into the field of HIV prevention and care learned as we went, figuring out solutions by trial and error, seeking advice from our clients, and being constantly amazed by their resilience. Now, as more of an academic than a practitioner, I feel a responsibility to share some of the practice wisdom we learned, so that the transition into HIV and AIDS work is less challenging and confusing for new social workers. This book contains many tips from the experts—social workers who learned HIV and AIDS social work in the trenches. The chapters are designed for practitioners who already understand how to practice social work. It is designed to fill the gaps with information about how the system works with respect to HIV, what to expect from clients, and how to be proactive with case advocacy, program development, and policy reform. The book is case based—that is, it uses stories to help make the content real. The cases are fictional, but most are composites of numerous clients who trained us over the years. Scattered throughout are questions to be used for personal reflection, public group discussion, or both. Thus, the book is suitable for use in a classroom, as a supplement for a course on medical social work, practice with populations at risk, or as a dedicated text for an HIV/AIDS elective. Beyond the classroom, we hope this volume will make it to the bookshelves of AIDS service organizations, and into the hands of front-line practitioners. All of the contributors to the book have worked in the field, and this volume is another way for us to stay connected to the important work going on.

We address the topic of religion head on with a chapter on integrating spirituality into HIV and AIDS care, and in a chapter on mobilizing the Black faith community for HIV advocacy. Sex also takes a front seat, with a chapter that unapologetically and directly discusses how sexual behaviors are related to HIV and AIDS. We don't avoid politics, either: there is a chapter on the changing landscape of AIDS policy and an assessment of the state of AIDS services in this season of change. Given the inequitable impact of HIV on minority communities, we pay attention to cultural competence in work with African Americans, Latinos, men who have sex with men, adolescents, young adults, and older Americans. In short, this book breaks all the rules on avoiding conflict and treading in uncomfortable territory. Therefore, it is a great fit for any social worker, or any professional or paraprofessional who thinks like a social worker, and who has an interest in providing the best interventions possible to address incredibly complex social issues. It is our hope that we are on the brink of a cure and the pandemic will retreat, but reason and history lead us to believe that, unfortunately, workers who focus on HIV and AIDS care and prevention will be necessary for a while. With hard work, however, we can aspire to put ourselves out of business and curb the epidemic in our country.

We share our very best wishes with each of our readers. Now go out, break the social rules, and change the world, one client at a time.

Acknowledgments

I would like to acknowledge all of the contributors to the text, for without your expertise the book would not have been complete. Thanks to David Follmer and his team at Lyceum Books. I was encouraged by your support and excitement about this project, beginning with our first meeting about the book proposal. I also owe much gratitude to a number of people who helped with editing versions of chapters, including graduate assistants Rebecca Stamler, Vanessa Leyton, and Lamont Holley. And special thanks to the best professional editor ever, Elizabeth Tornquist, whose sharpened pencil and kicks in the hind end kept this project moving in the right direction. Thank you to my colleague and chair, Professor Dennis Long, for allowing me the time to focus on professional writing.

Thanks to the members of my family for your support and specific contributions: to Robert, for helping to solve computer and printer problems; to Lacey, who helped with the timeline and typing in edits; and to Alec, who periodically and kindly asked how the book was progressing and then opened up video games for me, as a distraction. And, thanks to Bella the cat for hours of companionship while the book was being written—sleeping on the desk, playing fetch with paper clips, and stealing rubber bands. I am also grateful to Mom and Dad, and my sister, Jean, for patiently listening to me complain about the challenge of the week related to the book. You are likely all as glad to see it finished as I am.

Most of all, thanks to the numerous people living with HIV and AIDS who served as the inspirations for the composite case examples appearing throughout the chapters of the book. Your struggles, your courage, and your wisdom bring the content to life. You are the best teachers of social work. We learn from what you teach us.

—Diana Rowan

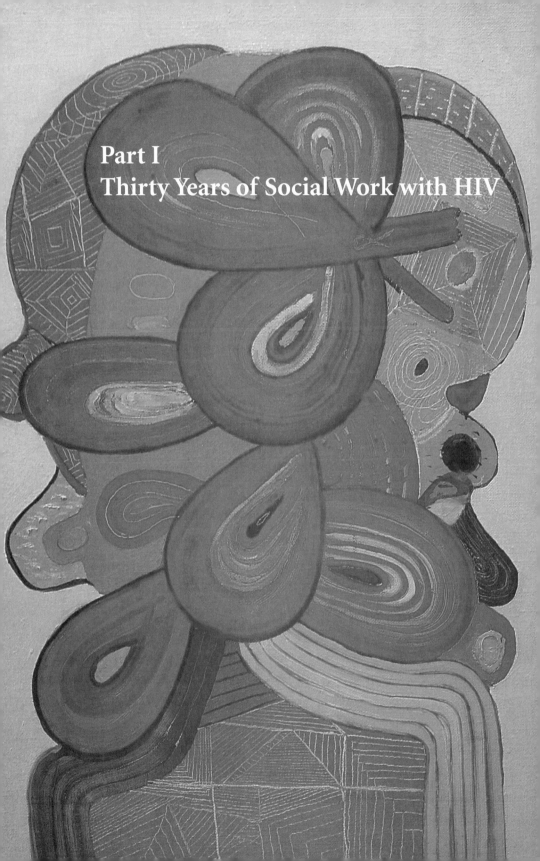

Part I
Thirty Years of Social Work with HIV

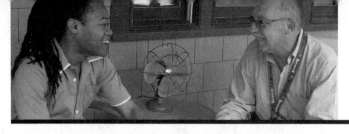

Social Work Practice with HIV and AIDS: The Current Landscape

Diana Rowan

> If you have come to help me, you are wasting your time; but if you have come here because your liberation is tied up with mine, then let us work together.
>
> **—Aboriginal activists group, Queensland, 1970s**

From a Death Sentence to a Chronic Disease

In 2006, Dr. Peter Piot, then executive director of UNAIDS, the joint program of the United Nations on HIV/AIDS, called for the global community's response to HIV/AIDS to shift "from crisis management to sustained strategic response." Although the focus of this text is not on international dimensions of the global pandemic, this perspective applies equally well to U.S. domestic responses. The societal perspective in the United States is largely that HIV is no longer a problem here, since it seems to be treated adequately with medications. AIDS had its thirtieth birthday on June 5, 2011, the anniversary of a report in *Morbidity and Mortality Weekly Report* (Gottlieb, 1981) on the first cases of what would become known as the AIDS epidemic. The virus called HIV (human immunodeficiency virus) and the clinical syndrome called AIDS (acquired immune deficiency syndrome) have evolved over the past three decades as social phenomena. Unlike the crisis climate around AIDS in its first decade, there is now little panic about the virus; many people who identify themselves as being at low risk are not concerned about HIV or AIDS, except perhaps when rock gods and movie stars appeal for money for AIDS in faraway African countries.

The advent of effective antiretroviral (ARV) medications that work to stop the replication of the virus is undoubtedly an overwhelming positive development in the story of AIDS in the United States. It is said that when AZT (azidothymidine), the first ARV, came on the market that people very ill with AIDS at the time got up off their deathbeds and started living again. This phenomenon, termed The Lazarus Effect, after the Biblical story of a man raised from the dead, changed the way the health-care community and society at large viewed AIDS.

One unintended consequence of the medical breakthrough of widely available ARV medications was that it encouraged development of apathy. When this social worker recently told an acquaintance what field she worked in, the acquaintance's response was, "HIV and AIDS . . . That's not something you hear much about anymore. Are there still jobs in that field?" This well-intentioned but naïve stance is not unique to mainstream adults. Even with many sexually transmitted disease (STD) prevention campaigns deployed on MTV and through other teen outlets, adolescents share a lack of awareness about the reality that almost no one is safe from HIV exposure and how unpleasant life spent on ARVs can be. It is not uncommon for social workers who interface with sexually active adolescents to report hearing that they are not concerned about getting HIV for one of two reasons. They report no concern, either because "It is something that only affects homosexuals and I don't do that stuff," or "So what if I get it? There are drugs for it and you can live as long as you want."

Unfortunately, another type of apathy about HIV infection in young adults is on the rise as well, though it is distinctly different. It is the viewpoint of some high-risk young adults, primarily young men of color who have sex with men, who believe the myth that HIV infection is inevitable and there is no reason to work hard to prevent it, since it will eventually happen despite one's best efforts. With this perspective can come a sense of fatalism, and even the belief that one deserves it, stemming from poor self-image and shame. All of these mindsets can be changed by targeted, culturally tailored education and counseling, interventions that align well with the skill sets of social workers. There is a delicate balance between being alarmist, inciting panic about HIV, and delivering a firm message paired with frank education about skills for staying safe. However, social workers are skilled at reading the needs of clients and communities well.

There are now effective treatments for suppression of HIV and AIDS. Still, no cure exists. Although many Americans die annually from AIDS, with proper care, excellent adherence to a medication regimen, and a healthy lifestyle, a person can live an indefinite length of time with the virus. Therefore, a growing consensus exists that HIV/AIDS should be treated as a chronic condition. Some assert that the time for crisis-level urgency has passed, and that efforts should be made to fold HIV/AIDS care into care for other chronic conditions that can be managed with medications. Yet others disagree, pointing out that AIDS will never be like other chronic conditions. "HIV/AIDS is not now, nor has it ever been, a purely medical issue; it is a social issue, a political issue, a cultural issue, an economic issue, and perhaps above all, a deeply personal issue" (Rowan & Honeycutt, 2010, p. 71). Consider serious chronic conditions such as diabetes or kidney disease. No one ever lost the love of family members over a diagnosis with either of these. No one has had guilt and shame over these diagnoses, nor have they had to restructure their sex life and body image due to them. No one has to park down the street from a clinic that treats hypertension because of fear that someone would spot their car in the clinic's parking lot. Stigma remains for those living with HIV disease, those who love them, and those who provide formal and informal care for them. HIV still carries the stereotype of affecting people with so-called bad behaviors that are outside the mainstream, such as irresponsible gay sex, sex for money, injection (or intravenous) drug use, or, perhaps in some cases, the tragic infection of what is considered a good person who was unknowingly infected by a philandering spouse or partner. People living with HIV and AIDS encounter stigma and discrimination at every turn. Other chronic conditions do not affect as many spheres of one's life as HIV does.

The Medicalization of HIV and AIDS Care

When AZT came on the market in 1987, the medical profession finally had an effective tool to fight the virus. Before that time, the work of AIDS care involved running lab tests to see how low T-cell counts would go, conducting unsuccessful clinical trials, gathering data on symptomatology, and providing palliative care. Social workers played an active role in providing psychosocial support, counseling, helping families and friends with grief and loss, combating stigma among helping professionals and the general population, and advocating for the rights of marginalized people. (For a compelling look inside the story of an AIDS social worker who began in the field at the start of the epidemic, see chapter 2, which describes the realities and struggles associated with social work with people living with HIV and AIDS over three decades.) With the advent of effective medications, the medical side of the health-care system took the lead in addressing the epidemic. Social work had its important role, but it was seen as supportive of care by an infectious disease physician.

As time passed, the federal legislation that provides funding for care of people living with HIV and AIDS, called the Ryan White Comprehensive AIDS Resources Emergency (CARE) Act, steered funds toward the provision of "medical case management" (Rowan & Honeycutt, 2010). (See chapters 2 and 17 for details on Ryan White and the act named for him.) This trend of shifting funds toward medical care led social workers to get creative in determining ways to provide services to clients for psychosocial and concrete needs. For example, if patients do not have transportation to a medical appointment, they will not stay in care. Similarly, if a newly diagnosed man decides to drive his car off a bridge rather than face a life in which he fears he will die of AIDS, there is no chance of getting him placed on an effective medication regimen. Social workers excel in areas where there is a wraparound approach to case management, including supportive counseling, creative linkages to other services, education, involvement of the client in a strengths-based care plan, and engagement of the natural support system. (See chapter 10 for more on social work case management with HIV.) A continuum of care has been shown to produce the best health outcomes and medication adherence for clients. (For more on the importance of and challenges behind medication adherence, see chapter 13.)

Enduring Themes

During the thirty years that AIDS has existed in the United States, some facts have changed while others remain stubbornly constant. In a classic text entitled, *HIV/AIDS at Year 2000: A Sourcebook for Social Workers*, Lynch (2000) identified five areas where, at that time, progress was needed. Of these five areas, each one remains elusive. Lynch (p. xv) said, "We do not yet: have equal access to all therapies for all people; have a cure; have a vaccine; know why some people respond to drug therapies and others do not; and, know how or why certain drug-resistant strains of the virus exist." Some progress has been made on the last two, but those goals are still not completely met. There remain several enduring themes with respect to social work and HIV prevention and care. Four are explained and illustrated with case examples below.

HIV continues to disproportionately affect communities that are already marginalized, and these vulnerabilities are intertwined with systematic poverty, discrimination, and lack of access to equal resources.

In his text, Lynch (2000, p. xiii) commented that at that time—more than a decade ago—there had been a slow decrease in AIDS deaths and new infections in the gay community, but there had been an explosion of HIV/AIDS in another so-called throwaway community—people of color, especially African Americans. It can be theorized that if HIV were affecting upper- or middle-class majority populations in a similar way that it is affecting gay men, people in poverty, and people of color, more resources would be dedicated to HIV prevention, improvement of access to care, and development of new treatments. HIV affects African Americans inequitably—at a rate that is seven times that of White Americans. African American women are the fastest-growing demographic for new infections, and young women of color are dying more from the disease than are White women. In a debate during the Democratic primary race for the 2008 presidential election, candidate Senator Hillary Clinton aptly stated, "Let me just put this in perspective. If HIV/AIDS were the leading cause of death of White women between the ages of 25 and 34, there would be an outraged outcry in this country." Institutional racism, discrimination, and White privilege continue to limit access to care and resources for marginalized people. (For more on HIV in the African-American community, see chapter 4; for more on social work practice with Latinos with HIV, see chapter 5.)

The social work profession places emphasis on intervening when marginalized populations are exposed to forms of social injustice such as discrimination and lack of access to quality health care and supportive services. The National Association of Social Workers (NASW) has stated the mission of social work as follows (2008): "The primary mission of the social work profession is to enhance human well-being and help meet the basic human needs of all people, with particular attention to the needs and empowerment of people who are vulnerable, oppressed, and living in poverty. A historic and defining feature of social work is the profession's focus on individual well-being in a social context and the well-being of society."

This enduring theme highlights the reality that those affected by HIV always have been and continue to be people who are "vulnerable, oppressed, and living in poverty." Therefore, it is essential that more and more social workers, not just those actively working in HIV/AIDS care, recognize and combat inequity evident in the disparities in who is being infected and affected.

The best models for care of people living with HIV and AIDS utilize a comprehensive approach, in which all systemic factors in a client, their family, and their community are addressed.

The profession of social work, by definition, is concerned with "helping people obtain tangible services; providing counseling and psychotherapy for individuals, families, and groups; helping communities or groups provide or improve social and health services; and participating in relevant legislative processes" (according to NASW, quoted by Zastrow, 1995, p. 7). If the best outcomes for people living with HIV and AIDS occur with a comprehensive approach to care, then social workers are well positioned to provide valuable contributions to improvement of care. One of the main orienting frameworks of social work practice is the Ecological Systems Model, which considers the multiple internal factors of an individual, as well as external environmental factors. Toward that end, social workers are trained to assess and address the following when designing interventions: subsystems of the individual (biophysical, cognitive, emotional, behavioral, motivational); interpersonal systems (parent–child, marital or couple, family, kin, friends, neighbors, cultural or ethnic reference groups, spiritual belief systems, and other members of social networks); organizations, institutions, and communities; and aspects of the physical environment (housing, neighborhood infrastructure, buildings, employment opportunities, resource access, and climate) (Hepworth, Rooney, Rooney, Strom-Gottfried, & Larsen, 2010).

A single focus does not work in HIV/AIDS care. Consider the following scenario, in which only the biophysical aspects of a person living with AIDS are considered:

An infectious disease physician with a narrow focus considers only the biophysical data for a patient, Willie. (This is an extreme hypothetical scenario, to illustrate a point. Fortunately, most infectious disease physicians are savvy enough to include other systemic factors when treating patients with HIV.) According to the medical history and laboratory results, she determines that Willie requires a particular combination of ARV medications. She writes the prescription, and tells him to be extremely compliant and follow the medication regimen carefully, lest he develop medication resistance. Willie was recently released from state prison, where he served a ten-year sentence for selling crack cocaine, after multiple prior arrests. The physician scolds him for not continuing on the regimen provided to him in the prison. (For more information on an HIV medical visit, see chapter 11; for more information on the importance of medication adherence, see chapter 13.) After stopping at the in-house pharmacy to have his prescriptions filled for the first month, Willie walks out of the clinic and heads for the homeless shelter. He had been unable to find a more stable place to stay because he is unemployed. With a 14 percent unemployment rate in the city where he lives, it is difficult for anyone to find work, and it is nearly impossible for anyone with a felony record to find work.

Willie believes he was infected with the virus while he was in prison. He considered contacting his family for financial help, but he didn't bother, since he had not heard from a single friend or relative during the last nine years of his sentence. In fact, the thought that even his mother does not care anymore breaks his heart. He had been very close to his mother since she shot and killed his father in self-defense during a domestic incident. After his father's death when he was twelve, he had to be "the man of the house" and take care of his mother and younger siblings. He wonders if she died years ago. As sad as that would be, it would be easier to accept than the fact that she chose for so long not to communicate with him.

Three weeks later at the shelter, someone steals Willie's backpack. It contains all of his possessions, including his HIV medications. Someone at the shelter saw him at the HIV clinic and outed his positive status around the community at the shelter. At breakfast, he notices that none of the women he was pursuing for a relationship will sit with him. He feels the same sense of stigma he felt when he was routinely convicted of drug offenses. He knows God will never forgive him for selling drugs to kids, and he knows that is why God gave him HIV. He knows he can't run from his past, but he tries by hitchhiking to the next city. Maybe he will find a good woman to love there.

Two months later, Willie is relieved to be living with Sherrie, a woman he met while she was tending bar in a club. He finds her very attractive and enjoys having sex with her. It makes him feel loved, and as if he belongs someplace. He does not disclose to her that he has HIV because he does not want to jeopardize the relationship or his free place to stay. In addition, his cellmate had told him that as long as he doesn't have anal sex with a woman, she can't catch it. He hopes his cellmate was right, but doesn't know whom else to ask. Sherrie has not suggested the use of a condom, so he figures she doesn't mind any risks. Plus, he loves her too much to put a barrier between them. Occasionally he thinks about the fact that he has HIV, but he is actually glad that he lost his medications. He hated to be reminded several times a day that he may die from AIDS, plus they gave him bad side effects. He has been feeling pretty good, so he doesn't search too hard for a free medical clinic. He also doesn't want to be scolded by another doctor for stopping his ARV medications.

Two months later Willie is in the emergency room, having collapsed. He denies having HIV to the nurse, who is suspicious when she looks at his lab results. He starts a fight with Sherrie while he is in the hospital bed, trying to chase her out before she finds out he is HIV positive and has AIDS. When he calls her a crack whore, she walks out and he knows he has seen her for the last time.

The emergency room physician admits him to the infectious disease unit. There he learns that he has developed resistance to several of the most effective ARV medications. He will have to be prescribed a combination that has more side effects. He is also warned that he must stay in care and be adherent this time—his life depends on it. He is linked with an HIV case manager named Tyrek, who works at an active AIDS service and advocacy center in this city. Tyrek visits Willie in the hospital and makes plans to meet with him immediately upon discharge. He tells Willie that he has some ideas about how to help him get his life together. Willie plans to try to push Tyrek away, but if Tyrek passes that test, Willie plans to trust him. Willie doesn't usually trust Black people, but Tyrek doesn't seem racist like the other Black people he has known. He hopes Tyrek might be able to help him find out what happened to his mother.

(For more information on case management, see chapter 10.)

This case example illustrates the importance of integrating multiple aspects of the client's life into his or her care. Stable housing improves HIV outcomes. (For more on housing and HIV, see chapter 16.) An assessment of Willie's spiritual concerns might have helped to alleviate the guilt and shame that were interfering with his desire to live healthily. (See chapter 14 for information on the importance of integrating spirituality into HIV care.) Willie is operating on false information about HIV transmission risks. No one provided him with a risk assessment and risk reduction education. (For more on conducting a risk assessment, see chapter 10.) Also, no one gave him a plan to ensure continuity of care should he leave town. He did not have a person to be accountable to for medication adherence. He would have benefitted from counseling about healthy relationships and assistance in telling Sherrie about his HIV status.

Questions for Reflection

1. So much has gone wrong with Willie's life. Despite these events, what are his strengths?

2. List decisions and events in Willie's life that had negative impacts on his well-being.

3. If the state prison had embraced a comprehensive approach to care and linked Willie with proper case management upon his release, what events might have been avoided?

4. What might have been the outcome if the state prison had offered an HIV-prevention program? Many prisons elect to not provide condoms to inmates in an effort to discourage sexual activity, yet many oppose this policy, stating that availability of condoms is a public health issue. Debate this issue, outlining the strengths and weaknesses of each side's arguments.

Unfocused HIV-prevention messages are often ineffective, and all levels of prevention are improved with targeted messages.

Social workers have been talking about the importance of understanding a client's culture and ethnicity since the origins of the profession a century ago. Since then, social work knowledge, values, and skills have evolved to more effectively deliver interventions to diverse populations. Culturally competent practice is now seen as a requisite for a social worker who is operating within the NASW code of ethics (NASW, 2008, Responsibility 1.05 Cultural Competence and Social Diversity in the NASW Code of Ethics). HIV-prevention messages, in order for people to effectively receive and efficiently absorb them, must be designed with a specific audience in mind. They need to be delivered in a mode that is suitable for the audience. For example, young people communicate through text messaging and are heavy users of social media sites. They do not read newspapers. People who are not proficient in English will not respond well to spoken or written messages prepared in English. Even if English messages are translated, they may not align well with the values of another culture. Posters and flyers placed in locations not frequented by the targeted audience will not effectively reach that audience. For example, one should not imbed television public service announcements aimed at people over fifty in shows for a younger adult audience, and vice versa. Furthermore, messages should be prepared in a way that is closely aligned with the unique vernacular, graphics, art work, and vibe of the target group.

It is not easy to prepare and deliver HIV-prevention messages. These messages should be culturally tailored with respect to age group, race or ethnicity, income level, region of the country, language use, and unique features of the subculture targeted. Furthermore, the goal of the message must be clear, whether it's providing impact at primary, secondary, or tertiary levels of HIV prevention. The content should reflect the goal—primary prevention (preventing infection), secondary prevention (getting tested early), or tertiary prevention (staying adherent to the ARV regimen).

HIV and AIDS disproportionately affect people of color, men who have sex with men, and others with risk factors such as marginalization, lack of access to health care, substance abuse, mental health problems, and poverty. Therefore, multiple chapters in this text focus on development of practice competence with specific types of diversity. Chapter 4 addresses the growing impact of the virus within the African-American community. Chapter 5 provides tips for practice with the Latino community. Chapter 6 provides more information on HIV prevention and the levels of prevention, as discussed above, but with an emphasis on men who have sex with men. As America "grays," increasing numbers of older adults are living with HIV and AIDS; chapter 8 discusses prevention and care for people over fifty. Another area of diversity where development of cultural competence is essential is the area of religion and faith. Two chapters focus on involvement of spirituality in social work interventions with HIV: Chapter 14 discusses the relevance of a client's spiritual life with respect to living with the virus and describes how social workers can leverage spiritual strength to achieve better outcomes. Chapter 15 takes a look at the involvement of churches from a more macro-level approach, with a focus on the African American faith community and homosexuality, HIV, and AIDS.

> **Box 1.1. What Is Cultural Competence?**
>
> Culture is an integrated pattern of human behavior that includes thoughts, communications, actions, customs, beliefs, values, and institutions of a racial, ethnic, religious, or social group.
>
> Cultural competence is the process by which individuals and systems respond respectfully and effectively to people of all cultures, languages, classes, races, ethnic backgrounds, religions, and other diversity factors, in a manner that recognizes, affirms, and values the worth of individuals, families, and communities and protects and preserves the dignity of each.

Culturally competent practitioners continually work toward

- Deepening awareness of their own cultural worldview,

- Checking their attitude toward cultural differences,

- Increasing knowledge of different cultural practices and world-views, and

- Developing cross-cultural skills.

Developing cultural competence increases one's ability to understand, communicate with, and effectively interact with many elements of diversity. Cultural competence is a lifelong pursuit, since it is never mastered, only developed. Pursuit of this type of sophisticated cultural competence does not come naturally to every social worker and requires a high level of professionalism and knowledge.

HIV/AIDS is a global pandemic but that does not excuse minimization of its devastation at home. Worldwide, it is estimated that 33.3 million people are living with HIV, with 2.9 million infected in 2009, and 1.8 million dying from AIDS that year. It is clear that HIV/AIDS meets the definition of a pandemic, and it has been called one of the greatest threats to humankind (Council on Foreign Relations, 2004). A 2005 United Nations Development Report concluded, "The HIV/AIDS pandemic has inflicted the single greatest reversal in human development" (Piot, 2006). HIV/AIDS affects all regions of the world, with 70 percent of cases concentrated in the countries of Sub-Saharan Africa.

It is true that poverty levels in countries and their rates of HIV infection are correlated, thereby justifying an energetic response by wealthier countries to assist developing nations with funds for prevention and care programs. In fact, President George W. Bush's PEPFAR program, The U.S. President's Emergency Plan for AIDS Relief, is the largest commitment in history by any nation to fight a single disease. By 2008, PEPFAR had spent more than $18.8 billion to fight the virus in fifteen focus countries. In 2008, Congress committed $48 billion more to be spent worldwide over the next five years. PEPFAR has massively increased access to ARV medications and therefore has greatly raised the number of people around the world who are able to live with the virus.

The ambitious commitment of the United States to partner with other nations to fight the global pandemic is admirable, and aligns well with the social work values of promotion of social justice and the dignity and worth of each person through human rights initiatives. Still, PEPFAR is not without its critics. One criticism is that although increased access to free ARV drugs was accomplished, the number of new HIV diagnoses has not gone down as expected. Many speculate that PEPFAR invested in programs that were not culturally appropriate for the regions where they were deployed, often pushing an Ameri-centric model. Faith-based agencies that received a large portion of PEPFAR funds used an abstinence-only approach to HIV prevention, which was not practical and that imposed social values on other cultures. Another criticism is that all or part of these massive allocations of U.S. funds could have been directed toward the domestic HIV problem.

The prevalence of HIV in Washington, DC, our nation's capital, is at least 3 percent. According to a 2008 report by the D.C. HIV/AIDS administration, this rate is higher than in parts of West Africa, and is on par with parts of Uganda and Kenya (Associated Press, 2009). In Washington, DC, Black men have the highest rate, at 7 percent HIV positive. The report warns that actual rates are almost certainly higher, since not all residents have been tested. With HIV-positive rates in the African-American community surpassing the rates seen in PEPFAR-funded countries, one must wonder why more funding is not directed to fight HIV in our own cities. One must wonder where are the fundraisers supported by rock bands and the Hollywood elite? Are these marginalized U.S. residents not worthy of the same crisis response? Or is it more glamorous to rescue the poor outside our borders?

While access to free ARV medications has increased through PEPFAR-funded programs around the world, we still have many people living in America who are denied access to life-saving ARVs. Although drug manufacturers have lowered the costs of generic ARV medications, they are still outside the reach of Americans living at lower-middle-class income levels or below. One might ask, don't we have a federal program to provide AIDS medications to uninsured Americans? Yes, we do: ADAP (AIDS Drug Assistance Program). (For more on ADAP, see chapter 17.) However, in September 2011, there were 9,066 Americans on an ADAP waiting list, hoping for a spot to open up so they could receive life-saving drugs. At this time, Florida has the longest waiting list, at more than 3,000 people. It is not uncommon for the following scenario to occur in one of the eleven states that currently have ADAP waiting lists:

An uninsured twenty-five-year-old woman receives the news at the county health department that she is HIV positive. She is not surprised because she has been feeling weak and is unable to hold a job because of exhaustion. She heard that a boyfriend from high school had recently been hospitalized and was told he had AIDS. The Disease Intervention Specialist (DIS) employed by the county health department instructs her to seek medical care. She is not insured, is currently underemployed, and is couch-hopping (staying with various friends and family members for short periods to avoid complete homelessness). The DIS directs her to a free neighborhood medical clinic where she learns that her CD4 count is 80 and her viral load is 300,000. She also hears the words, "You have AIDS." The physician at the free clinic tells her that she needs ARV medications right away. She states she is willing to take them but can't pay for them herself. The physician directs her to the clinic social worker who, he said, "works wonders" with finding resources and getting scarce resources for their patients. He states that the social worker will certainly have paperwork to get her access to these important drugs.

The social worker, upon learning of the problem, is dismayed. Though she does not regularly work with HIV/AIDS, she has heard that her state recently had to resort to a waiting list for the ADAP program, since all the funds for that fiscal year were expended and neither the governor nor the state legislature fought to secure an extension of funds. She networks with a case manager at a local AIDS service organization (ASO) and finds out how to get the client on the waiting list. The case manager at the ASO also suggests she pursue a charity program with a pharmaceutical company to provide the medications for free. The social worker knows she needs help in order to adequately serve this client. How will she learn which drug(s) the client needs? How will she know which pharmaceutical manufacturer to contact? How will she secure specialized medical care from an infectious disease physician for this client? The young, single woman is not on Medicaid; though she is diagnosed with AIDS, she has not yet been determined to be disabled. The client looks forlorn and weak. The social worker says, "We will keep working on this, but right now I don't know of a way to get you medications. Yes, I understand you need them to keep from getting sicker or even dying. Yes, we do have federal programs to help people with AIDS, but you either don't qualify, have to wait for someone to drop out to open up a slot, or wait for the paperwork to be processed for disability determination." The client blinks her eyes, stands up to leave the office, and thinks about planning her suicide. The social worker, feeling helpless, takes a break from her desk to check her favorite social networking site. A pop-up ad appears for a fundraising program for AIDS in Africa. She wonders why so much federal funding and money from charities goes overseas to fight AIDS when her client is possibly left to die from the same condition. She flippantly considers telling her client that she should move to Botswana where American ARV meds are free and widely available. Then her supervisor knocks on her door and asks her why she did not straighten up the Lego toys in the waiting room as asked an hour ago.

Questions for Reflection

1. Were you aware that the rates of HIV infection in Washington, DC, especially in Black men, are higher than those seen in many Sub-Saharan African countries?

2. Do you agree that people in the United States seem more willing to donate to fight AIDS in another country than in the United States? If so, or if not, why do you think it is that way?

3. In the case example above, what should be the next steps of the social worker at the neighborhood clinic?

4. What do you think the social worker might like to say to her supervisor when she is told to straighten up the waiting room? What should she say to gain the best results?

Introduction to the Text

These pages have briefly outlined the historical context of social work with HIV and AIDS, with respect to the movement from crisis management to strategic response. This chapter has acknowledged the systematic medicalization of treatment for HIV and AIDS, as well as the fact that some challenges in prevention and care have continued over the thirty years of the pandemic. Four areas that are enduring themes of the pandemic carry special concern for social workers, and these four areas produce the foundation for the chapters of this text. Throughout this chapter, the reader has been provided teasers, or references to content coming in subsequent chapters. In truth, each chapter could contain multiple links to others, since the body of knowledge is not in discrete silos of information. Still, for the sake of organization, the text is divided into four sections: Part I, HIV/AIDS and social work through time; Part II, selected population groups with high impacts of HIV; Part III, multiple issues in the practice of social work, from micro emphasis in the case management chapter to macro emphasis in the chapter discussing community organizing and the Black church; and Part IV, HIV/AIDS policy in the context of the current shifting landscape.

This book can be read from cover to cover, but since each chapter can stand alone, the reader can also use it as a reference guide. The primary audience for this book is those who are new to social work with persons who are living with HIV or AIDS. The authors wrote the chapters with practitioners in mind, those who understand the practice of social work but may not understand the complexities of HIV/AIDS prevention and care.

Throughout the book the reader may notice that some authors use the slash version—HIV/AIDS—sparingly, and instead, where practical, use the phrase "HIV and AIDS." This is purposeful: despite the common worldwide use of HIV/AIDS, HIV and AIDS prevention and care are distinct. The psychosocial needs of the two populations differ, as do their medical and supportive service needs. In fact, social workers in the field will find that expertise with one group may not transfer smoothly to the other. Therefore, living with the virus and living with the syndrome are recognized as distinct by the use of the phrase "HIV and AIDS."

Almost all chapters contain at least one lengthy case example to illustrate concepts presented in the chapter. Bringing both concrete and abstract concepts to life through depictions of clients or their social workers can heighten learning experiences for readers. The title of this text proves the importance the authors place on the use of the case illustrations.

The authors also provide questions for reflection, for both the solo reader and those who are reading as part of a group, perhaps in a classroom setting. Some will call for answers that are deeply personal, and others welcome public debate. Furthermore, readers may find that their answers may change as their levels of experience and knowledge change.

It is an exciting time to be working in the field of HIV and AIDS social work. So many facets of the landscape are changing. ARV medications continue to evolve, and more and more clients are being provided regimens that consist of one pill a day, an inconceivable reality even five years ago, making adherence easier (see chapters 11 and 13). Clinical trials continue to provide hope that early treatments and strong adherence greatly limit transmission of the virus. The Centers for Disease Control and Prevention's (CDC) list of DEBIs (Diffusion of Effective Behavioral Interventions) continues to grow, expanding the arsenal of best practices for both micro- and macro-level HIV-prevention strategies. The current version of Ryan White legislation is due to sunset in 2013, just as health-care reform initiatives are rolled out. As of 2010, our country finally has a national HIV/AIDS strategy and efforts are ramping up to meet the goals for reduction of new cases of HIV by 2015. (For more on policy evolution, see chapter 17.) And, our profession has a fledgling organization, called PASWHA, or the Professional Association of Social Workers in HIV and AIDS (no slash). A cadre of inaugural members is currently drafting action statements. Social work is part of the sustained strategic response to HIV and AIDS. This book explains how.

References

Associated Press. (2009, March 16). HIV-AIDS rate in D.C. "Higher than West Africa." *FoxNews.com*. Retrieved from http://www.foxnews.com/story/0,2933,509316,00.html

Council on Foreign Relations. (2004). Addressing the HIV/AIDS pandemic: A U.S. global AIDS strategy for the long-term. *Council Special Report, 3*.

Gottlieb, M. S. (1981, June 5). Epidemiologic notes and reports: Pneumocystis pneumonia—Los Angeles. *Morbidity and Mortality Weekly Report, 30*(21), 1–3.

Hepworth, D., Rooney, R., Rooney, G. D., Strom-Gottfried, K., & Larsen, J. (2010). *Direct social work practice: Theory and skills* (8th ed.). Belmont, CA: Brooks/Cole.

Lynch, V. (2000). Preface. In V. Lynch (Ed.), *HIV/AIDS at year 2000: A sourcebook for social workers* (pp. ix–xv). Needham Heights, MA: Allyn and Bacon.

National Association of Social Workers (NASW). (2008). *NASW code of ethics*. Washington, DC: Author. Retrieved from http://www.socialworkers.org/pubs/Code/code.asp

Piot, P. (2006). AIDS: From crisis management to sustained strategic response. *Lancet, 368*, 526–530.

Rowan, D., & Honeycutt, J. (2010). The impact of the Ryan White Treatment Modernization Act on social work within the field of HIV/AIDS service provision. *Health & Social Work, 35*(1), 71–74.

Zastrow, C. (1995). *The practice of social work, 5th edition*. Belmont, CA: Brooks/Cole.

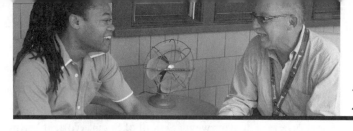

2

A Conversation with Alan Rice: Reflections on Twenty-Eight Years as an AIDS Social Worker

Diana Rowan and Alan Rice

One faces the future with one's past.

—Pearl S. Buck

Part of practice wisdom is gleaning lessons from those who have become experts in the field. One of those experts in social work is Alan Rice, who has been working on the front lines of the AIDS epidemic in New York City from 1983 to this writing in 2011. Alan Rice is currently serving as co-director of Social Work/Case Management, Center for Comprehensive Care, St. Luke's–Roosevelt Hospital AIDS Program, New York City.

This chapter summarizes a recent interview by Diana Rowan with Alan Rice at the 2011 National Conference on Social Work with HIV/AIDS held in Atlanta in May 2011. (For a more thorough look at the struggles of social workers during the formative days of AIDS care, see Willinger & Rice, 2003.)

> **Please describe your career path in doing social work with HIV in New York City.**
>
> It is important to understand that everything in my career is guided by what happened in the 1960s. It was an era of social justice and injustice, and a time of advocacy. The times you grow up in dictate what you do throughout your life. I love the field of social work. For the pure doing for people, there is no better profession. Getting an education in social work was very important. I graduated from high school in 1971 in Brooklyn and went to community college. Luckily, I had a high draft number or I would have gone to Canada. Five years after I finished my BSW [bachelor of social work] degree, I went back for a graduate degree. Going to school was very intense. Not only did I do it while working, I was married and had two small children. My wife was like a

single mother for two years. I went to a two-year MSW [master of social work] program at Wurzweiler School of Social Work at Yeshiva University, in a new specialized program for people who worked while going to school. It was such a rich opportunity to sit with people who had much more experience than me, since I had only worked for five years after my BSW degree at that point. The whole process of earning my master degree was very formative. I was never a great student, and the fact that I earned a master degree was monumental. Even more interesting is that I am now an adjunct professor at Wurzweiler School of Social Work and I have the opportunity to say to my students that I truly know what you are going through, because I sat in that very seat.

As a BSW, I had been working on the male drug detox unit at Beth Israel Medical Center in New York City as a social work assistant, which I always thought was a funny title, since I didn't assist anyone. It was a challenging position because lots of things were happening in the patients' lives that caused them problems. This job allowed me the opportunity to do intensive short-term work with patients. While in my MSW program, I had my first field placement in that program, but I had to do something distinctly different from my paid work. We started using a group modality in contrast to the individual modality I had been using, and in fact we discovered it worked a lot better.

My second field placement was doing social work on a unit for medically ill substance users, which was interesting but very challenging because my supervisor was tough. I equated our relationship at the time to the relationship between Richard Gere and Lou Gossett, Jr., in the film *An Officer and a Gentleman,* which was in the theatres at the time. But he was just what I needed. When you think you know it all and you really know nothing, you need someone to go in depth with you, which he did. While I was working on that unit, I learned a great deal about self-determination. I worked with a man named Leon who had a very serious leg wound that would not heal. He had maggots on it that were the only thing keeping the wound clean. But Leon just did not want to have his leg cut off, no matter how medically necessary it was. He eventually did, when given an ultimatum from the medical staff. However, in working with him, I learned that we must support what the client wants, regardless of what we think is best, or what we would do if in their situation. This was such a powerful part of my education that I wrote my final essay, which was something like a thesis, on self-determination. All of these learning opportunities would turn out to be critical in preparing me for my career in HIV and AIDS social work.

When I graduated with my master of social work degree, I had a fantasy that I would become an expert in some field, probably work with chronic substance users, and travel around and talk about it. However, right after graduation I decided to take a long break to rest and use up some of my accumulated vacation days. I planned to go back into my old position as a social work assistant, even though I was now overqualified with an MSW. Then, something very strange happened. One day I received a call from my supervisor at Beth Israel; he offered me a position as a medical social worker on a Med/Surg [medical/surgical] unit. I didn't have experience with that type of work, but my supervisor said, "You never know, maybe you'll like it." So there I was, a brand new MSW with no discharge planning experience, and I was overseeing three units. I had a social work assistant, which is what I was two minutes ago! So although it was bizarre, it was also fascinating. I never saw it as laborious or as having mundane paperwork. I found myself using all of my skills, including my clinical skills. To this day I still think you cannot do a complicated discharge plan without doing work that is very clinical. I think that is part of our problem in medical social work—we don't toot our own horn enough.

Still, I had the feeling something strange was going on. How did I get this job? I'm not that good! Then, about a month and a half after I started, I got a phone call from my supervisor again. He said he needed someone to work with the patients who had mysterious infections. It was the AIDS patients, but at the time we might have still referred to it as GRID [gay-related immune disorder]. It was 1983 and the epidemic was very new. Dr. Donna Mildvan was working at Beth Israel, and she was the one who diagnosed the first cases in New York City. I first heard of the mysterious cases in 1982 but I hadn't had any personal contact with them. You see, they had an agenda behind giving me that Med/Surg position. They had been through every medical social worker and nobody wanted to work with the GRID patients. No one else wanted to do it. But then there was me, with experience with drug addicts and medically ill people, and they thought I would be suited for it. The job would be to add on to my caseload about eight to ten GRID patients per day. Luckily, even in those early days, my supervisor recognized that there would be many psychosocial needs. His vision was to provide continuity of care and to keep sending any readmissions back to the same social worker, me. Most were so sick there was no discharge planning to do, just counseling. They didn't leave the hospital.

Box 2.1. Dr. Donna Mildvan and the First Identified AIDS Case at Beth Israel

Beth Israel Medical Center in New York City saw its first AIDS patient in July of 1980. The patient was a thirty-three-year-old homosexual male, originally from West Germany, who had recently worked in Haiti as a chef for three years. He went to New York City after he got very sick in Haiti with severe weight loss and uncontrollable bloody diarrhea. At the time, no one had heard of AIDS, and the human immunodeficiency virus (HIV) had not yet been isolated. In the chef's stool, Dr. Mildvan identified amoebic parasites that were not common but that had been recently identified in other homosexual men who were very ill. The man developed sores around his rectum and lost vision in one eye. It was suspected that the patient had a viral infection in his eye, but Beth Israel did not have a virology lab at the time. A sample of fluid from his eye was sent to a lab in the Bronx and was later identified as cytomegalovirus (CMV). This was surprising and confusing, since this virus is common but rarely causes a disease of this magnitude. Dr. Mildvan is quoted as saying,

We had nothing for the CMV. It spread to the other eye, and he lost vision. Over the next couple of months, he deteriorated neurologically. CAT scans showed his brain had shrunk. He stopped talking to us. He curled up in a ball, staring blindly into the distance. He was incontinent. And he died. It was frightening and horrible in a 33-year-old man, and it had an unknown cause. It was clear he had CMV, but why? . . . That's when it clicked. I bet this is a new disease (Tanne, 1987, para. 18).

To read the full article discussing the diagnoses of the first cases of AIDS (at the time called GRID) and Dr. Mildvan's role, see Tanne (1987).

I knew very little about the disease at the time. As I thought about whether I would take the job, I was less worried about bringing something dangerous home than I was about the reaction of other people. I had a long conversation with the doctors in the infectious disease department and they convinced me that they were very confident that this was not an airborne transmission. I believed they were the experts. So I was feeling okay, but I had to talk it over with my wife, Barbara. I told her, "If you say no, I will turn it down, but this could be the opportunity of a lifetime." She had lots of "what if's." We compared it to TB: even though it is airborne, it is very hard to get. I don't usually trust anything the government says, probably because I am a product of the 1960s. I hold the government at arm's length. I believed the infectious disease docs up to a point. I told my wife, "If I'm wrong and it is very contagious, then we're all dead anyway and so it doesn't matter." So I would be at the eye of the storm as far as exposure, but Barbara said, "Okay, it's your career." But she asked that I please not advertise what I did for a living around the neighborhood. I thought that was reasonable. I know how people are, and thirty years later people are still the same. I saw a recent national survey that said that 30 percent of people still believe you can get HIV from sharing a toothbrush. So that was the first step of a very good career move.

There it started. I worked all over the hospital, on eleven floors. Some floors had two isolation units, some had four. When someone was admitted with an AIDS diagnosis, I got the phone calls. My first patient was a Hispanic guy. I put on a mask, hat, gown, shoe covers, the whole bit, before I went into his isolation room. I sat down on his bed and that was the start of being an AIDS social worker. After I sat there and talked to him for a few minutes, he looked at me with tears in his eyes and said, "You are the first person to sit down on my bed since I've been here." All people wanted was for you to sit and talk for longer than five minutes.

At first, seeing the AIDS patients was an add-on to my Med/Surg job. When I got up to about fifty AIDS patients at once, it became my full-time job to cover all of the AIDS patients admitted to Beth Israel. The hospital didn't really want them, because it was bad for business if people found out who had what. There was so much fear at that time. That was the administrators' problem. I just had to do a good job.

What was "doing a good job"?

For me, it was getting housekeeping to come in and clean the room after a week of it not being cleaned. And that meant grabbing the housekeeping guy by the arm and saying "I'm gonna walk in there with you." A good job meant not letting the food trays pile up outside. That was advocacy. I stopped garbing up [wearing mask, hat, gown, and shoe covers] very soon after starting the job. That stopped within a year for me. There was no such thing as universal precautions yet; that came a bit later.

What were your job duties?

At that time, in 1983, we held the AIDS clinic for only a half day, once a week. I was present at the clinic during those hours, doing what I could. I was doing a group, and the care was pretty low level, almost palliative care. There were some clinical trials going on, so people were coming in to participate in those; they would come for monitoring, to get examined, something to give them hope. During that time I became very familiar with the inpatient and outpatient units all around the hospital. I became very aware of its structure, and that gave me legitimacy. I was known as "the AIDS social worker," once it was called AIDS.

One very awkward moment occurred when I went to see a patient and it turned out to be a hospital employee I knew. He saw me walk into his room and said, "What are you doing here?" He didn't know his diagnosis, and when I walked in the room it was like the grim reaper coming in. People knew what kind of patients I served. It was not a good thing if I came in your room. I told him I just got a referral and I would go check on it. I paged the doctor and said to him, "Did you forget to do something?" So I pulled him in the room and the patient was told. That was the most important thing I could do for him at that point. I tell the students in my classes that good social work is all about establishing relationships and meeting the client where they are. If the patient needs a cup of water, then get them one. Just help meet the need instead of worrying about transference/countertransference, because all of that will come later. There is plenty of room for that, but not now. That is the way I've always practiced. So if what they needed was for me to drag people in the room, all garbed up, then that is what I did. And plenty of people hated me for it!

The fear coming from other people has always been a factor. When people were discharged to go home, fear was always a big barrier. There was fear on one side and reality on the other. I used to work with patients to get them to compromise with the people in their lives, all the while understanding that it was irrational to be fearful of catching the disease. It's not what's in the literature and the studies, it's what people believe is true that matters. I had to help patients understand that in order for them to go home and live with family and friends, they had to sacrifice something, too. So, if they needed to use separate plates, just accept it. Otherwise they were not going to get what they ultimately wanted.

At this point I was seeing a caseload of eighty to a hundred patients with AIDS, and I was doing it by myself. The pace was incredible. I was running from floor to floor and I loved it. It was the most stimulating thing I have ever been involved in. What was I doing for the patients? Not too much, but I was doing what I could. These were really disenfranchised people. They were of lower income, and many had insurance issues. Some had housing issues, family issues, substance use issues. They had so many of the variables we were used to, but all at once.

Did what you do for a living ever get disclosed in your neighborhood?

It did. I promised my wife when I took the job that I would keep it quiet, so at first no one knew, except her family and mine. We were both raised in Brooklyn and we settled in Canarsie, and our children were enrolled in the local school there. We managed to keep the secret until 1985. One day after work my wife asked me to meet her at a PTA meeting at the elementary school. This was going to be an important meeting and all the parents were encouraged to attend. The place was packed, with standing room only. Now in 1985, this is the time when Ryan White was in the news for being banned from his school because he had AIDS. That whole issue came up. They started talking at the PTA meeting about precautions against children with AIDS and about ambulances coming to the school and things like that. Now, I am not the most sophisticated and PC person, though I have honed these skills over the years. But in 1985 I did not have them. I just couldn't keep quiet. I said, "You don't know what you are talking about. This is the way you get it." They said, "How do you know this?" And I had no choice but to say,

"Because I work with them every day and I am fine." And there was a huge hush in the crowd. I didn't have the nerve to look over at Barbara. She was not happy, but she understood I could not bite my tongue anymore. It was an issue of social justice. In the end there were no negative repercussions I could see, for any of us, including the kids.

Box 2.2. What Does PC Mean?

PC is a commonly used abbreviation for the term "politically correct." Political correctness is said to have had its origins in Marxist culturalism. PC is a term used for speech, writings, ideas, policies, and behaviors that others may view as supportive of elements of another's occupation, gender expression, race, culture, sexual orientation, religion, beliefs or ideologies, disability, or age, as well as other dimensions of diversity. Recently, the term has begun to take on a negative tone, reflecting fear to speak one's true beliefs, for fear of being denounced as insensitive at best or racist, sexist, homophobic, or offensive at worst. Now, some might say that being politically incorrect has taken on a more positive meaning than being PC, because it reflects being true to oneself and not being intimidated by society's imposed norms.

Questions for Reflection

1. On the continuum of political correctness to political incorrectness, where would you position yourself? How does this compare to your place on the continuum at other points in your life?

2. Think of a few social workers you admire. Where does their behavior appear to fall on this continuum? Were you aware of this before stopping to think about it? Why or why not might that be?

3. How do political correctness and incorrectness relate to social work values? Can you identify professional value positions that support both tendencies?

4. What are some perspectives regarding HIV and AIDS that could be considered PC or politically incorrect?

Box 2.3. Who Is Ryan White?

I know our agency receives funding to deliver AIDS care through federal money called "Ryan White funds," but who is this Ryan White?

This question is often asked by new and younger workers who did not follow the national news during the 1980s. So, who is Ryan White?

Ryan White was an Indiana teenager with hemophilia who contracted AIDS through a contaminated blood transfusion. He was expelled from his middle school because enraged parents and administrators were fearful that he would spread the infection, because little was understood about transmission of the disease at the time. The media coverage of his lengthy battle with the school system made him a national figure in the news, and attracted the attention of celebrities. Michael Jackson and Elton John became close friends of Ryan and his mother throughout his illness. He courageously fought AIDS-related discrimination and helped educate others across the country about the disease. Upon Ryan's death at age eighteen, Michael Jackson wrote the song "Gone too Soon" in honor of Ryan. Ryan White died on April 8, 1990, just a few months before the passage, with overwhelming bipartisan support from both houses of Congress, of the groundbreaking Ryan White Comprehensive AIDS Resources Emergency (CARE) Act. At that time, more than 150,000 AIDS cases had been reported in the United States and more than 100,000 people had died. The CARE Act was reauthorized in 1996 and again in 2000. It was reauthorized and renamed the Ryan White HIV/AIDS Treatment Modernization Act of 2006, and reauthorized and renamed again in 2009, this time as the Ryan White HIV/AIDS Treatment Extension Act. It is the largest federally funded program for people living with AIDS, and it seeks to improve availability of care for low-income, uninsured, and underinsured people living with AIDS (HIV/AIDS Bureau, 2011).

Ryan's autobiography, entitled *My Own Story*, was published in 1991. His mother, Jeanne White-Ginder, is still an active speaker and AIDS educator. She was present in the Rose Garden of the White House when President Obama signed the last reauthorization of the Ryan White legislation in 2009. To learn more and see clips of interviews with her, see HIV/AIDS Bureau (2011).

Did you see the AIDS population change?

Yes, and the way I know this is hysterical. At first I mostly saw gay men. I would walk in their room at two o'clock and Julia Child would be on channel 13. As the years went by, there were more and more cartoons on. I saw that the intellectual level was going down. That was connected to income level. You can call it the changing face of AIDS, though I hate that phrase. I hate "the changing face of AIDS" because to me it is just a disease and it doesn't matter what the person's face looks like. Another thing that changed was the workers. I was an initial member of the New York City Social Work AIDS Network and it also changed. A lot of us went on to do other things, and some of us stayed. You had newer and younger people coming in and I realized that was me in 1983. I understood that. But these were people without experience. When I was new, I looked to certain people for two things. One was that I needed to know the historical perspective. Another was that I needed someone to teach me what they knew, to be my mentor. These new people didn't want either of those things. They were more radical. That was the time of ACT-UP and all of that.

Box 2.4. ACT-UP

ACT-UP is an acronym for AIDS Coalition to Unleash Power. It is an international direct advocacy group dedicated to improving the lives of people living with AIDS, through influencing legislation, medical research, policies, and treatment of people with HIV and AIDS. ACT-UP traces its origins to March 1987 at the Lesbian and Gay Community Services Center in New York City, when AIDS activist Larry Kramer called for its formation. Kramer designed the organization to be leaderless and anarchist. Since then, ACT-UP has been credited with many effective demonstrations raising public awareness about AIDS and placing pressure on political and economic stakeholders to change policies.

ACT-UP, over the decades, has used civil disobedience, which is not a new idea. Civil disobedience can be defined as "a public, nonviolent and conscientious breach of law undertaken with the aim of bringing about a change in laws or government policies. . . . The persons who practice civil disobedience are willing to accept the legal consequences of their actions, as this shows their fidelity to the rule of law. Civil disobedience, given its place at the boundary of fidelity to law, is said to fall between legal protest, on the one hand, and conscientious refusal, revolutionary action, militant protest and organized forcible resistance, on the other hand" (Brownlee, 2010). Descriptions of some noteworthy demonstrations, illustrating various methods used by the protestors (www.actupny.org), follow.

- March 24, 1987. Two hundred and fifty ACT-UP members demonstrated in New York City at the corner of Wall Street and Broadway, calling for increased access to experimental AIDS drugs and a coordinated national policy to fight the disease. Seventeen members were arrested for civil disobedience. A year later, at a similar demonstration in the same location, more than a hundred people were arrested. Surprisingly, it was not until 2010, twenty-three years later, that the National HIV/AIDS Strategy (NHAS) was unveiled.

- April 15, 1987. In the years prior to electronic filing of tax returns, U.S. post offices would be overwhelmed with last-minute tax filers on tax day, April 15. ACT-UP demonstrators showed their media savvy by showing up at the New York City General Post Office near midnight, when the television media were filming the last-minute filers mailing their returns. This was the first time the famous poster with the words "SILENCE = DEATH" was used.

- January 1988. Women from ACT-UP protested an article published in *Cosmopolitan* magazine that said that in unprotected sex between a man and a woman the risk of HIV transmission was negligible, even if the male partner was infected. About 150 activists "shut down *Cosmo*" by protesting in front of the Hearst building, which housed the magazine's offices. They held signs saying, "Yes, the *Cosmo* girl CAN get AIDS!" Phil Donohue and other news outlets latched onto the story and *Cosmopolitan* was forced to print a retraction, since there was no scientific evidence that penis-to-vagina transmission was not possible.

• December 1989. A large-scale demonstration turned into negative publicity when protestors crossed a line with regard to sacred religious practices. Angered by the Archdiocese's position against condom distribution, about 4,500 activists protested at St. Patrick's Cathedral during a Roman Catholic Mass. A protestor threw a communion wafer that had been consecrated by the priest on the ground, an act considered blasphemy by Roman Catholics, as well as by others who respect sacred rituals. The protest was denounced by New York City Mayor Ed Koch and more than a hundred protestors were arrested.

• September 14, 1989. Seven ACT-UP members chained themselves to the balcony at the New York Stock Exchange, holding a banner that read, "Sell Wellcome." Burroughs Wellcome was the manufacturer of the first anti-retroviral (ARV) drug, AZT (azidothymidine), which was available at the time for a cost of $10,000 per patient, per year. Several days after the demonstration, the pharmaceutical company lowered the price to about $6,400 per year, which was still well out of the reach of most HIV-positive persons.

Currently, ACT-UP is a worldwide organization that provides a website education portal with information from more than sixty countries. It contains topics including "human rights and health as they pertain to the minority sexual experience" (actup.org). There are also numerous local chapters in cities such as San Francisco, Philadelphia, and San Diego. ACT-UP New York's website states their mission as a "diverse, nonpartisan group of individuals united in anger and committed to direct action to end the AIDS crisis. We advise and inform. We demonstrate. WE ARE NOT SILENT" (www.actupny.org). The chapter is working on the AIDS Activist Video Preservation Project. The videos, which offer a detailed history of the AIDS epidemic in the United States and the motivations of these change agents, can be viewed through their website (http://www.actuporalhistory.org/).

Question for Reflection

1. Read the following quote from Frederick Douglass, a former slave who became a social reformer and abolitionist. Do you agree or disagree with his words? Name some causes that might be considered worthy for the use of civil disobedience. What are the necessary circumstances (if any) for you to participate in civil disobedience?

If there is no struggle there is no progress. Those who profess to favor freedom and yet depreciate agitation, are men who want crops without plowing up the ground, they want rain without thunder and lightening [sic]. They want the ocean without the awful roar of its many waters. This struggle may be a moral one, or it may be a physical one, and it may be both moral and physical, but it must be a struggle. Power concedes nothing without a demand. It never did and it never will.

—Frederick Douglass, African-American abolitionist and orator, 1857

When people first started to talk about the "changing face of AIDS," they wanted to shift it to being a minority illness. I warned them not to do this, but my credibility was low, because I am a White male and was talking to minority people. I explained to them that as long as it stayed a White disease there would be more money and it would never stop, but if you made it a minority disease then you would get what they always get—nothing. And that of course is exactly what happened. If this had remained a disease of White people, gay or not, all of these cutbacks would not be happening—nor would the shifting of money over to Africa. It would not have happened as severely.

How do you understand the epidemic in a historical and social context?

I have always been interested in how things fit into history. I like to understand what happened before and its impact on the present and future. Perhaps that is due to my growing up in the 1960s. You have to understand the amount of change that took place then. No other modern decade has ever had that much social change, including the civil rights movement, women's rights, and people getting out and voting. It was actually the ten-year span from 1964 to 1974, to be really accurate. When I started my career, I knew I needed some history behind me. I think today's workers need this, also. It is ironic that now I am part of the history of social work and HIV and I am the first president of PASWHA [Professional Association of Social Workers in HIV and AIDS]. It is all part of the same story.

Box 2.5. Professional Association of Social Workers in HIV and AIDS (PASWHA)

Established in 2010, PASWHA has a mission statement of "energizing and supporting social workers and other professionals providing services to impact the infection through education, research, policy/advocacy, networking, and professional development."

PASWHA was formed after a small group of social workers in HIV and AIDS conducted a web-based survey of social workers and other professionals employed in HIV and AIDS care, prevention, and policy or advocacy work across the United States This small group surveyed their colleagues to see if there was interest in forming a professional association. After positive responses from the professionals surveyed, the group established a 501(c) 3 (nonprofit) organization to launch the effort. One of the main goals of the organization is to inform social workers about recent shifts in the landscape of HIV and AIDS services, such as the passage of the Affordable Care Act (health-care reform), the creation of the National HIV/AIDS Strategy (NHAS), and a move by the CDC [Centers for Disease Control and Prevention] to focus more on social determinants of health. The group will work to ensure that these systems and strategies address barriers to full access to care and treatment for those living with HIV and AIDS, and encourage efforts to decrease the risk of others becoming infected.

In 2011, members elected the first board of directors of PASWHA; the board convened the first meeting in May 2011 at the Twenty-Third Annual National Conference on Social Work and HIV/AIDS, which was held in Atlanta. The first elected president of PASWHA was Alan Rice.

For more information about the new organization, see their website at www.paswha.org/

How do you process your emotions and reactions from your work?

I tend to stay away from AIDS activities after work. I've never been to an AIDS walk, I've never gone to a funeral of anybody who died of AIDS—and I've met some unbelievable people, famous and not, and I've never gone to one funeral. And that decision was made very early in order for me to have some separation and to avoid burnout. I think you have to learn that. It is such a good thing I started that. Oh my, can you imagine? I'd have had to decide "Whose funeral am I going to?," and my work week would have been spent going to funerals. It was an easy decision. I have not been involved in any AIDS activism, I have not been an ACT-UP person. I just leave that to other people. It's not that I don't think it is important, because I do. I think we need the Larry Kramers of the world, but I don't think we have to do it together. I certainly don't want him doing my part. I do my thing and they do theirs and together it is tremendous. Each of us does our part, rather than doing a little of each.

Two nights ago I went to see the reprise of Larry Kramer's *The Normal Heart* on Broadway. It wasn't my idea—the tickets were a gift to everyone on the unit from our supervisor. I had to think it over to decide whether I would actually go, because I never did see the play when it was popular years ago. I'm a rock and roll guy, not a theater guy. It was such a high-impact play. You would have had to have been there twenty-five years ago to appreciate what went on up on that stage. You would have had to have been a gay male at the time, or maybe a social worker in the community. So, in retrospect I am happy I went. I do not regret it.

Box 2.6. *The Normal Heart*

The Normal Heart is a semi-autobiographical play by AIDS activist Larry Kramer that focuses on the rise of the AIDS crisis in New York City from 1981 to 1984. Opening in 1985, it ran successfully for 294 performances off-Broadway at The Public Theatre. It had its Broadway debut on April 19, 2011, for a twelve-week run at the Golden Theatre.

In answer to your question about how I process all of this, I must say I have fully come to appreciate the term "cumulative grief" and to understand what it is. Sometimes there is no time to process grief for each trauma or loss, and you have to wait for the right time to process in a cumulative way. At one of the conferences [National Conference of Social Work and HIV/AIDS] many years ago, there was an administrator speaking about how she helped her staff with this issue. She talked about leaving messages for her staff on their voice mail distribution system. This was in the days before there were computers on every desk, or email and Listserv. I thought it was an interesting idea. I had ten to twelve staff members at the time and I created a voice mail distribution list and started giving messages. On Fridays of every week, I would ask for a moment of silence for our patients who had died that week. I would actually wait the whole minute in the message so everyone would be forced to reflect and remember. That's how I was able to process grief better and not wait too long. Now we don't do that anymore. We are not accumulating as many deaths and losses as before, but we certainly still have them and I think it's important for people to know that. People still get hospitalized and some don't leave. We have to be very attuned to even the subtle losses that happen, and that people you have known a long time still die. We still have repeated hospitalizations. Our AIDS team at St. Luke's and Roosevelt hospitals still sees twenty-two to twenty-seven patients a day. So with all the medical advances and improved training, it's still a high number. You still need an AIDS team.

We are at an interesting fork in the road. As we try to standardize AIDS care, we still specialize in areas and eventually we will have to pick one. Do we want to remain a specialty or have everyone else join us? Should everyone be able to work with the HIV and AIDS populations? I'm very betwixt and between on this. I don't see any social workers breaking down our doors on the inpatient side to help us, and the last thing I want is to force people to do things they don't want to do. If that is the way it is going to be, I think we should continue with the system we have. I think it is unbelievably disgusting that the profession of social work has allowed for specialized AIDS social workers to continue working on their own for as long as we have. Everyone should share the burden. Say you are a social worker and you are sitting in a mental health clinic—AIDS is the last thing on your mind, and you aren't thinking about talking to the client about safer sex practices. I think it is time everyone joins up. Of course, I live in a very naïve world sometimes. I just wish people would volunteer to come learn about how to work with HIV and AIDS.

Is this issue of reaching out to a broad range of social workers something PASWHA will address?

One of the roles I view for the organization is to get all social workers to be aware of the issues even if they think they can avoid HIV. I think that HIV prevention is terribly lacking in our country and always has been. It makes me think about Larry Kramer and *The Normal Heart*. We are so puritanical in this country. I am saying this in 2011 and I said it in 1983. It is unbelievable to me that we still can't get a major safer sex commercial on at two o'clock in the afternoon. Enough said.

I hope the organization can help with this, so that thirty years from now we don't have Mr. and Mrs. Social Worker who believe they are going to avoid AIDS and sexuality and go to work "over there" to avoid these people "over here." We need to explain that you are never going to avoid it because sexuality is part of who we are, and condom negotiation is so critical for all women. Do social workers even know what that looks like? And what about the questions asked on assessments? Do they include a sexual history? As an administrator, I understand what time means, and I understand you are limited in the number of questions you can ask, because you have to move on to the next person. However, that doesn't forgive us for not asking our supervisor if we can add it to the assessment form, so they can in turn make that recommendation to their boss. How do you work with someone on intimate feelings and not know about them sexually and what they are struggling with? How can you possibly do that? I think that the organization will take a look at this when we increase our membership. Then we can increase our committees and reach out to non-HIV social workers. I think that is an important role we can play.

Describe how a diagnosis of AIDS and course of care in 2011 differs from what occurred in 1983.

In 1983, when someone was diagnosed in the hospital, in most cases it was determined based on having PCP [pneumocystis carinii pneumonia]. PCP could not happen any other way in the people we were seeing. Every opportunistic infection existed before—PCP, Toxo [toxoplasmosis], CMV. All of these OI's—opportunistic infections, meaning there is an opportunity for the infection to occur that normally would not become symptomatic but because of low immunity there was an

Figure 2.1. PWA Coalition Newsline

PWA Coalition Newsline

┏ ISSUE NO. 4 ★   PUBLISHED BY AND FOR   ★ SEPTEMBER ★

PEOPLE WITH AIDS & AIDS-RELATED CONDITIONS   1985

EDITORIAL POLICY

You hold in your hands the fourth issue of the **PWA Coalition Newsline** written for people with AIDS and AIDS—related conditions by PWAs and PWARCS and our healthy friends.

We continue to encourage ALL individuals--gay and non-gay--affected by AIDS to contribute articles. We hope this newsletter can be a forum for the expression of our diverse opinions. We encourage all PWAs and PWArcs to give us a piece of your mind!

If you are a person with AIDS or ARC and you would like to contribute, please contact one of us or send your submission to:

P.O. Box 197
Murray Hill Station
New York, NY 10156.

PLEASE NOTE: The articles contained in this publication are for information only and do not necessarily constitute an endorsement of any health or exercise regimen or general program or event. The publication of any name or image does not necessarily imply that that person has AIDS or ARC. Also, the opinions expressed by individual authors do not necessarily represent the opinions of all members of the PWA Coalition or any organization who may be mentioned herein.

∗ ∗ ∗

If you have events of interest to PWAs and PWArcs, you can now leave a message on our answering machine by calling (212) 242-0545. Please leave a detailed message including where, when, who and what cost (if any). We ask that you leave your name and phone number so that we can contact you to confirm and/or double check the information if need be. We reserve the right to determine which events to list on the calendar.

Enjoy!

Wolf Agress	Sam Alford
Mark Arnold	Mark Earley
Albert Graham	Griffin Gold
Andre Saint-Jean	Paul Lande
Ken Meeks	Les Simpson
Jane Rosett	Bobby Bloom
Michael Callen	Jack Steinhebel
Joey Colello	David Summers
David Garfield	David Goldstein
Max Navarre	

THE GROWING PAINS OF SUCCESS!
by Sam Alford

As the fourth issues of PWA Coalition Newsline is readied for publication, we are experiencing growing pains which are the direct result of an incredible response from our readers.

Rather than pretend these problems do not exist and place ourselves in the position of promising more than we can deliver, we wish to share with those of you who support us just where our operation presently stands.

It should be noted that this is not an attempt to rationalize for the brevity of this particular issue -- (after-

opportunity to be symptomatic. Who did we see PCP in before AIDS? Elderly people, patients having chemotherapy, anyone with depleted T-cells. KS [Kaposi's sarcoma] was very common at the time. Prior, we saw KS only in middle-aged Eastern European men, for whatever bizarre reason. At the time, researchers knew about T-cells and B-cells. That was how the diagnosis was made. I would say 75 percent of cases all, it is August)--or for delays in responding to letters, donations and requests from readers. It is, however, our way of providing readers with insights into the difficulties and demands thrust upon us by the sudden success of Newsline.

Four issues ago when we published the first Newsline, we estimated our audience to be in the neighborhood of 400 people. Providing monthly copies to those 400 seemed entirely within our capabilities.

What has subsequently happened, however, is a growing demand from all kinds of individuals and organizations wishing to contribute information for print, as well as requesting large numbers of copies for distribution to PWAs and PWArcs they encounter. Requests now total over 2,000 copies monthly.

Where we come up short and what is preventing us from being able to adequately supply enough copies to those making such requests is cash flow, staff and photocopying support.

First of all, we are still in the process of obtaining legal status as an organization. Since this step has not yet been completed, we are unable to cash personal checks forwarded to us as donations. While we expect to correct this situation shortly, it has created a snag we had not anticipated earlier.

Secondly, our staff is extremely limited. To date an average of only 10-12 persons have been responsible for the news collecting, writing, editing, typing and all production chores required to get us into print. Although many new faces appeared at our last organizational meeting, the primary work up to and through Issue NO. 4 has fallen on the shoulders of the same people. This has resulted in our not being able to respond as quickly as we would like to those who have made donations and who have requested to have their names placed on our mailing list. To all those readers whom we may have offended by not responding earlier, we apologize.

Monthly photocopying of Newsline has also become one of the most challenging and frustrating steps in the production process. Since actual publication depends entirely upon the availability of photocopying equipment at several organizations who generously allow us free use of their machines, publication deadlines have to be scheduled according to these organizations' convenience. This sometimes prevents us from getting the required 2,000 plus copies into PWA hands as quickly as we would like. We hope to remedy this situation by limiting the number of pages in future issues, and by establishing a more dependable production schedule.

Despite the difficulties we are encountering as a result of the unexpected degree of success we are enjoying, we will continue to publish Newsline on a monthly basis. Our goals remain the same: to provide information to people with AIDS and AIDS-related complex, to offer a forum for an exchange of ideas and to encourage those who need support to seek it out. We are grateful to all our readers who have helped us in the initial stages of establishing ourselves as a source of information and support. While growth is sometimes painful, we are certain the rewards are worth the effort. We ask for your continued support and inspiration.

 LETTERS TO THE EDITOR

An article announcing an AIDS Support Group at Beth Israel Hospital which appeared in Issue #2 has caused a stir. For the sake of clarity, we are reprinting the following letter which first appeared in Issue 3, along with two responses.

"Issue #2 of Newsline announced an AIDS Support group for "Gays Only" (your quotations) offered by Beth Israel Medical Center in Manhattan. What the Medical Center defines as a "gays only" group is in actuality a group for gay

had PCP. This determination was usually made with a bronchoscope, which is not an easy test to have performed. You have a tube inserted down your throat. You are sedated a little bit, but it is not a pleasant test. Besides enduring this test, these patients were deathly ill. Because people had waited until the last minute to come to the hospital, they were very sick. In 1983, people were not willing to acknowledge that this was what they had. Denial was easier, and very practical. You had a life expectancy of six to nine months, which of course we know meant men led by a straight, married, male social worker.

PWAs do not need to be subjected to discussing the complex and intimate sexual, psychological and social issues of being a gay PWA to a group leader without gay experience when there must surely be a qualified therapist who is gay on the hospital staff. I would caution your readers to take control of their treatment and know who your services providers are and what their qualifications are.

Other hospitals, such as Sloan-Kettering and Roosevelt, have groups led for gays by therapists who are gay. Beth Israel should either do it right, or not do it at all. But they should certainly not mislead PWAs and the gay community. It's like advertising a group for black people led by a white therapist.

Name Withheld"

KEN MEEKS (the author of the original notice) RESPONDS:

A letter in Issue #3 questioned non-PWA, non-gay leadership of the Beth Israel AIDS support group for gay men.

The issue is simple. The leader is a trained professional who is capable of dealing with issues, problems, feelings and services. Complete commonality with members of the group is not required; the "therapist," as the letter terms him, is NOT a member of the group.

Here we have a trained social worker who has wide experience dealing with support groups. Would the "Name Withheld" letter writer suggest a support group for adolescents be led by an adolescent? And if so, where would one find a trained adolescent social worker?

As one of the main promoters of the BI group, let me assure the letter writer that I HAVE taken control of my treatment: I choose to attend the BI group. I know who my service provider is and what his (and in his absence, her) qualifications are.

Beth Israel IS doing it right: Name Withheld is not forced to attend. Finally, the group was advertised for gay men; no one suggested the sexual orientation or health-status of the group leader.

—KEN MEEKS

VALERIO PANISI WROTE IN TO SAY:

Dear Editors:

I was disturbed after reading one of the "Letters to the Editor" in Issue No. 3 of the Newsline. It is the one regarding the Beth Israel AIDS Support Group.

First I think it's wonderful that there is such a group at Beth Israel. Second, it's even more gratifying that a straight, married male social worker (Does "Name Withheld" prefer a woman?) is leading the group. We should thank this man (His name is Alan) for giving us his help and support instead of criticizing him. It is not by criticism or rejection that we are going to get the help and understanding of straight people out there who are willing to give us help, love, caring.

I consider myself a human being first and gay second. As a human being I accept the help offered to me from other people, no matter what their color, sexual preference or position in life may be. One straight person leading a gay PWA support group does more for us than the hundreds of gay people who are hiding their heads in the sand, trying to ignore what is going on right now in the gay community.

Beth Israel is not trying to mislead or subject anybody to anything. It is only offering PWAs a hand, a caring hand to help us through a terrible illness and a difficult time.

I haven't attended the Beth Israel PWA support group because I go to Bellevue, and GMHC is providing me most of what I need right now and is closer to where I live. But, if I lived around the corner from Beth Israel, I would surely use that support group.

that patients never left the hospital. There were deathbed scenes all over the place. Many of the patients had families. I think it was a myth that many died alone. Some people's families came out of the woodwork. I guess blood is blood. Many of the drug users who had burned their families for years and years still had family come to their bedsides.

The two secrets that were there with the families were the patients' sexuality and their drug use. There are many stories I could tell about both. There was one gay man whose sister was his only living relative. Their parents had both died. The sister lived in Jersey somewhere and he kept

So, "Name Withheld," if you are a PWA, I wouldn't look too much into the horse's mouth. Take the help from wherever it comes.

In my support group all of us are men, but the leader of the group is a woman social worker. I thank God that she is there every week to share my tears, frustration, fears and rare moments of joy.

It is my personal belief that, while there is still no cure for AIDS right now, the best things to get me through this difficult time are love, understanding, a hug from a friend, and chemotherapy (in that order). My arms are open to the straight world out there, just as they are to you, "Name Withheld."

— Valerio Panisi

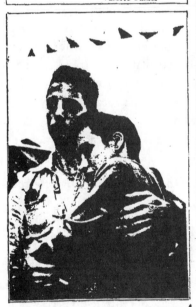

PWAs & PWArcs NEEDED TO LOBBY IN D.C.
by Sam Alford

Mobilization against AIDS (MAA), a San Francisco-based group with whom several New York PWAs and PWArcs lobbied in Washington, D.C. last May is calling for more PWA and PWArc volunteers to join them when the group returns to Washington September 26-October 3 in order to present a Nine-Point Program on AIDS to President Reagan and significant Congresspeople.

One of the group's goals is to have representatives from as many states as possible join in this second lobbying effort. A five-day vigil in front of the White House and a "Day of Accounting" scheduled for September 30 are just two of the activities planned during this Washington visit.

Any PWAs and PWArcs interested in joining the New York delegation, and any persons who might wish to represent New Jersey, Connecticut or other Northeastern states, may contact Sam Alford at (212) 255-9260 for further information. It should be understood that all those who participate in this effort will have to cover their own expenses for the trip. It is hoped, however, that if a large enough delegation forms from the New York area, expenses can be diminished by the sharing of automobiles, hotel rooms, etc.

I encourage those of you who feel the need to become more politically active to call me as soon as possible.

**ACUPUNCTURE ON TUESDAY:
CALL BEFORE COMING!**

The Lincoln Hospital Acupuncture Clinic has announced that due to staff shortage, it may be closed Tuesday nights starting August 6th. They apologize for the inconvenience, but suggest that those seeking acupuncture on Tuesday nights should call before coming: (212) 993-6850; (212) 993-6847; or (212) 993-6879.

4

This newsletter, "People with AIDS Coalition Newsline," published by and for people with AIDS and AIDS-related conditions, was started in 1985 to offer information and resources in New York City. It was written by volunteers, all living with AIDS, who received their care at a variety of medical facilities around NYC, including private physicians' offices and clinics. In one of the features in this issue, Alan Rice was at the forefront of a controversial exchange of letters to the editor.

telling her that he had lymphoma—regular cancer. She and I would speak on the phone from a discharge planning point of view because he was planning to go live with her. She would ask, "Can you tell me what kind of cancer he has?" Apparently, Cancer Care or whoever wanted to know so they could set up care. I had to tell her I couldn't talk to her, and that she would need to ask him. I went down to his room and I said, "Your sister is planning your aftercare based on a lie. You don't even have cancer. It's not even like you have the cancer part of AIDS." He didn't know what to do. We talked about it and then he said, "You know, I'm gonna call her. I'm just gonna tell her." Now, this scenario still happens. It doesn't come up as often, but it still happens.

Overall, the world of AIDS in New York City is much different today. Fortunately, today if you have AIDS you get benefits. You get a lot of benefits, such as ARV medications, housing benefits, money benefits, other benefits. Today it is a different diagnosis. Sometimes it is almost like, "Thank God I have it. Now I can live!" I think it is a poor statement of who we are that you have to get a disease *like this* in order to think that this is the best moment of your life. We know for sure that some people try to get it. We know for sure that there is fraud, and I don't necessarily blame the individuals. I blame the system that set this up. It is on society. So that is another big difference. Years ago it was difficult to give people the news. In fact, in some cases the docs would avoid it. Now, you don't get that severe "oh my God" reaction when people are told. It is not a death sentence.

What do you want your students to know about what you have learned in your work?

Back in the 1980s I had a tough role. I didn't want to be the grim reaper, but I think it is essential that as social workers we are realistic. I talk to my students about this as well, especially those who work with chronic drug addicts. They usually want to do these long, projected treatment plans, when really what you need to concentrate on is very short term. That is the way I helped patients and preserved myself. I went day to day. My treatment plans were about tomorrow. I did not talk about a month from now or six months from now. Two weeks, maybe. I always wanted to give hope that people were leaving.

Here is a story from well into my career that shows the impact of not thinking carefully before speaking. I get a call at four o'clock on a Friday from a nurse on a unit, saying that I need to see a guy who was admitted that morning because he's almost psychotic. And remember, I'm seeing the same patients over and over again. It is not like in an office where you're coming to see me once a week. However, it is a bit like that because they keep returning, and unfortunately the time since they were last discharged is not that great. So our work was often a continuation. I walk into this guy's room and he's there with a friend and he's pacing around the room. He's pacing, like a lion. I try to calm him down. He is saying, "You don't understand, I am dying and I need you to do this for me." I don't even remember what it was he wanted me to do because it isn't relevant to the point of the story. He pleaded with me and out of my mouth came, "But you aren't dying tomorrow. It can wait." Then he did die over the weekend. So the lesson is that you can't discount how someone is feeling. He felt like he was dying tomorrow and part of me just wanted to go home. It was 4:30. I regret what I said and I know you need to be careful what you say. I don't even remember what it was he wanted from me. I guess it was just recognition that it was over for him, and it helped me realize that if somebody is agitated, you need to find out what it is about. If you can help him, fine. If you can't, it's okay, too. You can't do everything for everybody. But it's these little snippets and vignettes that always help ground me. They bring me back to knowing that in this work it can be very short term. He really needed something given to him and I didn't give it because it was Friday afternoon and I wanted to go home. If I made the decision to go up to the unit, then I really should have been there. So when people ask me how I have done it all these years, with people dying, it's just a matter of the moment. What do they need from me now.

People ask how I can stand being around all these death scenes, and what I say is, "It's my job." And I don't mean that as "It's only a job." I mean it as "This is my job." My wife always wants to know why I can't be as sensitive at home as I am at work. She was visiting me one time on a day when it was my day on the rotation to see walk-ins from the outside. I was on call in my office that day. There was an elderly man who needed something. Barbara, my wife, was sitting in my office and I asked her to wait next door. I brought the man in and he was almost deaf. I had to talk very loud for him to hear me. So, then this unbeliev-able sensitivity flowed out of me and Barbara could hear me through the wall. When she saw me, she said, "Who the hell are you?" And I said, "Listen, this is my job and I am trained to do this." Clearly it must be the training, because I am not normally a sensitive guy. I have skills to listen and respond and I told her, "I can't do it in both places." It's a skill set—it's not my personality.

The main difference between the 1980s and now is discharge planning. People go home now and live their lives. We now do long-range planning and the struggles we have today are with those who are healthy enough to go back to work. They don't want to lose their social security disability benefits, which would make them lose their Medicare, and they don't know whether their insurance will be picked up by an employer. There are so many things that affect the payments, and I'm not sure yet where health-care reform fits into that. I think we are keeping people disabled because of uncertainty. Yes, the preexisting condition clauses are gone, but not really. I know a case where an insurance company denied admission to a twenty-eight-day treatment program based on an assessment that showed it was not a severe enough problem. So the man ended up in the Bellevue emergency room, passed out from drinking too much. I'm not sure what else they want. I equate that to an oncologist trying to get approval for radiation and being told the tumor is not big enough yet—come back when it's huge. This is frightening. Obama is trying his best, but there are loopholes all over.

We have 6,000 people in our clinic system, and not all of them can go back to work. Some have never worked a day in their lives because they have lived on public assistance. We know this is generational and I think it is unfair to expect something different from people. When Clinton passed welfare reform in 1996 and mandated that people go to work after five years on welfare, they did not realize that this is unrealistic for untrained people. But it happened. Now that we have fewer people on public assistance, I am not seeing more money as a taxpayer. What happened?

Another difference is that in the early days we never talked about sex, drugs, or any of the other behaviors that may have gotten people where they were. This is because people were deathly ill and it was the last thing on their mind. When the ARVs started, obviously it was an overnight sensation. We didn't know what kind of impact they would have. So many people gave up right before the ARVs came out. If they had hung in there, they might have really lengthened their lives.

AZT was pretty rough. A lot of people decided not to be on it; they went the alternative medicine route. People died. The only people who lived were the outliers, the nonprogressors. When the cocktail took off in 1996, we were caught with our pants down. We did not realize that when people began to feel better, they would want to be normal. "Normal" means returning to their previous behaviors, such as sexual acting out. Drug use continues. Mental illness arises. Problems in relationships pop up where one partner was just waiting for the other to die instead of just separating, because the relationship is no good. Other consequences I saw were the decision to sell your life insurance policy, and now you have no money. Another was the decision to charge up a storm and now you're in debt. How about the decision to not declare yourself legally, and now you can't get student loans, for example. This was all because people thought they were going to die. We were unprepared.

Box 2.7. The Lazarus Effect

According to the Biblical story, Jesus raised Lazarus from the dead. When highly active anti-retroviral therapies [HAART] became available to patients with AIDS, medical professionals and other workers claimed they were quickly pulled back from the jaws of death, like Lazarus. Recently, as HAART has become available in regions of Sub-Saharan Africa with high rates of HIV infection, the term "Lazarus effect" has been used more prominently.

In May 2010, HBO [Home Box Office, Inc.] premiered a documentary that follows four HIV-positive residents of the country of Zambia, showing how ARV medications have changed their lives. According to the film, ARV drugs in Zambia dropped in cost from $27 a day in 2002 to 40 cents a day at the time of filming. The reduction in price was due to support of The Global Fund, and the U.S. President's Emergency Plan for AIDS Relief [PEPFAR].

See www.pepfar.gov for details of how the United States financial support is being allocated and evaluated.

See www.theglobalfund.org to view videos showing programs funded by that international nongovernmental organization.

Box 2.8. Emotional Impact of Client Losses on Social Workers

There is no avoiding the fact that service to others is stressful. In the field of social work, clients are dealing with multiple social problems, chronic, severe mental and medical illnesses, trauma, and suffering. The professional work of caring requires that workers prepare themselves to withstand the stress of helping, for their own good as well as that of their clients (Zellmer, 2005.) Issues related to stress and loss responses in professional helpers are briefly described below.

- Compassion fatigue (originally called secondary traumatic stress) is the term used to identify the emotions and behaviors that result from knowing about a traumatizing event experienced by someone close to the person (Figley, 1995). It stems from helping or wanting to help the traumatized or suffering person.

- Burnout is commonly defined as a syndrome of emotional exhaustion, depersonalization, and reduced personal accomplishment that can occur in individuals who do "people work" (Maslach & Jackson, 1981). Burnout is seen as a psychological reaction to working in difficult conditions that often involve difficult client relationships. It is widely understood that qualities of the work environment also affect the level of burnout seen in workers.

- Vicarious traumatization causes unhealthy changes in the workers' inner experience that result from empathic engagement with clients' trauma material. It is thought that continuous exposure to graphic accounts of suffering may leave the worker open to "emotional and spiritual consequences" (Trippany, White Kress, & Wilcoxon, 2004). Workers with continued exposure to clients who have experienced trauma have been shown to experience some similar effects, such as alterations in ability to trust; anxiety, unexplained anger, and irritability; disrupted sense of meaning, connection, and worldview; and decreased capacity for intimacy (Trippany et al., 2004).

- Grief is a normal process of reacting to a loss. The loss may be physical (such as a death or loss of fertility), social (such as a relationship), or occupational (such as a job or ability to support oneself). Normal grief reactions include anger, guilt, anxiety, sadness, and despair. Normal physical responses include changes in appetite, sleeping patterns, or illness.

- Cumulative grief occurs when someone experiences multiple or continual losses, with little time allowed for separate grieving. This can happen with a helping professional when working in high loss settings. When the worker hides the grief, or the worker does not openly express the grief because there is no outlet for it, the grief accumulates and becomes internalized (Clark, 2011). Just becoming experienced with death or other types of loss does not equip a worker to avoid cumulative grief. Losses must be processed and expressed or they will accumulate.

- Complicated grief is identified by the length of time of one's grief reactions, the severity of the reactions, and the degree to which they interfere with normal daily activities. Grief complications can include adjustment disorders such as depression, anxious mood, and suicidal thoughts or acts. Complicated grief, which is sometimes called unresolved or prolonged grief, should be treated with medications, therapy, or both.

- Collective grief is what a community, society, or nation experiences in response to a traumatic event. It is a shared experience, which diminishes the sense of aloneness and isolation that can be felt during an individual loss. Those who are deeply and not so deeply affected derive comfort from experiencing the same feelings alongside others. Events that can trigger collective grief include natural disasters, such as the tsunami in the Indian Ocean; incidents of terrorism, such as the attacks on September 11; the death of a high-profile person, such as Princess Diana; or the accidental drowning of a neighborhood child in the local pool. For a while, people of the community, nation, or world are united in common emotional reactions.

Questions for Reflection

1. What practice settings or fields in the profession of social work might be prone to cumulative grief? Why?

2. Think of any recent instances when you have been part of a communal instance of collective grief. Did knowing others felt similarly help you work through your grief? Or did the fact that others were also suffering add to your grief?

3. Are you now or have you ever been burned out? You can take a quick fifteen-question Burnout Self-Test online for no cost. Visit http://www.mindtools.com/stress/Brn/BurnoutSelfTest.htm. For a more rigorous, validated test, the Maslach Burnout Inventory is highly respected and is available for purchase through Mind Tools.

4. The AIDS Memorial Quilt continues to be hugely popular, with more than 18 million visitors worldwide. Why do you think people continue to travel to view sections of the quilt? Why are new memorial squares continually being submitted for inclusion by loved ones? What is the pay-off for these visitors, friends, and family members?

We don't talk about sexual histories and other sensitive areas. If you are into mental health, you ask a page of mental health questions. If you are into HIV and AIDS, you ask a page full of sexual history questions. If not, maybe it's two questions. I think people's sexual behavior, more than any other part of the assessment, can tell you everything you need to know about the person. But you have to ask the questions, even if it makes you feel uncomfortable. You need to ask if they are insertive or receptive, if and when they have anal sex, and if so, whether they like it, and whether they achieve orgasm that way. This is important because it gives insight into how likely they are to practice safer sex. From the statistics I have read, more women than one would think have anal sex. But you have to ask all the questions and be open to listening to the answers. All of that will tell you who you have in front of you, and that will tell you if they will be adherent to their treatment and follow after-care plans.

What do you think will happen to the Ryan White funding stream as a consequence of health-care reform?

I think from a money point of view this is all going away. I think Ryan White money will be melded into something else. The money itself won't disappear, but the management will not be handled the way it is now. I think it's bad on one hand and good on another, opening up some doors that have been closed. For example, I said earlier that I think we can play a tremendous role in HIV prevention and all we need to do is learn how to get some money for it. If Ryan White is about AIDS and AIDS care, then ABC Agency that does not do AIDS care is not interested. But say you are ABC Agency that has nothing to do with HIV, but you have a ton of people who certainly have a need for STI [sexually transmitted infection] education, then this is an area you can get involved in.

That brings up the issue of chronic illnesses. There are many chronic illnesses out there. I will always be on record saying that AIDS is like no other, for all of the psychosocial reasons. You don't lose your housing because you are diabetic. You don't lose your job because you have a chronic heart condition. You don't lose family because you have cancer. You never did. Cancer in its worst time just caused some isolation, and not very much. With it you never lost your job, your home, you never lost your insurance. So that will always make AIDS stand above. However, if it is truly a chronic illness, which I believe it is for a significant part of the positive population, then we have a lot to teach other social workers about other chronic illnesses that have not had such a good success rate. A couple of years ago I looked at the statistics about AIDS deaths and diabetes deaths in a particular year so that I could compare them. Ten times more people died from diabetes than AIDS. So we think we have the power of numbers behind us, but really we don't. In terms of mortality from the disease, what we bring to the world of chronic illness is a particular area of expertise. If we continue to wait for the American Diabetes Association to come to us, we will be waiting forever.

What expertise do you think AIDS social workers have to offer workers dealing with other chronic illnesses?

We have an understanding of the totality of the patient. The ecological model of care has everything. We have an appreciation that just because somebody has an illness with a known success rate and treatment, it still might not be successful. Even if the patient is 100 percent compliant all of the time, their outcome may not be great. And more likely, high compliance is not always the case. Diabetics still get amputated no matter how well they do. We know how to identify the barriers that get in the way of someone doing well. You must appreciate that not everybody's going to have a big success. I think that's what we've learned over the last thirty years.

Do you think burnout is a common problem for social workers who work with HIV and AIDS?

Burnout? I don't believe in it. I do believe in vicarious trauma and collective grief. I think it's another reason that it is probably time to get more people on board to work with patients so that we don't take the whole burden on ourselves. We know about vicarious trauma from the Red Cross, who first identified it in disaster relief workers. They started to notice that the people who went all the time started to behave the same way as the people they were treating. I think no matter how much therapy one gets, it's not really going to take it away. The only way you can move away is to expose yourself to less—not to no exposure, but to less and less. And so, the question is what can we do to bring on board those social workers who are not working in trauma, to help us. I don't think that's going to happen, so unfortunately support groups and all the things we were involved in internally, either in our job or professional network, are all gone because all of that requires time and money which are things we don't have. Self-care is not billable.

Box 2.9. Healing Collective Grief from AIDS

The NAMES Project Memorial AIDS Quilt is an example of a collective effort to process grief over the loss of so many individuals who have died from AIDS-related complications. The Quilt can be viewed not only as a vehicle to heighten political awareness of the pandemic, but also as a therapeutic tool (Lewis & Fraser, 1996). Each square in the quilt solidifies the nation's collective memory of those who were lost in the fight against AIDS.

Founded in 1987 by AIDS activist Cleve Jones, the Quilt now comprises more than 91,000 squares, each one created in memory of a person who died of AIDS-related complications. The quilt is now too large to display in its entirety. Sections of the Quilt travel for public viewing. The last display of the entire quilt was in October 1996, when it covered the entire National Mall in Washington, DC. The Quilt was nominated for a Nobel Peace Prize in 1989 and remains the largest community art project in the world (www.aidsquilt.org).

What do you know now that you wish you had known early in your career?

For me, probably not much. I am a big proponent of self-determination. In a hospital setting that is a rough stance to take. Think about it. We work with doctors who are doers. We work with nurses who are task oriented, and then you have us, who are for self-determination of the client. You remember I told you about my long-time patient, Leon. Leon was my first teacher about the importance of self-determination. If you are in health care and are working in a multidisciplinary setting, I think the role of the social worker is always to represent the ego of the patient. You always have to advocate for your patient's right to self-determine. That is not a popular stance, especially as we become more and more aware that the medications will work and more aware of patients who don't want to take them. Now it's going to be even more of a controversy given the statistics out there that transmission rates will decrease if meds are given right from the get-go. Get an early diagnosis, get on the medication, and you will transmit to fewer and fewer people. All of that is wonderful. I will not make any negative comment about all that. However, you cannot force people to take the treatment unless they are ready—if they are ever ready. It is something we need to appreciate and not force them into treatment by jumping on the bandwagon with everyone else.

What do you see as the most pressing area for reform in the way we deliver HIV and AIDS services?

I have a concern about whether hospitals and clinics can sustain personnel doing services for which they cannot recoup money. That is a huge question today. I am fortunate to work for somebody who understands that you need a lot of soft money to run a program with many supportive staff members. Grant money will always be out there. The question is will it have to be reframed. For instance, we have a grant-funded program called Coming Home, which is intended for formerly incarcerated HIV-positive patients. We also know there are some formerly incarcerated people who are not HIV positive who also need help. Some have other chronic illnesses such as hepatitis, for example. We applied for an additional grant to take care of these patients as well. If they have insurance, we can bill. But think about it. We are an HIV clinic taking care of HIV-negative patients. That's the way to go. What's the danger? That you become a non-HIV clinic? Well, let me ask, if you find a niche and you can sustain yourself, isn't that good? We will never become a non-HIV clinic. But in New York City, for example, we are all vying for the same patients. The managed care part of health-care reform will stop patients from hopping from clinic to clinic. I think getting a grant to serve non-HIV-infected patients is a great way to sustain. This was a perfect way and the hospital allowed us to do it. It has created a tremendous boost to our numbers.

It is a very bad idea to not look at care delivery from a business point of view, and social workers are as guilty of this as anyone. We need to become as expert at the business side of care as we are with our clinical skill set. That idea of losing your moral character when you see it as a business is a bunch of B.S. We have to be business savvy. We can't be walking on financial eggshells. You can do both. You can take care of patients with a dedication and compassion second to none and still keep your head above water—and that is what is going to be required. If you show administrators that you are self-sustaining, they will leave you alone. They will consume you into the regular mainstream if you don't fight for autonomy. To do that, we must speak their language.

If we continued this conversation in five years, what might we be discussing?

In five years I would be discussing my retirement! Actually, I have always tried not to look that far forward into the future. Five years is a long time for me. My plan is to retire in eight years. That doesn't mean I will stop working, but I will stop the craziness I am involved in now.

I think PASWHA will have a role in the future but it probably will not be within my own vision for it. With Medicaid reform, we are already seeing the need for prior authorization for tests. This has never happened before. I think it's good. I think the abuse of the Medicaid system needs to be curtailed. That is something we will be discussing. In five years if you are still alive with HIV and you've lost your rent supplement and you need to go to work, it will be interesting to see what the stress of it will do to your condition, since we know stress is not good. What I have always told my patients to consider when making decisions about whether to go on disability or work, is, "What will cause you the least amount of stress? Will it be staying at work or the lack of money you will have if you don't work?" You need to think about your health. Do you want to live in substandard housing, or do you want to try to get yourself a job? That's still what we'll be discussing in five years.

Thank you.

It has been my pleasure to share.

References

Brownlee, K. (2010). Civil disobedience. *The Stanford Encyclopedia of Philosophy.* N. Zalta (Ed.). Retrieved from http://plato.stanford.edu/archives/spr2010/entries/civil-disobedience/

Clark, E. (2011). Grief and loss tip sheet: Understanding professional grief. *Social workers: Help starts here.* Retrieved from http://www.helpstartshere.org/mind-and-spirit/grief-and-loss-tip-sheet-understanding-professional-grief.html

Douglass, Frederick. [1857] (1985). "The significance of emancipation in the West Indies." Speech, Canandaigua, New York, August 3, 1857; collected in pamphlet by the author. In John W. Blassingame (Ed.), *The Frederick Douglass Papers.* Series One: Speeches, Debates, and Interviews (Vol. 3, pp. 1855–1863). New Haven, CT: Yale University Press, p. 204.

Figley, C. (1995). Compassion fatigue: Toward a new understanding of the costs of caring. In B. Stamm (Ed.), *Secondary traumatic stress: Self-care issues for clinicians, researchers and educators* (pp. 3–28). Luterville, MD: Sidren Press.

HIV/AIDS Bureau. (2011). *Who was Ryan White?* U.S. Department of Health and Human Services (DHHS), Health Resources and Services Administration (HRSA). Retrieved from http://hab.hrsa.gov/abouthab/ryanwhite.html

Lewis, J., & Fraser, M. (1996). Patches of grief and rage: Visitor responses to the NAMES Project AIDS memorial quilt. *Qualitative Sociology, 19*(4), 433–451.

Maslach, C., & Jackson, S. E. (1981). *Maslach burnout inventory: Research edition.* Palo Alto, CA: Consulting Psychologist Press.

Tanne, J. H. (1987, January 12). Fighting AIDS: On the front lines against the plague. *New York Magazine.* Retrieved from http://nymag.com/health/features/49240/

Trippany, R., White Kress, V., & Wilcoxon, S. A. (2004). Preventing vicarious trauma: What counselors should know when working with trauma survivors. *Journal of Counseling and Development, 82,* 31–37.

Willinger, B., & Rice, A. (Eds.). (2003). *A history of AIDS social work in hospitals: A daring response to an epidemic.* Binghamton, NY: Haworth Press.

Zellmer, D. D. (2005). Teaching to prevent burnout in the helping professions. *Analytic Teaching, 24,* 20–25.

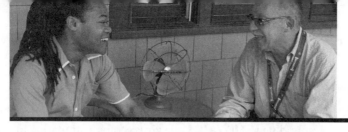

3

Seasons of Change: Exploring the Future of HIV/AIDS Social Work

Michele Rountree, Marsha Zibalese-Crawford, and Maestro Evans

Let no one be discouraged by the belief there is nothing one person can do against the enormous array of the world's ills, misery, ignorance, and violence. Few will have the greatness to bend history, but each of us can work to change a small portion of events. And in the total of all those acts will be written the history of a generation.

—Robert F. Kennedy (1966)

This tradition [of innovations during the Progressive Era and the New Deal] was very much in evidence as social workers like Diego Lopez in New York, Judy Macks in San Francisco, Caitlin Ryan in Atlanta, David Aronstein in Boston, Bill Scott in Houston, and Anthony Hill in London pioneered the design and delivery of the first psychosocial services for people affected by AIDS.

—Key Informant (May 19, 2009)

Social work, once in the forefront of the fight against AIDS, is now at a crossroads. Social workers are increasingly turning to private practice (Specht & Courtney, 1994), and as a direct impact there are fewer social workers entering the HIV/AIDS (human immunodeficiency virus and acquired immune deficiency syndrome) field. Although there is no cure, with medical advances HIV is now considered a chronic disease (Clarke, 1994), and funding for HIV/AIDS, both public and private, has been steadily declining over the past few years (Kaiser Family Foundation, 2003). At the same time, HIV continues to spread among a variety of populations and the virus continues to change, enabling it to become resistant to current interventions. If there are to be enough HIV/AIDS social work providers ready to meet the needs of clients in this decade and beyond, we must ensure the sufficiency and quality of this frontline workforce (NASW, 2005).

The search for new medical treatment appears to be cyclical: although the medical profession is responding to HIV/AIDS, the virus is rapidly mutating in response to the most recent remedies science can produce. Social work with public health has become increasingly clinical, however, and follows the direction of the medical profession's response to HIV/AIDS. It appears that social work can contribute as an appendage of the medical profession (NASW, 2005).

Throughout the history of the profession, it has been uncharacteristic of social workers to follow others' lead. Is this new role a suitable one for the world we live in, or should social work reassume a leadership role in the fight against HIV/AIDS, and make a contribution unique to social work? Should social workers partner with others, rather than follow them?

Social work must revisit its history and use that history as a way of exploring social work today in relation to HIV/AIDS in order to clarify its agenda. How did we confront the issues of the past? How do we deal with the concerns of today? Where are we going? What will be our vision for the next two decades?

This chapter discusses an agenda for social work in the HIV/AIDS arena. This chapter is divided into three parts: first, the history of the HIV/AIDS epidemic; second, how social work's history affects its future; and third, clarification of concerns for the future of our work. With vision ultimately comes action.

The History of an Epidemic
Inauspicious Beginnings

The challenges of the current AIDS era required bold action in the field of social work. The extent to which social workers have been on the forefront of these campaigns has varied (Linsk & Keigher, 2002). Among early efforts, social workers, in many cases serving as unpaid volunteers, demanded that nursing staff take food trays into hospital rooms of people with AIDS instead of dropping them off outside the door, and that these workers not allow patients to wallow in their own excrement because they are too fearful to change the linen. Edith Springer, a professional social worker and recovering narcotic addict, pioneered AIDS prevention outreach to intravenous (or injection) drug users by teaching them how to clean needles and use condoms in the crack dens and shooting galleries in Manhattan's Lower East Side (Evans, 1987).

The HIV/AIDS epidemic and social work's response to it have changed radically since the identification of the disease in the early 1980s. Because our past provides a context for social work practice today and influences the future, it is important to understand the history of the epidemic, and to present an overview of the challenges social workers have faced.

Between 1979 and 1981, physicians began documenting a pattern of young, gay men in three urban areas—New York, Los Angeles, and San Francisco—being diagnosed with rare forms of cancer (e.g., Kaposi's sarcoma) and pneumonia (e.g., Pneumocystis carinii pneumonia [PCP]). These diseases were accompanied by severe weight loss, diarrhea, high fever, swollen lymph nodes, and oral and anal thrush that were characteristics of suppressed immune systems. This pattern was unusual, as typically only elderly people or those taking drugs with immunodepressive side effects suffered from a weakened immune system. As the number of documented cases increased, physicians and public health officials became alarmed. What was this strange development that seemingly targeted young, gay men? On July 4, 1981, the Centers for Disease Control and Prevention (CDC) published a report in *Morbidity and Mortality Weekly Report*: "Kaposi's Sarcoma and Pneumocystis Carinii Pneumonia among Homosexual Men—New York City and California." The report painted the picture of the unusual nature of these two diseases and warned physicians to "be alert for Kaposi's sarcoma, *Pneumocystis carinii* pneumonia, and other opportunistic infections associated with immunosuppression in homosexual men" (as quoted in Grmek, 1992, p. 8).

This new disease became known as "gay cancer," "gay pneumonia," "gay-related immune deficiency" (also known as GRID), or "gay compromise syndrome" because it affected gay men, almost exclusively, in the early years. These names are "interesting precisely to the extent that they reveal medical error and . . . moral prejudice" (Grmek, 1992, p. 32). By 1982, the universality of the disease was recognized as it continued to spread to heterosexual men and women. Replacing inaccurate names such as GRID, four new initials, A.I.D.S. (acquired immune deficiency syndrome), was used to label the disease at a CDC meeting in Atlanta in the summer of 1982. Due to the wide dissemination of research studies in CDC publications, "AIDS" became widely accepted as the new name for the disease. Not until 1984—two years after the naming of AIDS—did scientists successfully isolate a retrovirus from the lymph node of a thirty-three-year-old man with AIDS. After discovering that this virus actually killed cells (differentiating it from the other two known retroviruses), they were able to show that it caused AIDS. In 1986, the CDC named this the human immunodeficiency virus (HIV).

The Early Response

As the AIDS epidemic emerged as a primary concern in the medical community, hospitals were at the forefront of the response to the AIDS epidemic and became involved in AIDS diagnosis and treatment. Hospital staff, including "nurses, residents, social workers, technicians, dietitians, and orderlies" faced their personal fears and, in most cases, overcame them and persevered in the field (McKenzie, 1992, p. 271). In addition to the medical response, community-based organizations (CBOs) quickly emerged to meet the medical and psychosocial needs of people living with HIV and AIDS (PLWHA). People who had watched their friends die, and who, after attending funeral after funeral, decided they needed to respond, organized these early AIDS CBOs. These emerging AIDS CBOs were grassroots in nature, made up of community volunteers—people living with AIDS and their family members, friends, and advocates.

One example of such a CBO was the Gay Men's Health Crisis, founded by six men in 1981 to raise funds for research and provide information to an increasingly alarmed population (McKenzie, 1992). Beginning with a crisis hotline, Gay Men's Health Crisis was different from traditional social service organizations or medical service providers in that the Gay Men's Health Crisis were "more like the help that a family or close-knit community would offer someone in need" (McKenzie, 1992, p. 543). Gay Men's Health Crisis developed both therapeutic and practical support services. Primary services included crisis intervention as well as a buddy program, wherein volunteers were matched with a person living with AIDS to provide support. Gay Men's Health Crisis became a model for other CBOs as well as future government programs. AIDS CBOs—also referred to as AIDS service organizations (ASOs)—grew to offer a wide variety of programs, including "public health education; psychosocial counseling; practical support, particularly help with day-to-day activities, e.g., cooking, cleaning, laundry, shopping, and transportation; home health-care services; housing; government benefits advocacy; legal protections, e.g., fighting employment and housing discrimination; access to health care, including providing referrals and access to clinical trials and experimental drugs" (McKenzie, 1992, p. 569).

The gay community's rapid response to the epidemic was made possible by the foundation of a decade of organizing by gay groups in the 1970s, including organizing as national political groups, advocacy groups, and thousands of community groups (Altman, 1986). Thus, ASOs were hybrid agencies offering a combination of both service provision and activism. Gay Men's Health Crisis not only raised funding for research and provided services, but also worked in political lobbying efforts.

The Social Environment

Although community organizing and service provision was occurring at the grassroots level, the epidemic was spreading fear in the minds of the American people, particularly with the realization that the disease could be transmitted through blood transfusions and the growing realization that AIDS was not a disease that affected only gay men. The Reagan administration was largely in denial of the AIDS epidemic and its impact on the American people. Congress pressed to pass legislation providing funding for AIDS research. Funds for AIDS research to the CDC, National Institutes of Health (NIH), and others increased from $5.5 million in 1982 to $96 million in 1985.

Socially and politically, AIDS was unlike many other medical concerns because it was treated as a moral issue as much as a health issue, if not more so. For example, an editorial in the *Southern Medical Journal* claimed, "Might we be witnessing in fact, in the form of a modern communicable disorder, a fulfillment of St. Paul's pronouncement: 'the due penalty of error'?" (Altman, 1986, p. 13). This moral treatment of AIDS, seen as a penalty, created an environment where people blamed the victims of AIDS and did not see it as a human disease. On the other hand, although many in the political and even medical sphere blamed AIDS patients for their illness, there were others who advocated for them and actively sought treatment for the disease.

Changes in Medical Treatment

In 1987, a major medical breakthrough occurred with approval of the first drug for AIDS treatment. Azidothymidine (AZT) is a nucleoside reverse transcriptase inhibitor (NRTI). NRTIs are incorporated into the virus's DNA, making the virus ineffective. With the introduction of AZT, AIDS was no longer an immediate death sentence; the medication significantly increased the lifespan of individuals living with AIDS. There are, however, limitations to the use of AZT. First, AZT has toxic side effects. Over prolonged periods of use, AZT can lead to the death of red blood cells, or anemia. Second, AZT is not a cure: ultimately, it is unable to halt the progression of AIDS because of the way HIV can mutate in the body, developing AZT-resistant strains of HIV. Third, AZT is very expensive, about $3,500 per year for one person (Fan, Conner, & Villarreal, 2002).

Not until 1995 did the Food and Drug Administration (FDA) approve a different kind of drug, called a protease inhibitor. Protease inhibitors work differently from NRTIs: they inhibit the protease enzyme, which is responsible for the maturation of HIV. This is important because immature HIV particles are not infectious (Fan et al., 2002). A drug that inhibits protease will ultimately stop the production of infectious HIV. With the availability of protease inhibitors, so-called triple combo therapy became the standard of care in 1996. Triple combo therapy was a combination of two NRTIs and a protease inhibitor. In 2002, highly active antiretroviral therapy (HAART) replaced triple combination therapy (this term was shortened to ART, or antiretroviral therapy).

Since the discovery and use of NRTIs and protease inhibitors, other classes of drugs have also become widely accepted as a part of ART. They include nonnucleoside reverse transcriptase inhibitor (NNRTIs), maturation inhibitors, integrase inhibitors, and entry inhibitors, some of which are still being developed. It is important to remember that these differing types of drugs inhibit different functions of HIV, each making the body unable to produce new infectious HIV in the body. The development of new medications is critical to increasing the life spans of individuals living with AIDS, because of HIV's capacity to mutate rapidly, which enables it to develop resistance to drugs over time. Although combining three drugs at once is an improvement in this regard, HIV can become resistant to a drug cocktail. The more drug combinations that are available for people living with AIDS, the greater the length of survival after diagnosis.

The Evolving Response of Public Health and Social Work

Alongside the growing medical response to the AIDS epidemic was a similar growing response in the fields of public health and social work. A major aspect of this response included the development of standard practices, ranging from prevention to testing, counseling and referrals, and partner services. The CDC published the first set of guidelines for testing and counseling in 1986, highlighting the "importance of offering voluntary testing and counseling and maintaining confidential records" (CDC, 1999). The CDC developed a new set of guidelines in 1994, covering

- encouraging availability of anonymous as well as confidential HIV testing;

- ensuring that HIV testing is informed, voluntary, and consented;

- emphasizing access to testing and effective provision of test results;

- advocating routine recommendation of HIV counseling, testing and referral (CTR) in settings (e.g., publicly funded clinics) serving clients at increased behavioral or clinical risk for HIV infection;

- recommending use of a prevention counseling approach aimed at personal risk reduction for HIV-infected persons and persons at increased risk for HIV; and

- stressing the need to provide information regarding the HIV test to all who take the test (CDC, 1999)

Officials with the CDC updated these counseling, testing, and referral guidelines in 2001, demonstrating that as the epidemic changes and new challenges emerge, the response needs to change as well.

In 2003, the CDC implemented rapid testing. This was important because it removed many of the barriers to testing, making it possible for a person to take an HIV test and receive the results on the same day. It enabled the CDC to launch the campaign, "Advancing HIV Prevention," which was targeted toward reduction of barriers to early diagnosis of HIV and increasing the access to quality medical care, treatments, and ongoing prevention services" (CDC, 2003).

In 2006, *Morbidity and Mortality Weekly Report* reported new counseling, testing, and referral guidelines for medical settings, including guidelines for patients in all health-care settings and for pregnant women. In an article discussing the guidelines, the CDC reported,

- HIV screening is recommended for patients in all health-care settings after the patient is notified that testing will be performed unless the patient declines (i.e., opts out of screening);

- Persons at high risk for HIV infection should be screened for HIV at least annually;

- Separate written consent for HIV testing should not be required; general consent for medical care should be considered sufficient to encompass consent for HIV testing;

- Prevention counseling should not be required with HIV diagnostic testing or as part of HIV screening programs in health-care settings;

- HIV screening should be included in the routine panel of prenatal screening tests for all pregnant women;

- Repeat screening in the third trimester is recommended in certain jurisdictions with elevated rates of HIV infection among pregnant women. (CDC, 2006, p. 1)

In 2008 the adoption of partner services and confidential name-based reporting were substantial breakthroughs. "Partner Services is a range of medical, prevention, and psychological and social services that are offered to individuals with HIV or other STDs and their sexual or needle-sharing partners. . . . By identifying infected persons, confidentially notifying their partners of their possible exposure, and providing needed services, public health professionals and health-care providers can improve the health not only of the individuals, but also of the community" (CDC, 2009, p. 1).

We Are Makers of History

Social work has demonstrated remarkable successes in response to the challenges of the HIV/AIDS crisis. Social workers made important, often pioneering, contributions in responding to the disease. Unfortunately, AIDS is a persistent, mutating virus; regardless of the formidable efforts of social workers and others in related fields, the AIDS crisis remains with us.

The Praxis: Issues and Concerns

In "The History of an Epidemic" of this chapter we reviewed the history of social work and AIDS. Now we will examine the issues that remain from the past, and clarify our concerns for the future of our work. AIDS has changed what social workers do. We must decide what our work will look like in the future. The social work profession must understand the issues and concerns that confront us in order to begin to create a vision for the future of the profession and our work with HIV/AIDS.

Issues that Persist

Two issues of importance that have developed out of our history and that remain are the role of social workers in HIV/AIDS, and the failure of primary prevention.

Social Work's Role. As noted above, the extent to which social workers were at the forefront of campaigns against AIDS has varied (Linsk & Keigher, 2002); many have responded to the needs of the most vulnerable and least influential. Following the outbreak of AIDS, social workers struggling in hospitals against AIDS were in the right place at the right time (Willinger & Rice, 2003). This was primarily because of the profession's willingness to rise to the occasion when no other profession would do so. Although this has often been the case in the face of new—sometimes dangerous—challenges, the social work profession as a whole appears less willing to rise to the challenges.

Social work's fight against AIDS started as a grassroots movement but shifted over time to focus on professional accountability—but accountability for what? We are locked into the original model of care (e.g., HIV testing), although the complex needs of those suffering from HIV/AIDS demonstrate that more could be done. This professionalizing of HIV/AIDS care and treatment in social work and the successful introduction of HIV/AIDS prevention services have led to a decline of leadership by social workers in the fight against AIDS. Some say that leadership has been replaced by apathy, that job stress has left us with a lack of innovation and a sense of hopelessness (NASW, 2005). How can this shift be explained?

In spite of occasional increases in government funding for HIV drugs, resources have remained extremely limited (Linsk & Keigher, 2002). The lack of a nationalized health program in the United States has taken its toll on clients and social workers alike. Social workers have learned to live with the imbalances that characterize our distribution of health-care-related prevention, treatment, and care (Linsk & Keigher, 2002). To be content with less than what many of our predecessors would have worked for—to settle for what is given us—has had its costs. There is less professional activism today than there was fifteen years ago.

Social work's leadership in the fight against HIV/AIDS has been replaced by leadership within the medical profession. This is particularly unfortunate because those in medical fields too often fail to recognize the best plan for each person with

HIV (Linsk & Keigher, 2002). With its successful development and use of science and technology, U.S. medicine has become the authority regarding disease and the treatment of the disease (Linsk & Keigher, 2002).

The focus of colleagues in other professions is most often guided by scientific process alone; important scientific and medical findings have resulted. Social work also includes scientific methodologies, but social workers focus on the humanity of the individual in need and we share professionalism and humanity through our work (NASW, 2008). A more nuanced approach of dealing with the client is what social workers bring to partnerships.

Prevention. Primary prevention is the prevention of the disease. Primary prevention has proven to have limited efficacy in the fight against HIV/AIDS, therefore we need secondary prevention. Secondary prevention aims to detect and treat disease that has not yet become symptomatic. Tertiary prevention is directed at those who already have symptomatic disease in an attempt to prevent further deterioration, recurrent symptoms, and subsequent events. The need for all three levels of prevention has greatly increased. Social workers have been in the best position to provide these services because we view and assess people within the context of their environments and their strengths. Indeed, we have claimed that providing effective and sustainable behavioral change is one of the hallmarks of the profession. However, as HIV/AIDS continues to spread, it is clear that we have yet to develop the necessary proficiency in providing services for people living with HIV and AIDS.

More than thirty years into the AIDS epidemic, the one truth that we can count on is that knowledge of how HIV is transmitted does not translate into a behavioral change that will prevent the transmission of HIV. There is a disconnect between knowledge and behavior. Social workers do not yet fully understand all the factors that affect behavioral change. We have not learned to work with clients on how to best use their cognitive and interpersonal skills for sustainable behavioral change in reducing or eliminating their risk of infection.

Other Current Concerns

Micro Social Work. Social workers at the micro level of practice work with people who are infected with and affected by HIV/AIDS: the client and those in a relationship with the client, most often family members. This involves general care, specific treatment, and provision of knowledge and resources to prevent the client from acquiring new strains of the virus or other sexually transmitted diseases (STDs). A defining feature of social work has been the profession's focus on individual well-being in a social context and on the well-being of society.

Fundamental to social work is attention to the environmental forces that create and contribute to problems for persons living with HIV/AIDS (NASW, 2008). Individual clients are not islands unto themselves: we must address the dynamics that come into play in the life of the client and in the lives of those who interact with the client (e.g., family members) while maintaining and observing the confidentiality of the family member living with HIV or AIDS.

Treating the Client as a Whole Person. Today's social worker often is trained to assess the client as a whole person and to include assessments of contributing factors in the client's environment. A number of issues work against the social worker in this respect, including oversized case loads and a lack of follow-through by the agency. For a number of reasons, society as a whole too often refuses to view our clients in a constructive way. It is important that the social work profession provide clients with a holistic assessment and treatment plan.

Family Dynamics. In most people's lives, the primary support system is the family. When a person is in crisis or needs someone for support, they typically will look to the family. Family support, however, often comes with conditional love. Thus, as social workers we must explore the family dynamics of each family affected by this virus to determine the functional and dysfunctional coping mechanisms in play. We must be observant of the unspoken and spoken rules. What are the communication styles within the family? What role or function does each member provide for the family? What are the alliances? We must determine if this is a family of origin, a blended family, an adoptive family, or a family of creation. Is this family bicultural, biracial, or bilingual, or a combination? All of these factors will aid the social worker to serve the person living with HIV and AIDS, and her or his family.

Cultural Competency. Social work research needs to examine the complex issue of culture and cultural competency when providing HIV/AIDS services. Research should examine and expand our thinking and practices as people begin to live longer with HIV and AIDS. We need more research on HIV/AIDS and the elderly, and HIV/AIDS in the workplace. Social workers need to be more open and observant when applying the culturally competent interventions.

Spirituality. Spirituality involves a person's belief in something greater than himself or herself, something greater than the sum of our physical earthly experience and that transcends immediate reality. Clients faced with life-or-death illnesses often search for meaning in their lives. If a social worker understands the client's belief system, her or she can assist in helping the client identify their strengths. Identifying spirituality as a strength can increase the client's self-efficacy and assist that person in making sustainable changes. This belief system may or may not be part of organized religion. Many social workers avoid discussion of religion when doing assessments with clients. According to Gray and Lovat (2008), the social workers must ask themselves, What is the relationship among spirituality, religion, and the applied values inherent in day-to-day social work practice?

Macro Social Work

Macro-level social work practice provides services for large groups, organizations, and communities affected by HIV/AIDS. This area of social work involves advocacy, policy, education, awareness, and community mobilization. We have already seen some success in influencing policy decisions as demonstrated by the Ryan White CARE Act programs. Access to policy decisions may be easier to achieve than many social workers have been willing to admit (Linsk & Keigher, 2002). When we look at the bigger picture, we see that social workers are in a prime position not only to drive the profession in dealing with HIV/AIDS, but also to influence other disciplines.

Collaboration. Mobilizing the Community. As a profession, social work must seek opportunities to collaborate, and create networks to implement innovative programs, strategies, and best practices. We also must create opportunities to form unlikely partnerships. These unlikely partnerships will include persons or organizations with which we typically have an adversarial relationship. Social work collaboration needs to involve respectful planning and implementation based on principles of awareness, acceptance, and action. Social work should encourage collaborations that (1) accept the implications of culturally derived preconceptions; (2) act intentionally, based on realistic expectations for the partner's contributions; and (3) sustain momentum over the long haul (Abell & Rutledge, 2009). Social workers should not only look to government entities (e.g., CDC, Health Resources and Services Administration [HRSA], NIH, and Substance Abuse and Mental Health Services Administration [SAMHSA]) for funding opportunities, but also should create new types of opportunities for partnering and collaborating. Social workers also can drive policy by collaborating with our usual partners but in a non-typical fashion, such as training the medical profession (from research to practice) on the importance and use of the biopsychosocial model.

In order to effectively mobilize communities and increase awareness, social workers must begin to incorporate the following types of organizations into our mobilization efforts: political actions groups or politicians, social or civic groups, faith or spiritual groups, all forms of media, public or private school systems, as well as public or private colleges or universities and schools of all faith traditions. With community support, social workers can become more effective in influencing vital policy issues. Those most directly influenced by policy, namely those in communities with few resources, should have a strong role in the making of policy decisions at all levels.

Compassion Fatigue. We must address the issue of compassion fatigue, a form of caregiver burnout. We must develop our skills in building personal and professional resiliency. We must examine and explore how to create a balanced life space, both personally and professionally.

Advocacy. We need to become a driving force in government and private policy-making decisions. To begin we can affect policy that develops an HIV/AIDS nomenclature that is easily understood and recognizable by all persons. It is incumbent upon us to drive policy that will make sexual health assessments universal in all health-care settings (e.g., medical, mental; public, and private).

We must advocate for ourselves so we can better advocate for our clients. The pharmaceutical firms should not be the primary decision makers. Should only those with the means to purchase the drugs have access to them? We must be able to take an empowered role in addressing the dilemmas in HIV, which include questions of access, allocation of funding, and client advocacy (Linsk & Keigher, 2002).

Social Work Education

The grassroots advocacy of HIV/AIDS lost something along the way to professional accountability. Apathy and complacency seem to have become the norm. Strong social action has disappeared. Therefore, it is important to institute a call to action in all levels of social work education. The development of a social work reinvestment initiative for HIV/AIDS among schools of social work can be the impetus of this call. The Council on Social Work Education can aid this project by strongly recommending this initiative.

Field Education. Schools of social work typically seek out internships and practicums with ASOs and CBOs that provide HIV/AIDS services for their students. Social work students see the variety of roles that social workers play in the broad spectrum of HIV/AIDS services. Students may have the opportunity to work and learn about implementing HIV-prevention strategies from a national perspective while learning how to increase the capacity of individuals and organizations to implement these prevention strategies. Social work professionals demonstrate to the students how national policy shapes the development of these intervention strategies from a multidisciplinary approach and how social work has an impact on the development of policy.

Mentoring. It is imperative that we are able to demonstrate the importance and value of these modalities to our multidisciplinary teams. We demonstrate this to other disciplines by emphasizing and stressing elements such as the client's strengths, personal belief system, social support system, and faith tradition. Furthermore, it is our obligation to the profession of social work to use the same or similar modalities when mentoring new social workers or social work students who are considering working in HIV/AIDS treatment and prevention.

Mentoring is an opportunity to pass the profession to the next generation. If you do not have a mentor, seek one out, no matter your years of experience or practice. Likewise, offer to be a mentor for someone who has less experience than you.

The literature on mentoring in social work education is sparse. Using a variety of terms (e.g., sponsorship, networking, coaching, and role modeling), mentoring has become a strategy used by employees for upward mobility. Lacking a generally agreed-upon definition, social workers usually discuss mentoring within the context of functions. Psychosocial and career functions are thought to collectively provide protégés with the skills, knowledge, opportunities, and support needed for successful careers and advancement in organizations (Simon, Perry, & Roff, 2008).

Unlike career mentoring, which functions at the organizational and systems level, psychosocial mentoring functions operate at the interpersonal level. One such example of social mentoring is the START (Social Workers Today Achieve Retention Together) mentoring initiative at Wayne State University School of Social Work in Detroit, Michigan. The initiative assists students in establishing a professional social work network for improving student retention at Wayne State University. The program assigns a master of social work mentor who is a graduate of the school to each participating student. The mentor assists the student in building his or her professional, educational, and leadership potential and encourages that student to continue pursuit of higher education in social work.

Developing a New Agenda

According to Linsk and Keigher (2002), the social work profession must define its domain as social workers, case managers, health educators, and counselors before other professions claim these roles as their own. We must claim our place in making decisions about programs, clinical guidelines, policies, and programs. HIV service providers are open to the participation of social workers as members and observers. We must watch the legislative and budgetary process and provide input, testify, educate, and encourage a consumer-driven response to current changes in HIV treatment and care. But how do we begin?

- Social work needs an agenda to address the emerging dilemmas in HIV/AIDS (Linsk & Keigher, 2002).

- Social work's contribution to the AIDS epidemic must be more focused (Linsk & Keigher, 2002).

- Policies and programs for HIV testing and counseling, mental health services, service coordination and case management, and HIV-prevention education have too often been designed and implemented by professionals in public health, nursing, medicine, and public administration, and by the new hybrid, the ASO administrator (Linsk & Keigher, 2002).

Let us now answer the question, How do we develop this agenda?

The planners of the 2009 Annual National Conference on Social Work and HIV/AIDS recognized that often-overwhelming challenges still face professionals in today's AIDS arena, especially in the field of social work. With the intention of using the conference as a venue in which to actively explore HIV/AIDS and social work, conference planners decided on the theme of the future, with the title, "Defining the Future of HIV/AIDS Social Work: What is YOUR Vision?" Moreover, the conference planners decided to commission a study to lay the groundwork for answering this question. Their objective was to provide conferees and social workers with a starting point for establishing a vision for social work in the HIV/AIDS arena.

In general, the conference planners wished to answer the question, What are the major characteristics of social work today in relation to our work with populations suffering from HIV/AIDS, and where is social work going in regard to HIV/AIDS? In short, what is our vision for the future of HIV/AIDS social work? The conference planners turned to the authors of this chapter to take the lead in searching for an answer. The conference planners and authors agreed that the findings of this study would be widely distributed. In large part, this chapter is the result of the study findings.

Methodology

The social work profession takes pride in its development and use of practical scientific methods. Even before commissioning the study, the conference planners wanted to use the conference venue and the expertise of the conferees to contribute to the development of a new vision. They wished to use an unprecedented process as part of the activities of the conference itself. The conference planners informed the researchers that they would use the SWOT (strengths, weaknesses, opportunities, and threats) evaluation process (Valentin, 2001) to inform the analysis. The conference planners reasoned that a SWOT analysis would be a practical, participatory activity to collect the richness of the participants' ideas.

In this section of the chapter, we examine the process and the findings of the study. When conducting the study, the researchers focused on these questions: What does the future hold for social workers in relation to the rapidly changing face of the HIV/AIDS crisis? And what would our best strategy look like in dealing with HIV/AIDS in the future? In short, what is our vision for the future of HIV/AIDS social work?

The SWOT Analysis

The researchers agreed that the application of the SWOT analysis at the conference was appropriate, because the SWOT analysis fulfills the following functions (Valentin, 2001):

- Acts as a stimulus to participation in a common group experience

- Provides information (i.e., data) and the organizational framework for identifying and analyzing SWOT

- Establishes a platform for assessing core capabilities and competences

- Develops the evidence (i.e., data) for the need for change, and provides direction for a plan

- Helps balance idealism and practicality

The basic steps included in the SWOT analysis process were (1) gather necessary data, (2) apply content analysis, (3) transfer coded data to SWOT format, and (4) analyze SWOT outcomes.

Gather Data. At the conference, the researchers documented the activities in the plenary sessions. Each conference participant was asked to complete a questionnaire. The researchers asked each participant to (1) examine the external factors that affect HIV/AIDS social work, and (2) explore the internal resources and capabilities that affect HIV/AIDS social work. Within each of these two broad areas, the responses would correspond to the components of the SWOT analysis: (1) opportunities and threats (i.e., external factors), and (2) strengths and challenges (i.e., internal resources).

After the conference, the researchers collected data from three additional sources: (1) notes on the plenary session, which the researchers reviewed independently, after which they identified common themes in the notes; (2) responses on the completed questionnaires; and (3) thirty semi-structured interviews with macro and micro practitioners involved in various capacities of HIV and AIDS social work.

Applying Content Analysis to the Data. The researchers used content analysis to identify and code common themes in the various sources. Content analysis is an iterative process; therefore researchers read the data through repeatedly, data were modified or old categories discarded while new categories were developed.

Transfer Coded Data to SWOT Format. The authors transferred the coded data to the SWOT analysis table and then developed subcategories in order to interpret (analyze) the findings (Royse, Thyer, Padgett, & Logan, 2000). Table 3.1 presents a sampling of the findings.

Analyze the SWOT Outcomes. The SWOT analysis provided much insight from a micro perspective. Conferees discussed a range of issues, such as leadership, volunteerism, HIV/AIDS stigma, cultural competence, training, internal organizational cohesion, integration of services, lack of financial health in HIV/AIDS organizations, the changing practice contexts (particularly the aging of the HIV/AIDS population), job stress, and a growing sense of hopelessness amongst social workers.

Table 3.1. SWOT Analysis Findings

Strengths	Weaknesses	Opportunities	Threats
The history of social work and HIV/AIDS provides a strong foundation of experience, knowledge, and motivation. Comfortable working as leaders in the field. History of Volunteerism.	Social work not perceived as a profession but as a "soft science." Need to "brand" the profession.	Create new ways to deal with stigma. Move our knowledge base to deal with other chronic illnesses.	Downturn in economy tends to hurt underserved people even more than those in privileged economic positions. Cuts in funding. Stigma of AIDS remains.
Comfortable working as part of multidisciplinary team or project. Attention to cultural competence.	Lack of innovation or creativity; working "outside the box"; too complacent; locked into old model of care, e.g., HIV testing. Burden of job stress. Sense of hopelessness.	Increased service integration. Collaboration or partnerships.	AIDS viewed as disease of the past.
Understand the spectrum of HIV/AIDS from beginning to now. Success of orientation and training.	Little glamour working with underprivileged people.	Social work practice adaptability and creativity. Constant scientific developments in medicine.	Too much focus on international AIDS epidemic, need increased attention to domestic issues.
Social workers are client centered. Internal organizational cohesion.	Short-term tactical planners. Not long-term strategic planners.	Population is aging. Create change in practice to meet the new context.	Lack of medical coverage—especially prevention—and difficulty of compromise between the political left and political right. Power of pharmaceutical lobby.
Understand avenues, network of accessing needed benefits, services, resources.	General public losing interest in AIDS.	Increased service integration. New technologies and innovative strategies in social work, e.g., entrepreneurial ventures.	Lack of time or value to maintain record keeping, data, and complete program assessments.

However, the researchers noted important gaps in information, such as program development, programmatic structure, bureaucratization of social work agencies, what social work looks like as a profession, and the need for more research. The participants often discussed an issue only from the perspective of the practitioner (e.g., the micro perspective) and not from the point of view of the administrator or planner (e.g., the macro perspective).

The Need for More Data: Addressing Macro Concerns

As a result of the SWOT analysis the researchers determined that their methods had shortcomings, namely that the surveys they used and the time frame of the conference prevented the participants from providing more than limited responses. How could we define our vision for the future of HIV/AIDS social work if we do not include the macro perspective? As a result, the researchers turned to another established methodology for social workers: key informant interviews.

The researchers first divided the question into two queries: (1) What are the major characteristics of social work today in relation to our work with populations living with HIV/AIDS? And (2) Where is social work going in regard to HIV/AIDS? The SWOT analysis had produced adequate data for answering the first query, so the researchers focused on the second query by further subdividing it into two questions: (a) What does the future hold for social workers in relation to the rapidly changing face of the HIV/AIDS crisis? And (b) What would our best strategy look like in dealing with HIV/AIDS in the future? As a result of the SWOT analysis, the researchers found that the responses to the components that dealt with "the business of HIV/AIDS social work" and "our best strategy . . . in dealing with HIV/AIDS in the future" were inadequate. Key informant interviews would provide more data in these areas and provide more detail specific to macro issues.

Key Informant Interviews. Researchers chose key informant interviews as the best mode of data collection to complement the SWOT analysis. Key informant interviews do not restrict the participant's response or require strict adherence to a set procedure. Key informant interviews facilitate broader and deeper input from the participant, particularly facilitating a focus on underlying issues and assumptions. The researchers developed a key informant interview tool that included six broad questions:

1. Outside of any social work impact, what do you see as some of the most important sociocultural influences on the HIV/AIDS arena taking place over the next half decade?

2. What do you see as the most urgent priority in the development of agency and community roles related to HIV/AIDS?

3. What are some key administrative factors (e.g., marketing, business plan, technological applications) that you would suggest for greater focus in the profession?

4. How do you view the development of the social work profession in relation to HIV/AIDS over the next five years?

5. What are your suggestions regarding sustainability in the field?

6. What do you see as your role in the next phase of social work and HIV/AIDS?

The researchers used convenience sampling to recruit key informant participation from conference participants (Royse et al., 2000). Six key informants participated. The researchers conducted interviews with individuals who attended the conference and who possessed knowledge and interest in the next phase of social work and HIV/AIDS, especially those involved in macro social work. Discussions, by telephone, were confidential. The researchers typed and reviewed interview notes. The researchers devised a coding strategy to develop subcategories of themes in order to interpret the findings (Royse et al., 2000).

The researchers integrated the findings of the key informant data analysis into the findings of the SWOT analysis. The researchers quoted participants when possible and set these responses in quotes to substantiate their interpretations.

Study Findings: An Agenda for Addressing the Dilemmas in HIV/AIDS

The findings of the SWOT analysis and key informant interviews highlighted three major themes that ran throughout the responses:

• Collaboration is needed, particularly between disciplines.

• Our greatest strength is the social work profession's history across three decades in the HIV/AIDS arena.

• The social work profession needs to regain its proactive leadership role.

To better guide the reader and facilitate discussion of the findings, the researchers organized the discussion of the concerns into the following categories, with some overlap: (1) findings that apply to micro social work, (2) findings that apply to macro social work, and (3) those that apply to social work education.

The reader should not consider these findings to be exhaustive because additional actions unique to a particular agency or community are likely to be reported. The following pages include a brief discussion of the findings of the SWOT analysis and key informant analysis.

Micro Findings

Job Stress. The findings present a picture of disillusioned social workers who have realized over time that the AIDS crisis exposed faults in our current social and economic order. In particular, the impoverished are less likely than the wealthy to know about or use advanced (and expensive) medical procedures or to participate in experimental drug trials. Economically challenged people who develop AIDS, mostly intravenous drug users and inner-city minorities, lack private health insurance and access to university medical centers where the experimental treatments are being offered. As a consequence, poor people and other disadvantaged people with AIDS tend to live a shorter time and in a more debilitated state of physical, psychological, and social health, and in environments that foster further decline and early deaths from infection. In the opening plenary, a number of presenters stated that AIDS poses challenges to all aspects of professional social work by providing the opportunity to work with some of the most disenfranchised segments of our society, and that social workers in community organizations must continue to hold large providers such as Medicare, Medicaid, and private health insurance companies to the highest standards of equity for all people with AIDS.

Directly related to the above discussion is the issue of stress on the job. Myriad factors contribute to job stress in the field of HIV/AIDS social service work, including limited resources, too much work and too many roles, the psychological and emotional hardship of dealing with illness and death, HIV stigma, issues with confidentiality, legal and ethical dilemmas, and the overwhelming severity and intensity of the epidemic. This job stress can lead to burnout and feelings of hopelessness, in turn resulting in social workers providing poorer service to consumers, who may not feel listened to, cared for, or respected.

The findings demonstrate that we must challenge hopelessness and other barriers to good practice. Social workers must be better prepared to empower ill and dying clients by maximizing their options to live or to die how they choose. To accomplish this crucial clinical task with clients, professionals must feel empowered in their work.

Mid-level management and front-level employees must take the lead by creating a supportive work environment where it is safe for all employees to express feelings, and by providing supportive supervision and allowing for flexibility in work schedules, as well as using positive reinforcement of work completed.

Public Perception. The findings demonstrate that public perception of AIDS as a curable disease influences our work in a variety of ways. This perception affects safe-sex practices and reduces funding for the service demands of the illness. Some social workers, particularly those who are too young to have participated in the early years in the fight against HIV/AIDS, believe that AIDS is no longer a terminal illness. Social workers express feelings of less urgency now about the disease, as well as apathy about taking measures to prevent its spread.

Social workers have transferrable skill sets that are useful in the areas of community mobilization, community organizing, health communications, and public relations. As a profession, we are in a position to aid in reshaping the public's perception of persons infected and at risk of contracting HIV.

We can shape general public perception that (1) HIV is a complex, chronic disease that can be managed with medications, or that (2) HIV is a preventable and curable disease. Should only those with the means to purchase the drugs have access to them? Social work can shape public opinion in favor of access for those who are most vulnerable and the least influential.

Social workers and public health workers must address the barrier of misperception about AIDS no longer being a terminal illness. We must form strong messages that HIV/AIDS, if treated, is a chronic disease, and that without treatment it is still a life-threatening disease. It is still paramount to protect oneself, others, and the community from transmission.

Behavioral Change and Prevention. Social work has a long way to go before we can prove our claim of making effective behavioral change in our HIV/AIDS clients. Educating the client does not translate into action. Until we learn to understand behavior adequately so that we can make consistently predictable behavioral change in clients we will continue to fall short in our prevention efforts.

Social workers are in a prime position to provide behavioral change intervention as long as we view and assess people within the context of their environments and their strengths. Unfortunately, we do not yet know enough about behavioral change to reliably influence behavior that will prevent transmission of the disease. Social work could contribute much to facilitating individual decisions and improving quality of life.

First, we must understand the factors and processes that affect behavioral change. We must work with clients on how to best use their cognitive and interpersonal skills for sustainable behavioral change in reducing or eliminating their risk of acquiring the virus. Social workers must adapt and tailor methods for each individual client, taking into consideration such elements as risk factors, lifestyle, readiness to change, and culture. We must also take into account group and other environmental factors, and use group- and community-level interventions to create lasting behavioral change. Social work, with its long-standing hybrid of intervention and assessment processes incorporating the environment and the person, should steer at the helm of this mission (Linsk & Keigher, 2002).

Treating the Client as a Whole Person. In the area of prevention, public health resources dedicated to HIV testing continue to rival those used for education, needle-exchange programs, long-term counseling programs, and other initiatives (Scott, 2003).

Because testing is but one link in a larger chain of discourse and extradiscursive experiences, we might question the wisdom of making testing the centerpiece of HIV-prevention education. Other prevention efforts such as outreach education and ongoing peer counseling may hold more promise for subverting the national pedagogy than a two-part test counseling session. Although the development of better testing protocols is an important local intervention, we must approach intervention as an ongoing, comprehensive, and holistic process (Scott, 2003).

The fear of stigmatization, the fear of rejection or abuse, low self-esteem, poor communication skills, contrasting peer norms, resignation (e.g., infection is inevitable), and a number of other factors may act as barriers to safer sex. If we want to fully facilitate safer sex, we need to connect clients to resources and services outside test-based counseling. Such services might include partner counseling and referral services, reproductive health services, drug or alcohol treatment, domestic abuse services, and what the CDC now calls prevention case management (Scott, 2003).

Programmatic Structure and Program Development. The findings demonstrated that, in the words of one respondent, "Social workers [do not support enough] the development and implementation of programs that include educational and prevention strategies that meet the needs of diverse population segments of society."

Social workers have the best skills to conduct community psychosocial assessments, contribute to adherence to medication plans, assess the effects of other social and environmental factors, and estimate the consequences of marginalizing specific groups. At a minimum, social workers need to understand both the clinical and the policy dilemmas that have emerged in response to new drug therapies.

The findings demonstrated the following:

- Social workers should promote economic sustainability for resource-poor adults and their children through ensured academic and/or vocational education opportunities.

- Social workers should support science-based, comprehensive sexuality education programs for youth and adults that are culturally sensitive and promote culturally competent practice.

- Social workers should encourage the implementation of voluntary counseling and testing services and ensure that they are accessible and either free or affordable in resource-poor settings. Social workers should ensure access to the full range of substance use services, focusing on harm reduction models that include needle-exchange programs.

Volunteerism. Volunteerism was a major asset in the beginning of the epidemic, maximizing the potential of talented individuals in innovative advocacy, prevention, and treatment. This is no longer the case, although volunteerism continues to play a role.

The findings demonstrate the need for volunteerism to regain its momentum in the HIV/AIDS arena. ASOs will benefit from investing in their volunteer programs, recognizing the value of a variety of volunteer roles, and providing the training and structure needed for successful volunteer programs. Agencies must provide volunteers with the training and incentives needed to work hand in glove with paid employees and also pay particular attention to avoiding burnout among volunteers.

Cultural Competency. The findings demonstrate that cultural competence poses another challenge when it comes to the AIDS epidemic because AIDS affects a diverse group of individuals. At the beginning of the epidemic, the response was primarily headed by gay, White, middle-class men who had the resources to help and advocate. Thus practitioners have a great deal of competence when working with at-risk and HIV-positive gay, White, middle-class men.

The face of AIDS is changing. It is important for the response to the epidemic to be culturally relevant to women, racial and ethnic minorities, and people with limited access to economic resources. To become more culturally competent, not only do ASOs need to be aware of the diversity in the population they are serving, but also they need to reflect on their own internal diversity—or lack thereof. In addition, agencies should provide workers with the opportunity to attend workshops on cultural competency and how to develop skills, such as how to acknowledge one's own biases, practices, and beliefs.

Changing Practice Contexts. The changing social context in which the epidemic exists also poses a great challenge to social workers in the field. The AIDS epidemic has rapidly shifted in the past twenty-eight years. The disease is significantly affecting a growing population, with increases in the number of heterosexuals, non-drug-users, women, older adults, African Americans, and Latino(a)s.

The HIV/AIDS population is living much longer than was true in earlier decades. Rapid changes in medical technology have changed AIDS diagnosis from a death sentence to a terminal illness. With this change, survival and end-of-life issues are no longer the first priority of those living with HIV/AIDS; rather, meeting daily needs and quality of life have taken precedent.

According to Poindexter (2007, p. 10), "ASOs that were founded with buddy programs, hospital visitors, support groups, and peer counseling are moving into food banks, laundry service, and housing assistance" to meet daily needs of clients. Social workers must learn how to empower clients with hope. The hope may be not only for a cure, but also to stay healthy long enough for the next generation of medical breakthroughs to occur. Improved longevity of clients allows social workers more time to encourage people with AIDS to hope for and work toward improved relationships with estranged family members or friends.

Stigma. The findings demonstrate that the stigma that surfaced in the beginning of the epidemic is still a major problem for social workers in the field today. Service providers at ASOs work with one of the most stigmatized populations. Those with HIV/AIDS are stigmatized because of the associated fear with death and disease, fear of contracting HIV, taboo topics such as sexuality and drug use, and homophobia.

Social workers in the field must personally face this stigma, and at the same time must be continually aware of their own biases and prejudices.

Macro Findings

We now focus on the big picture of social work—the managerial, policy-making, and planning work—today and tomorrow, in relation to HIV/AIDS. We also include what study participants had to say about macro social work.

Internal Organizational Cohesion. An additional challenge for ASOs concerns the divisions that may occur within the organization between managers and direct service workers, staff and board members, staff and volunteers, and groups "based on gender, sexual orientation, HIV status, level of physical functioning, educational level, role in the agency, or pay status" (Poindexter, 2007, p. 21). When internal conflicts surface, an agency will often do its best to hide them from the public, funders, the media, and recipients of services.

Keeping tensions out of conversations will only deepen the problem, and often will keep emotional tension high. Addressing tensions and disagreements as they arise, rather than avoiding them, will provide an environment that is safe for healthy debate and critical thinking. This will mitigate oppression, increase the respect for diversity, and, ultimately, lead to agency growth.

Leadership. Participants agreed that leadership in the HIV/AIDS social work field is not currently effective and that there are specific actions or factors that should occur in order for the profession to be branded and, as one respondent put it, "play a role in the business of health care and HIV/AIDS." Key informants were concerned that the profession and society have made a shift in their thinking—specifically, that AIDS is no longer a terminal illness. The perception that AIDS is not a terminal illness affects safe-sex practices and reduces funding for the service demands of the illness. The general population and many social workers express feelings of less urgency now about the disease, as well as apathy about taking measures to prevent its spread.

The capacity of resource-challenged ASOs to mobilize support is compromised by other health-related issues such as growing rates of poverty. Despite notable success in the global fight against HIV/AIDS, worldwide 7,500 individuals contract HIV every day, and at least 6,000 people die of AIDS every day. Management must formulate messages that HIV/AIDS, if treated, is a chronic disease, but that without this vital treatment it is still a life-threatening disease and that protecting oneself, others, and the community from transmission is paramount.

Social work leadership needs to guard against donor and supporter fatigue; it is critical to integrate HIV/AIDS programs with other health and development programs. The mainstreaming of HIV/AIDS programs is also necessary because of the well-known health and development consequences of the pandemic. The mainstreaming of HIV/AIDS programs should start at the highest levels of executive and legislative decision making of national governments. It should also be a part of the highest-level decision making in the private sector as health and development strategies are developed (Kaisernetwork.org, 2008).

People who have AIDS have long been the heart of the AIDS response, bringing consumers of services to the table in making decisions about the services provided. Although this is a valuable and necessary asset to the work of ASOs, it is not always easy to bring consumer voices into decision-making processes. Doing so requires time and training to keep stakeholders up to date with relevant concerns and practice issues in the field, as well as commitment to capacity building. Moreover, working with people living with AIDS can be a challenge if there are physical limitations due to the illness. Building awareness in ASOs of the importance of the partnership and the reasons for its necessity, as well as providing education on the challenges of living with AIDS and the requirements of the Americans with Disabilities Act, are important steps for leaders in ASOs.

Professionalism, Evaluation, and Quality Control. Like other movements, ASOs began at the grassroots and have slowly become more professional and bureaucratic. Although this change can have many positive aspects, such as standardized care and professional legitimacy, it also poses a number of challenges. The larger, more-bureaucratic ASOs may have a slower response time and more red tape— making them similar to what they were trying to avoid in the early days of the epidemic. In addition, although professionalism allows them to access grants, they may struggle to stay aligned with the mission of the organization and fitting funders' expectations. ASOs face the challenge of finding the balance between the grassroots enthusiasm and activism efforts on the one side, and financial stability and institutional legitimacy on the other.

According to Poindexter (2007, p. 18), "All levels of the ASO, from board members to service recipients, should be involved in periodic strategic planning discussions regarding the guiding values of the agency," and "ASOs should make decisions regarding what principles cannot be compromised, even for funding."

At the program level, decision makers should focus on verifiable evidence of integrated HIV/AIDS, health, and development programs for specific target populations and communities. The global effort to promote universal access to drugs for the prevention and treatment of tuberculosis and malaria in resource-challenged environments is a good template for mainstreaming HIV/AIDS into regular health and development programs.

The majority of participants also reported that leadership should

• Enter into respectful community and consumer partnerships with people living with HIV/AIDS, with due regard for basic social work values such as self-determination, dignity, and acknowledgment of the respect for the worth of the individual;

• Identify, strengthen, and support the role of people living with HIV/AIDS and the community response to the pandemic;

• Work with people living with HIV/AIDS and people who are HIV positive and their self-help organizations and networks and provide assistance where appropriate;

• Ensure protocols that address the unique biomedical needs of women, children, and adolescents, and the psychosocial and spiritual needs of all people affected by HIV/AIDS;

• Integrate quality assurance procedures throughout the organization at all times; and

• During the program planning stage, ensure evaluation processes are an integral part of programming.

Prevention and Behavioral Change. The HIV/AIDS disease has not gone away and, through its ability to morph into new forms, continues to spread to new populations. Unfortunately, primary prevention has had limited efficacy in the fight against HIV/AIDS, therefore the need for secondary and tertiary prevention has greatly increased. The professionalizing of social work has not improved prevention of HIV/AIDS.

Prevention is most often a direct result of behavioral change. Social workers are in the prime position to provide behavioral change services because we view and assess people in the context of their environments. Social work could and should exert leadership in many dimensions of the AIDS epidemic, including determining how to advance HIV care and protect communities.

Social work can learn how to influence behavioral change through research. With social work taking the lead, universities must focus on behavioral change and involve a variety of disciplines. Effective program evaluation is necessary to identify best practices and to ensure programmatic follow through. Management must be consistent in insisting on program evaluation and quality assurance at all levels.

Financial Health. ASOs have struggled with financial resources since the beginning of the AIDS epidemic. At the beginning, they survived without the help of government, foundations, or corporations, functioning solely from private donations and a small mix of grants. The temporary nature of this funding caused additional stress and worry that compounded the taxing nature of HIV/AIDS work. Years later, even after larger funding sources began to contribute to ASOs, competition for limited resources has remained a significant concern. Leaders and managers of ASOs often spend a significant portion of their time concerned with staying afloat economically.

To establish and maintain financial health, organizations should diversify their funding sources so that they are not relying too heavily on one type of income. A variety of government grants, foundation grants, personal giving, special events, fundraisers, and capital campaigns can help an organization establish this balance of funding sources. A chief financial officer and board committee that are directly responsible for development are also useful tools. In addition, many ASOs are developing new sources of income, such as thrift stores, or using the Internet for fundraising. The term "social entrepreneurialism" will become commonplace with creative income solutions dominating income discussions.

Collaboration and Service Integration. Because of the grassroots nature of the HIV/AIDS response, a number of individual CBOs evolved rather than a single, nationwide network. These CBOs can cause problems with duplication of services: a number of ASOs (and often people living with AIDS) may have multiple case managers from multiple organizations. Often, there is a lack of coordination and communication among different ASOs.

However, compared to other professions, social workers are comfortable working as part of multidisciplinary teams or projects. ASOs can collaborate with one another and other service agencies, continually advocating for the best for their clients, forming partnerships where they bring their specialty to the table.

Advocacy. Social workers have long advocated on behalf of clients with some success. However, specific issues have not fared well, including prevention services and social work education. Social work must advocate for the resources to implement effective preventive services. As Linsk and Keigher (2002) remind us, a principle of civil rights is that oppressed and disadvantaged people cannot be left to advocate for themselves. Social workers have the opportunity to demand that all have equal access to life-saving formulas. Who should have priority for care and services? Our medical colleagues will ensure that those whose medical situation enables them to respond best to treatment and the economic means will have priority access. And who is most likely to adhere to a plan of care? Those likely to live longest? Those who can pay at least a copayment? As for who will decide the above, social workers' understanding of human behavior and their skill in conducting both comprehensive psychosocial assessments and interventions confirm that they have a legitimate role in this decision-making process (Linsk & Keigher, 2002).

Marketing the Social Work Experience. The history of social work and HIV/AIDS provides a foundation of experience, knowledge, and motivation. The findings demonstrate that there is an opportunity for the profession to create a market niche by promoting the client-based multidisciplinary models developed for meeting the needs of the HIV-positive clients and people living with AIDS. These models would be applicable to the work of other professions.

HIV/AIDS is dominated by the case management model. Social workers are taught to be case managers. Case management is a social work product and we must learn to market this product to other disciplines. We must determine how the case management model is implemented and used. We now have the opportunity to create a role for ourselves as the leaders driving the process of case management. We can build social work and case management into clinical care and behavioral prevention teams. HIV/AIDS prevention is dominated by evidence-based interventions. Social workers must collaborate with researchers to ensure that the social determinants are assessed correctly for each target population. Social workers also need to be at the forefront of the implementation of evidence-based interventions to ensure the fidelity of their use among providers. Social workers have the skill set to provide clinical supervision to providers implementing such interventions.

Social Work Education

Nothing could be more relevant to this discussion than education. It is education that will assist us in creating a vision and determining a road map for the future of the profession. With education, new generations of social workers can revisit the history of the profession in relation to HIV/AIDS and participate in creating a new vision. The following is what the study participants had to say about social work education.

Curriculum. According to findings, social work education should include more curricula that address HIV/AIDS from the perspective of the profession's core values. As noted above, it is necessary for social workers to continuously update their knowledge about all aspects of HIV, including new prevention strategies, treatment and care models, medications, research, and policies. Conference participants found social work education curriculum falling short in a number of areas, including theory, evidence-based interventions, and collaborations.

Many social workers are unaware of the many theories and modalities available to us. For example, few social workers use systems theory, the strengths perspective, the holistic approach, and the person in environment model and their practical application with clients. If they do not study and understand theories, social workers may overlook the opinions of people very different from themselves in relation to ethnicity, culture, gender, sexual orientation, and other forms of diversity. Being unfamiliar with a variety of theories leaves the social worker with simplistic modalities with which to address the client's complex needs.

Social workers on the front lines of HIV/AIDS need to partner with social workers from academic institutions and think tanks to facilitate and conduct research. To ensure this inclusivity, it is imperative that social workers be a major part of the teams that are recruiting for and conducting clinical and vaccine trials for HIV/AIDS treatment and cure. In addition, social work education must

• Promote full funding for research that identifies effective primary and secondary prevention and educational strategies, service delivery models, and the impact of related policies. Research protocols must include people living with and affected by HIV/AIDS.

- Promote fully funded research, development, and distribution of microbicides and HIV/AIDS vaccines.

Assessment. The study findings demonstrate that more needs to be done in client assessment and in viewing each client as a whole person. A dying young person can challenge personal and societal myths of immortality and what constitutes a good death. AIDS challenges social workers to change themselves by dealing with their feelings about pain, illness, death, and the illusion of personal immortality.

Management should understand and promote the understanding that meeting the AIDS challenge professionally means carefully assessing clients to see them as individuals and not categorize them as being "at risk" or "not at risk." Because anyone may become infected with HIV, social workers should not make assumptions about a client's risk status for HIV infection. The heterosexual married man with children may also have a history of having sex with men.

Cultural Competence. Although social workers, in comparison to other professionals, tend to be more culturally aware, more needs to be done to continuing to build our capacities in this area. The findings demonstrate that management should provide opportunities for and support social workers in attending workshops on cultural competency and how to develop skills, such as acknowledging their own biases, practices, and beliefs.

Research. Social workers do not do enough research, especially in the area of prevention. Through the Professional Association of Social Workers in HIV and AIDS (PASWHA), we can begin to examine the importance and the value of social workers participating in and conducting HIV/AIDS research. Social workers provide the best qualitative research because we begin with the client, whether individuals, families, groups, organizations, or communities. We need to include more qualitative and quantitative research to evaluate current practice, which will lead to the publication of best practices and lessons learned.

- Management should ensure protocols that address the unique biomedical needs of women, children, and adolescents, and the psychosocial and spiritual needs of all people affected by HIV/AIDS.

- Management should promote full funding for research that identifies effective primary and secondary prevention and educational strategies, service delivery models, and the impact of related policies. Research protocols must include people living with and affected by HIV/AIDS.

• Management should promote fully funded research, development, and distribution of microbicides and HIV/AIDS vaccines.

Conclusion

The authors see the discussion presented in this chapter as a framework for an agenda within which we can discuss our future as a profession and, we hope, arrive at a consensus about our vision. The profession will continue to be challenged by the changing demographic, political, and organizational context of HIV/AIDS interventions, with practice issues also affected by stigma and discrimination, issues of access and care, and the allocation of scarce resources (Giddens, Ka'opua, & Tomaszewski, 2000). Yet, through our diverse practice skills as clinicians, educators, and advocates, social workers have the opportunity to provide awareness and prevention information to our clients. In addition, mental health care continues to play an important role in the spectrum of care for individuals living with HIV/AIDS (O'Connor, 2003). Therefore, it is critical that we stay current about HIV disease progression and medication options, the role of adherence, and the connection of substance abuse histories and mental health status with a client's risk of HIV/AIDS.

Every day social workers continue their critical role helping clients gain access to services, applying for financial and care assistance, and understanding service guidelines. There is great competition for limited funds in the current economy. The fiscal challenges presented by policies such as abstinence-only initiatives, the focus on medical services at the possible expense of overall health and mental health services, the continued lack of access to all forms of health-care or basic medical services, and related health-care disparities make the future increasingly challenging to social workers and allied health-care professionals working to ensure clients' rights to access care and treatment.

With multiple demands and compelling—and sometimes competing—social and political pressures, it is difficult for us to stay current on funding and policy issues. Yet, three decades into this pandemic, there is new urgency to stay informed, to understand the implication of policy, to analyze funding priorities and formulas and their impact on services provision and reimbursable services, and to remain focused on our roles as advocates, educators, and clinicians for clients and the communities in which we work. As critical social welfare needs reach crushing proportions, the complexities of decision making also overwhelm us. Tension escalates as the jockeying and endless competition in the face of limited resources becomes even more complex. Our leaders attempt to guide funding streams that affect us and our service populations—without our input. Social workers, both as individuals and as members of a profession, must be at the negotiating table to determine priorities and to identify strategies that benefit the vulnerable and the powerless.

The history of our profession demonstrates that many social workers have traditionally taken a proactive role on behalf of the underserved. We have been among the leaders in planning, advocacy, and translating knowledge of social welfare needs into practice solutions. It is hoped that this generation and the next will eradicate HIV/AIDS. Unfortunately, the HIV/AIDS pandemic is still very much a part of our work. The tragedy of AIDS weighs particularly heavy on the poor and other disenfranchised populations. Social workers will be able to ameliorate the suffering caused by the HIV/AIDS pandemic only if we remain scientifically and technologically current, advocate fervently for our clients, provide feedback and guidance to social leaders (e.g., elected and appointed officials), and artfully negotiate professional and other partnerships and collaborations within the social systems in which we work. We must not only continue to acquire knowledge, develop strategies, and improve health and related services and accessibility for our clients, but also we must, at times, show others the way. Exactly how this will be done will be determined in large part by our vision for the future.

References

Abell, N., & Rutledge, S. E. (2009). Awareness, acceptance and action: Developing mindful collaborations in international HIV/AIDS research and service. *British Journal of Social Work, 40*(2), 656–675.

Altman, D. (1986). *AIDS in the mind of America: The social, political and psychological impact of a new epidemic.* New York: Anchor Press.

Centers for Disease Control and Prevention (CDC). (1999). Revised guidelines for HIV counseling, testing and referral. *Morbidity & Mortality Weekly Report.* Retrieved from http://www.cdc.gov/mmwr/preview/mmwrhtml/rr5019a1.htm

Centers for Disease Control and Prevention (CDC). (2003). Advancing HIV prevention: New strategies for a changing epidemic—United States, 2003. *Morbidity & Mortality Weekly Report.* Retrieved from http://www.cdc.gov/mmwr/preview/mmwrhtml/mm5215a1.htm

Centers for Disease Control and Prevention (CDC). (2006). Revised recommendations for HIV testing of adults, adolescents, and pregnant women in health-care settings. *Morbidity & Mortality Weekly Report.* Retrieved from http://www.cdc.gov/mmwr/preview/mmwrhtml/rr5514a1.htm

Centers for Disease Control and Prevention (CDC). (2009). *HIV, hepatitis, STD and TB partners: Prevention resources for our partners and grantees.* Retrieved from http://www.cdc.gov/nchhstp/Partners/index.html

Clarke, A. (1994). What is a chronic disease? The effects of a re-definition in HIV and AIDS. *Social Science & Medicine, 39*(4), 591–597.

Evans, H. (1987, October 4). Spread word—not disease: Fighting AIDS in the street. *New York Daily News*, p. 29.

Fan, H. Y., Conner, R. F., & Villarreal, L. P. (2002) *AIDS: Science and society* (4th ed.). Sudbury, MA: Jones & Bartlett.

Giddens, B., Ka'opua, L., & Tomaszewski, E. (2000). Ethical issues and dilemmas in HIV/AIDS. In V. Lynch (Ed.), *HIV/AIDS at the year 2000* (pp. 33–49). Boston: Allyn & Bacon.

Gray, M., & Lovat, T. (2008). Practical mysticism, Habermas, and social work praxis. *Journal of Social Work, 8*(2), 150.

Grmek, M. D. (1992). *History of AIDS: Emergence and origin of a modern pandemic* (R. D. Maulitx & J. Duffin, trans.) Princeton, NJ: Princeton University Press.

Kaiser Family Foundation. (2003). *Global funding for HIV/AIDS in resource poor.* Publication no. 6D51–02, Menlo, CA. Retrieved from http://www.kff.org/hivaids/6051-02.cfm

Kaisernetwork.org (2008, August 6). XVII International AIDS Conference. *Looking to the future: The epidemic in 2031 and new directions in AIDS research.* Retrieved from http://www.thebody.com/content/art48289.html

Linsk, N., & Keigher, S. (2002). Of magic bullets and social justice: Emerging challenges of recent advances in AIDS treatment. *Health & Social Work, 22*(1), 70–74.

McKenzie, N. F. (1992). *The AIDS reader: Social, political, ethical issues.* New York: Meridian.

National Association of Social Workers (NASW). (2005). *Assuring the sufficiency of a frontline workforce: A national study of licenses social workers. Preliminary report.* Washington, DC: Author.

National Association of Social Workers (NASW). (2008). *NASW code of ethics.* Washington, DC: Author. Retrieved from http://www.socialworkers.org/pubs/Code/code.asp

O'Connor, N. (2003). A personal journey to improve access to HIV-related mental health services. In B. Willinger & A. Rice (Eds.) *A history of AIDS social work in hospitals: A daring response to an epidemic* (pp. 247–254). Binghamton, NY: Haworth Press.

Poindexter, C. C. (2007). Management success and struggles for AIDS service organizations. *Administration in Social Work, 31*(3), 5–28.

Royse, D., Thyer, B. A., Padgett, D., & Logan, T. K. (2000). *Program evaluation: An introduction* (3rd ed.). Boston: Thomson/Wadsworth Publishing.

Scott, J. B. (2003). *Risky rhetoric aids and the cultural practices of HIV testing.* Carbondale: Southern Illinois University Press.

Simon, C. E., Perry, A., & Roff, L. L. (2008). Psychosocial and career mentoring: Female African American social work education administrators experiences. *Journal of Social Work Education, 44,* 9–22.

Specht, H., & Courtney, M. (1994). *How social work has abandoned its mission: Unfaithful angels.* New York: Free Press.

Valentin, E. (2001). SWOT analysis from a resource-based view. *Journal of Marketing Theory and Practice, 9*(2), 54–69.

Willinger, B., & Rice, A. (Eds.). (2003). *A history of AIDS social work in hospitals: A daring response to an epidemic.* Binghamton, NY: Haworth Press.

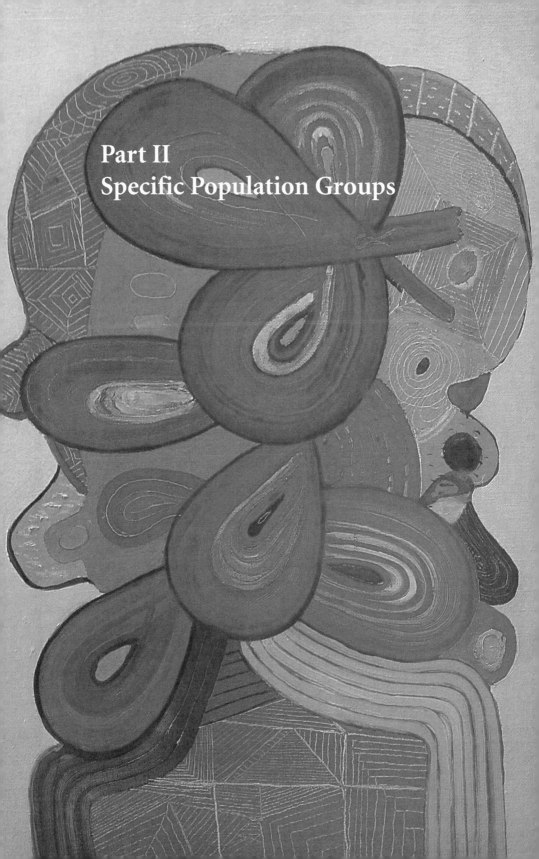

Part II
Specific Population Groups

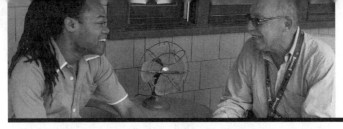

4

The Growing Impact of HIV among African Americans

Michele Rountree and Meredith Bagwell

HIV's racial divide is not new. Each year when national surveillance data are released, we see the ever-increasing toll the AIDS epidemic is taking on the African-American community. Each year, we ask the same question: Why is AIDS hitting Black Americans hardest? While much of the existing literature focuses on quality of care, health care access or individual risk behaviors, we believe that the HIV/AIDS epidemic in African-American communities results from a complex set of social, individual and environmental factors.... Homelessness, housing conditions, risk of incarceration and the concentration of poverty in communities of color are more than just "complicating factors" for people being treated for HIV/AIDS. They are the forces that produce marginalized communities and marginalized people.

—Robert E. Fullilove, *African Americans, Health Disparities, and HIV/AIDS*
(2006, pp. 7–8)

The growing impact of the HIV/AIDS (human immunodeficiency virus and acquired immune deficiency syndrome) epidemic among African Americans calls for attention, strategic planning, and action: African Americans are carrying the greatest burden of HIV/AIDS compared to other racial groups in the United States. Although African Americans make up 12 percent of the U.S. population, they comprised 46 percent of all HIV cases through 2005 and accounted for 51 percent of those diagnosed with HIV/AIDS in 2007. If you picture Black America as its own country, its population of HIV-positive people would rank sixteenth in the world (Centers for Disease Control and Prevention [CDC], 2009a).

This fact may be shocking, as there is significant attention on the global pandemic but little awareness of the impact of AIDS on the African-American community. For example, President George W. Bush launched the United States President's Emergency Plan for AIDS Relief (PEPFAR) in 2003 to combat the global AIDS epidemic. This public health initiative has been described as "unparalleled in size and scope" (Stolberg, 2008). Between 2001 and 2008, PEPFAR awarded $6 billion to provide treatment, prevention, and care for those affected globally by HIV/AIDS. Although this contribution is needed given the extent of the global pandemic, we must not lose sight of the growing crisis of HIV/AIDS among African Americans in the United States. Figure 4.1 compares HIV and AIDS diagnoses by race/ethnicity.

Questions for Reflection

1. What are some of the complex factors that contribute to African Americans having the largest rate of new infections?

2. What factors do you think lead to a shorter survival time after AIDS diagnosis among African Americans compared to people of other races or ethnicities?

Figure 4.1. A Comparison of Total U.S. Population in 2007 to HIV/AIDS Diagnosis by Race/Ethnicity

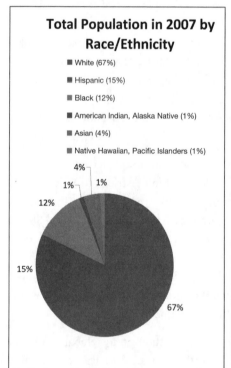

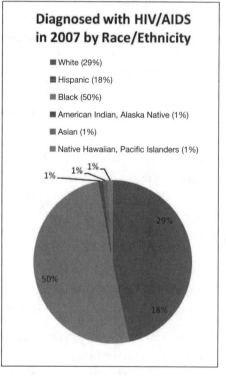

Sources: CDC (2009b); U.S. Census Bureau (2008).

3. Do these numbers make you think differently about the AIDS epidemic? Why or why not?

A Health Crisis

Prevalence. One in sixteen African-American men and one in thirty African-American women will be diagnosed with HIV in their lifetimes. Estimates indicate that nearly 25,000 African Americans were diagnosed with HIV in 2006. The infection rate of African-American men is six times that of White men and three times that of Hispanic men. Even more disproportionately, the infection rate for African-American women is fifteen times that of White women's and almost four times that of Hispanic women's. Among babies who were perinatally infected with HIV in the United States during 2005, 65 percent were African American. Likewise, 63 percent of the children under the age of thirteen who were diagnosed with HIV/AIDS in thirty-three states in 2005 were African American.

In addition to higher HIV infection rates, African Americans face a shorter period between HIV diagnosis and AIDS diagnosis, a shorter survival time after AIDS diagnosis, and a greater likelihood of dying with AIDS. AIDS is the first leading cause of death among African-American women between the ages of twenty-five and thirty-four, and the second leading cause of death among African-American men between the ages of thirty-five and forty-four. Since the beginning of the epidemic through 2007, approximately 226,879 African Americans have died with AIDS. This is 41 percent of all AIDS deaths in the United States. For 2007 alone, the amount was an even higher 45 percent, showing an increase in the proportion of African Americans dying with AIDS.

This trend is more compelling when compared with the change over time among Whites. Cumulatively, 44 percent of those who have died with AIDS over the course of the U.S. epidemic were Whites. Compare this to numbers gathered in 2007, when Whites made up 27 percent of those who had died with AIDS. This shows a major shift: at one time, White Americans made up the greatest percentage of those dying with AIDS; now, African Americans make up the greatest percentage, as portrayed in figure 4.2.

Changes in the Epidemic among African Americans. Trends over a decade (between 1997 and 2007), demonstrate that the epidemic among African Americans is changing:

Figure 4.2. Comparison: Percentage of Those Who Died with AIDS Cumulatively with Those Who Died with AIDS in 2007, by Race/Ethnicity

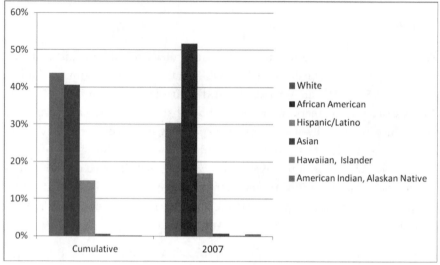

Source: CDC (2009b).

Note: Cumulative is the percentage of people who have died in the United States since the beginning of the pandemic.

- Increase in the proportion of women infected with HIV. In 1997, 25 percent of African Americans infected with HIV were women. By 2007, 33 percent were women.

- Increase in the proportion of transmission by heterosexual contact. In 1997, heterosexual contact made up only 13 percent of HIV infection. By 2007, it made up 43 percent. In 1997, there were 4,530 reported cases of transmission by heterosexual contact. This number had more than doubled by 2007, with 9,390 reported cases in that year.

- Decrease in the number of perinatal, mother-to-child transmissions. In 1997, there were 261 cases of mother-to-child transmissions. In 2007, there were 92.

- Decrease in the number of intravenous drug use transmissions. In 1997 there were 8,005 reported cases of AIDS being transmitted through intravenous drug use. In 2007, there were 2,819 cases.

Questions for Reflection

1. What are the trends over time in figure 4.3?

2. What do they tell you about the changes in the epidemic over time in terms of transmission?

3. How do you think trends should inform prevention efforts?

Figure 4.3. Transmission Categories in the United States by Gender, 2004–2007 (All Racial/Ethnic Groups)

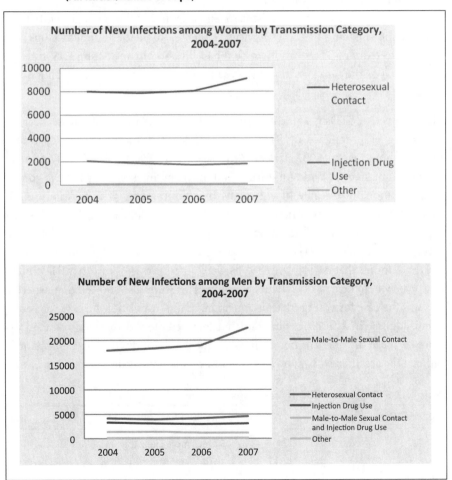

Risk Factors for HIV

African Americans face unique risk factors for HIV infection. These risk factors include the prevalence of sexually transmitted diseases (STDs) among African Americans, sexual relationships within racial or ethnic groups, a stigma associated with HIV/AIDS, sociopolitical risk factors, and testing and prevention challenges.

Prevalence of STDs among African Americans. STDs increase the chance of contracting HIV because of physical changes in the body, including lesions in the genital region that increase the likelihood of transmission through blood, vaginal fluid, or semen entering the bloodstream, and a change in the genital tract that can enhance the shedding of the HIV virus (Gullette, Rooker, & Kennedy, 2009). In fact, the presence of STDs can increase the likelihood of contracting HIV three to five times. For the same reason, the presence of STDs increases the likelihood of spreading HIV.

The presence of STDs is a particularly salient risk for African Americans because of the higher prevalence of STDs compared to other racial or ethnic groups. Reports show that in 2007 African Americans were five times as likely to have syphilis compared to White Americans and nineteen times as likely to have gonorrhea. Additionally, the rate of chlamydia infection among African Americans is eight times that of White Americans (see table 4.1; Gullette et al., 2009). A study supported by the National Institute on Drug Abuse, a component of the National Institutes of Health (NIH), U.S. Department of Health and Human Services (DHHS), found that African Americans were at risk for HIV or other STD infection, even when their risk behaviors were low. This study also showed that, whereas this was the case for young African-American adults, it was not the case for young White adults. These findings illustrate that "marked racial disparities in the prevalence of these diseases are not exclusively affected by individual risk behaviors"; rather, they are affected by a host of "environmental, institutional and contextual"

Table 4.1. STDs among African Americans

Type of STD	Likelihood of Contraction
Syphilis	5 times more likely than White Americans
Gonorrhea	18 times more likely than White Americans
Chlamydia	8 times more likely than White Americans

Source: Gullette et al. (2009).

risk factors (National Institute on Drug Abuse, 2006). The high rates of STDs in the African-American community contribute to the higher risk for HIV infection in that population.

Sexual Relations within Racial or Ethnic Groups. Individuals have a tendency to have sex with partners in their own racial group—a sociological trend called assortative mixing. Unprotected sexual encounters pose risks for HIV exposure. This tendency may be a contributing factor to African Americans' contracting HIV or other STDs as reflected in figure 4.4.

Compounding this risk may be the disproportionate male-to-female ratio among African Americans. There are more African-American women than men available for intimate relationships because of numerous factors such as high incarceration rates and early deaths among African-American men. Because of this ratio, African-American men have their choice of more sexual partners among African-American women, while African-American women have fewer African-American men from which to choose. A 2006 qualitative study at a historically Black college or university found that the gender ratio imbalance leads to men having more sexual partners during the same period, and to women complying with men's preferences with regard to condom use (Ferguson, Quinn, Eng, & Sandelowski, 2006).

A Stigma Associated with HIV/AIDS. AIDS-related stigma is defined as "prejudice, discounting, discrediting, and discrimination directed at people perceived to have AIDS or HIV, and the individuals, groups, and communities with which they

Figure 4.4. Cycle of Impact of HIV Prevalence

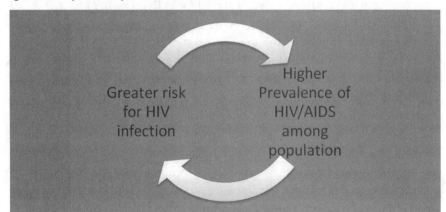

are associated" (Herek, 2009, p. 1). There are high levels of stigma surrounding HIV/AIDS for several reasons. First, there is a stigma because of the disease itself—a fear of transmission, a fear of suffering and death, and a fear of the burden of caring with someone with AIDS (Maman et al., 2009). Along with this stigma of the disease itself, the primary modes of transmission—high-risk sexual contact and intravenous drug use—are taboo topics in society. In African-American communities, the topics of sexuality—especially men who have sex with men (MSM)—and intravenous drug use are often kept private.

Box 4.1. Roots of Stigma

Fear of transmission

Fear of suffering and death

Fear of the burden of caring for someone with AIDS

Taboo topics of drug use and sexuality

Homophobia

Distrust of research and medical community

Societal norms that favor heterosexuality can contribute to AIDS-related stigma. Homonegativity (or homophobia) "reflects a lack of positive beliefs about being gay, about valuation of the larger gay community, and about the morality of being gay" (Shoptaw et al., 2009, p. S78). Because heterosexuality is dominant in society, it places people that are in same-sex relationships in the minority group. Not only does this group have less power, but also they face discrimination because of their sexual orientation. In relation to this orientation, there is fear of disclosure. Coming out as gay or bisexual, or as an MSM, would be putting oneself at odds with the rest of society. Among some African Americans, "homosexuality is seen as a taboo subject that clashes with race, gender role expectations, definitions of masculinity, community norms relating to sexuality, and is perceived of as sinful and unnatural. Homosexuality is also seen as a weakness or an embarrassment to the African American community" (Brooks, Etzel, Hinojos, Henry, & Perez, 2005, p. 738). Because African Americans often share a spirit of collectivism, valuing the group as a whole, coming out could result in being ostracized by the community, which would ultimately be very isolating (Brooks et al., 2005). The desire to prevent this isolation perpetuates a culture of silence.

Heterosexism is linked to HIV-related stigma because in the early epidemic HIV/AIDS was largely seen as a White gay-related illness due to the high impact of AIDS among gay men (Herek & Capitanio, 1999). This leads to an environment where getting tested for HIV and becoming aware of one's HIV status is stigmatized rather than normalized.

Box 4.2. The Down Low

Researchers have paid a great deal of attention to a phenomenon among African-American MSM called the "down low," in which men are in heterosexual relationships yet secretly have sex with other men. There has been a trend to link the growing rates of HIV among African Americans to men who have sex with both men and women (and especially with men on the down low). However, some researchers claim that there is no evidence-based research indicating that men on the down low engage in more risk-taking behaviors than those who are not. They further assert that attributing the spread of HIV to men who are on the down low is a type of discrimination and stigmatization. Sandfort and Dodge (2008, p. 676) state, "Demonizing Black male sexuality has been a staple of American culture since slavery, where our role was to work and breed, and the Mandingo stereotype of a hyper-sexual Black man with an insatiable appetite for White women was created.... We distort the truth about HIV in the Black community to divert our attention from the real 'down low' issues of oppression, racism, low self-esteem, sexual abuse, substance abuse, joblessness, hopelessness, and despair."

In addition to the stigma around the disease itself and its modes of transmission, African Americans have a historical distrust of medicine and the scientific community—with due reason. One of the most well-known abuses of human rights in the name of medical research occurred in what is known as the Tuskegee syphilis experiment. In this experiment, 355 African-American men with syphilis, most of them sharecroppers from a poor county in Alabama, were told they were being treated for "bad blood." In fact, the medical researchers and nurses involved in the experiment were purposefully withholding both the true diagnosis and its treatment. What was the purpose of this deception? It was to collect data from their autopsies and observe the degenerative effects of untreated syphilis. This experiment, conducted by the U.S. Public Health Service, lasted for forty years, from 1932 to 1972, and involved doctors, nurses, the Tuskegee Institute, and the United States government, including the surgeon general, before negative publicity from whistle-blowers and the media were able to put an end to it. The legacy of the study is a strong feeling of distrust of the medical community, researchers, and the government among African Americans.

A 2001 study on African Americans' views of research and the Tuskegee syphilis study found, "In relation to medical research, there was consensus that African Americans should generally avoid involvement given knowledge of past abuses and the inability to be certain that abuses would not reoccur" (Freimuth et al., 2001, p. 802). Participants in this study also brought up conspiracy theories about AIDS—another legacy of the Tuskegee experiment—such as the belief that AIDS is a disease created in a laboratory to annihilate Blacks. This distrust may contribute to difficulties in recruiting African Americans for research studies related to HIV treatment and prevention.

Sociopolitical Risk Factors. Sociopolitical risk factors such as poverty, limited access to health care, higher rates of incarceration, homelessness, poor housing conditions, drug use, and barriers to education uniquely magnify the risk of HIV in African-American communities.

- In 2006, the poverty rate for African Americans was 24.3 percent, compared to 8.2 percent for White Americans. This is significant because poverty puts people at greater risk for HIV infection (Krueger, Wood, Diehr, & Maxwell, 1990).

- Also in 2006, the percentage of African Americans without health insurance was 19.5 percent, compared to 10.4 percent of White Americans. Lack of health insurance limits an individual's access to medical care, which may in part explain the discrepancies between African Americans and White Americans in getting treatment for HIV/AIDS and having access to antiretroviral (ARV) drugs.

- In mid-2008, the incarceration of African-American males in state and federal prisons and local jails was 4,777 per 100,000 (Bureau of Justice Statistics, 2009) compared to 258 per 100,000 for the overall U.S. population (Minton & Sabol, 2009).

- In 2000, 83.6 percent of White students had graduated high school or more, compared to 72.3 percent of African-American students—an 11.3 percent difference (Bauman & Graf, 2003).

• Drug and alcohol use are linked with the spread of HIV/AIDS. It is most commonly known that sharing needles leads to blood-to-blood transmission; other recreational drugs and alcohol play a significant role in HIV infection, however, because their use increases an individual's risk-taking behaviors by altering judgment and decreasing inhibition. Figure 4.5 presents the percentages of the population to use illicit drugs and alcohol by race/ethnicity. For 2008, the rate of illicit drug use among Blacks ages twelve and up was higher than that of other races or ethnicities: 10.8 percent, compared to 9.5 percent for American Indians and Alaska Natives, 8.2 percent for Whites, 7.3 percent for Native Hawaiians, 6.2 percent for Hispanics, and 3.2 percent for Asians. The rate of alcohol use was lower compared to other races: 41.9 percent compared to 56.2 percent for Whites, 43.3 percent for American Indians or Alaska Natives, 43.2 percent for Hispanics, and 37 percent for Asians (Substance Abuse and Mental Health Services Administration [SAMHSA], 2009).

To better understand the relationship between these factors and race, it is important to look at racial discrimination and consider the historical context for these

Figure 4.5. Percent of Population to Use Illicit Drugs and Alcohol by Race/Ethnicity

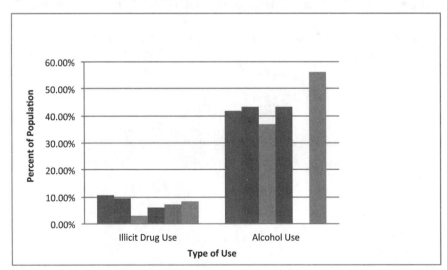

Source: SAMHSA (2009).
Note: Due to low precision, estimates for Native Hawaiians or other Pacific Islanders are not shown for alcohol use.

gaps that put African Americans at a disadvantage. Racial discrimination is still a prevalent problem in the United States. More hate crimes are committed against African Americans than against any other minority group (U.S. Department of Justice–Federal Bureau of Investigation, 2008). Although great strides have been made since the achievements of the civil rights movement, significant gaps still leave African Americans at a disadvantage.

Questions for Reflection

1. Do you see racism around you either overtly or covertly? How so?

2. Do you think structural or institutional racism is related to HIV/AIDS trends? Why or why not? If so, how?

Testing and Prevention Challenges. African Americans are more likely to get tested for HIV/AIDS than are other racial or ethnic groups, as reflected in figure 4.6. A Kaiser public opinion poll found that, in 2009, 68 percent of African Americans have been tested, compared to 57 percent of Latinos and 42 percent of White Americans (The Henry J. Kaiser Family Foundation, 2009). Moreover, this same survey showed that African Americans were more likely to talk to their health-care providers and their intimate partners about HIV/AIDS than were White and

Figure 4.6. Percent Who Report Ever Being Tested for HIV, by Race/Ethnicity

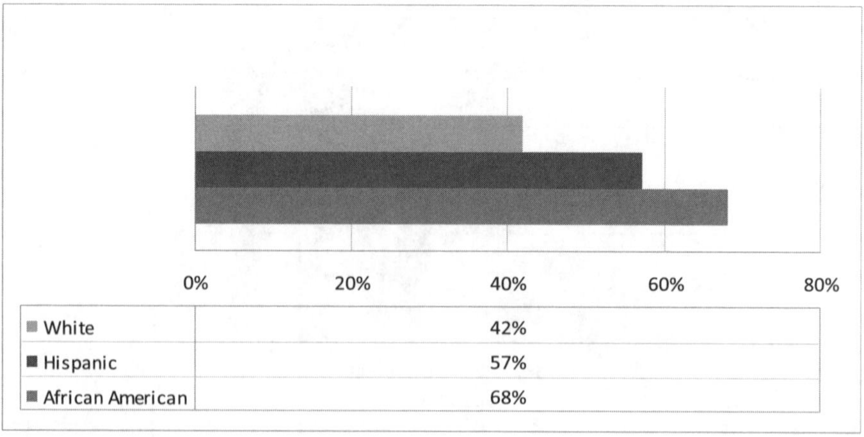

■ White	42%
■ Hispanic	57%
■ African American	68%

Source: Rountree et al. (2009).

Latino Americans. The paradox is that, although African Americans are getting tested at a higher rate, they still have higher rates of HIV infection. Likewise, Rountree, Chen, Brown, and Pomeroy (2009), in a study of the HIV testing rates among Whites, African Americans, and Hispanics, found that African Americans report higher testing rates. These authors suggest that testing alone will have limited efficacy in prevention without the addition of culturally and contextually relevant prevention strategies.

Heightened National Response to the HIV/AIDS Crisis among African Americans

As outlined in the article "Fighting HIV among African Americans," the CDC, along with leading African Americans in the field and other partner organizations, launched a comprehensive HIV program in 2009 directed toward fighting the epidemic in African-American communities (CDC, 2009a). This program, called the Heightened National Response to the HIV/AIDS Crisis among African Americans (HNR), provides approximately $300 million annually (about half of CDC's prevention budget) for preventing the spread of HIV among African Americans.

There are four main focal points of HNR:

1. Expand HIV prevention outreach.

2. Increase opportunities for HIV diagnosis and treatment.

3. Develop new, effective prevention interventions.

4. Mobilize broader community action.

Expand HIV Prevention Outreach. Of all the HIV-prevention funds designated for African Americans, the largest portion (about 83 percent) is spent on implementing prevention programs that have been proven effective. Despite this emphasis, many people still are not receiving these effective prevention programs. A study by the CDC found that in fifteen cities 80 percent of all African-American MSM had not been reached by proven HIV-prevention programs. In response, the CDC is disseminating evidence-based HIV-prevention programs more widely and expanding the number and types of organizations that offer these programs (table 4.2).

Table 4.2. Proven HIV-Prevention Programs for African Americans

Program	Target Group	Program Description
BART St. Lawrence, Brasfield, Jefferson, Alleyne, O'Bannon, & Shirley (1995).	High-risk youth	BART, or Becoming a Responsible Teen, is a group-level intervention using education and behavioral skills training to reduce risky behaviors and improve safer sex skills.
Be Proud, Be Responsible Jemmott, Jemmott, & Fong, (1992). Jemmott & Jemmott (1996).	High-risk youth, inner city	The focus of this small-group-based intervention is to increase knowledge of HIV/AIDS and other STDs, while changing attitudes toward risky sexual behaviors.
Enhanced Negotiation Sterk, Theall, & Elifson (2003).	Heterosexual HIV-negative adults, inner-city drug-using females	Through this enhanced negotiation training, four sessions of individualized counseling are provided to participants to explore HIV/AIDS risk in the context of daily life, including gender-specific behaviors, norms, attitudes, and race- and gender-related dynamics.
Focus on the Future Crosby, DiClemente, Charnigo, Snow, & Troutman (2009).	Heterosexual adult, male	This one-time, individual-level intervention is directed at reducing common errors and multiple problems that arise when using condoms, increasing African-American men's ability to use condoms correctly and consistently.
FOY + Impact Stanton, Li, Ricardo, Galbraith, Feigelman, & Kaljee (1996). Galbraith, Ricardo, Stanton, Black, & Feigelman, (1996). Stanton, Fang, Li, Feigelman, Galbraith, & Ricardo (1997). Li, Stanton, Feigelman, & Galbraith (2002).	High-risk youth, male and female	Focus on Youth + Impact is a two-part intervention. The first part reaches youth, working on reducing risky sex and drug behaviors. The second part reaches out to the youths' guardians, emphasizing communication and parenting.
Horizons DiClemente et al. (2009).	High-risk youth, female	Horizons is a group-based, two-session prevention intervention that focuses on gender and ethnic pride, increases knowledge of HIV and STDs, and enhances communication and negotiation skills.
3MV Wilton, Herbst, Coury-Doniger, Painter, English, Alvarez, et al. (2009).	MSM	Many Men, Many Voices (3MV). This seven-session group-level intervention is designed for African-American MSM who may or may not identify as bisexual or gay. It focuses on social, cultural, and religious norms, the interaction of other STDs with HIV, dynamics of sexual relationships, and the effects of racism and homophobia on HIV risk behaviors.

Program	Target Group	Program Description
SiHLE DiClemente et al. (2004).	High-risk youth, female	Sistering, Informing, Healing, Living, and Empowering (SiHLE). Using interactive discussions, SiHLE focuses on gender and ethnic pride and healthy relationships while increasing knowledge of HIV and STDs, preventing STDs and pregnancy, and enhancing HIV-prevention behaviors.
Sister to Sister Jemmott, Jemmott, & O'Leary, (2007).	Heterosexual adult female	Sister to Sister is a one-time intervention that can take place with either an individual or a group. It aims to increase self-efficacy of effective condom use and negotiation, emphasizing that protecting themselves is not only good for women personally, but also good for their families and the community.
WiLLOW Wingood, DiClemente, Mikhail, et al. (2004).	HIV-positive women who are sexually active	Women Involved in Life Learning from Other Women (WiLLOW) focuses on HIV transmission reduction among women living with HIV. This skill-based intervention emphasizes gender pride and the importance of social networks and communities of support. It focuses on skills for communication and condom negotiation, as well as how to differentiate between healthy and unhealthy relationships and how to recognize domestic violence.

Increase Opportunities for HIV Diagnosis and Treatment. Many African Americans do not know their HIV sero-status. Often, when they do get tested, it is late in their diagnosis and past the time when treatment programs are most effective. Estimates indicate that most cases of HIV transmission occur when the HIV-positive partner does not know his or her status; therefore, increasing HIV diagnosis and treatment through testing is a key prevention strategy.

Box 4.3. Steps to Increase Access to Testing

• Train health-care providers.

• Expand number of testing locations.

• Find new ways to motivate African-American men and women to be tested.

Steps for increasing access to testing include training health-care providers in routine HIV screening, expanding the number of locations in health-care and community settings that offer HIV testing, and finding new ways to motivate African-American men and women to seek out testing opportunities. In 2007 and 2008, the CDC devoted $70 million to increasing the testing efforts across the United States, specifically in African-American communities. Additionally, they have increased the variety of community settings in which rapid HIV testing is offered, such as minority gay pride events, historically Black colleges and universities (HBCU), and churches. They also have launched an HIV testing campaign targeted toward African-American gay and bisexual men between the ages of eighteen and twenty-four.

Develop New, Effective Prevention Interventions. Given the diversity within the African-American community, it is important to have a comprehensive range of culturally competent HIV-prevention programs that reach different segments of the population. There is still a significant need to create effective prevention interventions for MSM, as well as to create interventions that address larger sociopolitical factors that impact HIV/AIDS transmission and infection. HNR supports investigative studies on new interventions for high-risk African Americans, including women, MSM, and incarcerated individuals. To complement this effort, the CDC is researching the larger structural and system-level impacts on African Americans' HIV/AIDS infection rates to inform new prevention interventions that address these macro-level issues. The CDC is making additional efforts to increase the involvement of African-American researchers in studies on HIV prevention as well as efforts to more quickly implement newly developed interventions.

Practical applications of these efforts can be seen in several HNR initiatives. The CDC is developing and investigating the feasibility and effectiveness of HIV-prevention interventions for African-American MSM in Milwaukee, New York City, Baltimore, and Chicago. It is also researching ways that underemployed and unemployed African-American women can reduce their risk for HIV by changing their environment; the intervention focuses on getting them out of poverty through educating them to develop skills and abilities to start their own businesses. Finally, the CDC is financially supporting the work of African-American and Hispanic researchers, providing $2 million a year for research in communities that are most vulnerable to the AIDS epidemic.

Mobilize Broader Community Action. Engaging the African-American community, from business leaders to faith-based organizations, will be a key element in putting an end to the HIV epidemic among African Americans. Only through partnerships and collaboration will education and prevention efforts become widely disseminated throughout the community, decrease the amount of stigma around the topic, and inform people that the epidemic is indeed a community problem rather than an individual problem. Currently, the CDC is developing partnerships with African American–owned businesses, prominent African-American leaders, and faith leaders. Forums among these groups will gather stakeholders together to problem solve and develop substantial solutions for increasing prevention efforts.

Cultural Competence

A key to social work practice in the area of HIV/AIDS and African Americans is cultural competence. Cultural competence in social work entails being aware of one's own worldview while learning about the worldviews of the individuals we work with as social workers and professionals in the field of HIV/AIDS. Practitioners providing services to the African-American community must understand the Afrocentric worldview.

Awareness of One's Worldview. We all see the world through the lens of our experiences and the environment in which we live. Many factors influence our worldview, such as our cultural heritage, race or ethnicity, gender identity, sexual orientation, religious or spiritual beliefs, the presence or absence of a disability, political preferences, and level of education. These factors inform our identities and the perspectives from which we approach life events and the situations around us. They also affect our daily personal relationships.

It is important to be self aware and to understand our identity and how it is formed. What shapes who you are? What choices inform your identity? What are the biological and environmental factors—in other words, factors that you did not choose—that inform your identity? How does your identity affect your HIV risk level and knowledge, attitudes, and beliefs regarding HIV infection?

Reflecting on these questions leads to a new perspective with which to view the AIDS epidemic, its influence on your life, and its impact on African-American communities. Only by understanding our own worldview can we look into the worldview of others with some level of understanding.

Questions for Reflection

1. What shapes your identities?

2. What shapes your worldview?

3. How do you see yourself continuing to change?

4. Is this course on HIV changing your perspectives on the world? Why or why not?

5. How can deepening your self-awareness help you work with individuals with, or at risk for, HIV?

Power and privilege are important factors in our self-identities. Based on the dominant and minority groups in society, people will find themselves on either the advantageous or the disadvantageous side of power. Because people are complex, there may be some areas in which they have power and others in which they do not. For example, an affluent African-American woman with her master's degree in finance will find herself in more positions of having or not having power than will a lesser educated African-American woman. She is a minority in terms of her gender and her race, yet she has power based on her class and level of education.

Box 4.4. Activity: Power and Privilege

Reflect on your own life. Write about a time when you felt as though you were privileged and in a position of power based on a social identity. What were the benefits? How did it feel to have power? How does this privilege and power influence your everyday life?

Now write about a time when you felt as though you were at a disadvantage, without power based on a social identity. What are the benefits you missed out on by being in a position without power? How does that experience shape who you are?

The Afrocentric Worldview. While we should remain mindful of the diversity of African Americans' thoughts and experiences, looking at the Afrocentric worldview can help us to understand some of the core values of the African-American community. According to Hatter and Ottens (1998, p. 473), "An *Afrocentric* worldview is described as a holistic perspective assuming a spiritual/material unity and the interconnectedness of all things (Myers, 1988; emphasis added). It is centered in a spiritual and kinship connection to African culture (Robinson & Howard-Hamilton, 1994). . . . Examples of values inherent in this worldview include cooperativeness, cohesiveness, oneness with nature, spirituality, positive interpersonal relationships, and a flexible time orientation (Jackson, 1986; Kambon, 1992; Myers 1988)."

This definition of Afrocentrism emphasizes

- Collectivism through relationships, cooperation, and cohesiveness;

- Spirituality, the connectedness of all things, and a oneness with nature; and

- Connection to African culture.

Box 4.5. Nguzo Saba: The Seven Principles

There are seven principles defined by Dr. Maulana Karenga, the creator of Kwanzaa, that are rooted in African-American identity.

- Umoja (unity)

- Kujichagulia (self-determination)

- Ujima (collective work and responsibility)

- Ujamaa (cooperative economics)

- Nia (purpose)

- Kuumba (creativity)

- Imani (faith)

The Afrocentric worldview is based on empowerment—it celebrates the strengths of African-American families and the roots of their culture. The author R. B. Hill (1971, 1999) describes five strengths of African-American families (Waites, 2009): strong achievement orientation, a strong work orientation, flexible family roles, strong kinship bonds, and a strong religious orientation. These strengths have grown out of the historical and cultural context in which African Americans have lived their lives, including the harshness of slavery, Jim Crow laws, segregation, and racism. Joining together over celebrated strengths and looking at the rich history of overcoming hardship gives African Americans tools for combating the problems they face today, including the AIDS epidemic.

Afrocentric principles are important to performing outreach and developing HIV-prevention messages for African Americans. Research studies have indicated that Afrocentric approaches to behavioral change can be highly effective, including decreasing substance abuse, depression, and risky sexual behaviors (Gilbert & Goddard, 2006). By using empowerment as a foundation, Afrocentric-based programs help increase pride in ethnicity and racial identity. They employ spirituality and emphasize the collective group by showing that taking care of one's own sexual health can actually benefit the participant's family and community. This way, prevention messages are meaningful to their recipients. Rather than being seen as countercultural, being tested for HIV can become acceptable as mainstream and as an indicator of how well one respects oneself and one's community. One important aspect of this type of intervention and outreach is its use of peer educators. Peer educators may help participants feel less embarrassed and more comfortable talking about their experiences. This approach is both empowering to the peer educator and inspiring to participants.

Questions for Reflection

1. How can the Afrocentric perspective inform professionals working with African-American communities affected by HIV/AIDS?

2. How do you think the Afrocentric worldview could shape HIV-prevention messages?

Approaching the Epidemic Holistically

Addressing the HIV/AIDS epidemic among African Americans is an important component of fighting the AIDS epidemic in the United States and globally. We can now see the disproportionate impact of HIV/AIDS on African-American communities, why this is an indicator of broader social issues, and some appropriate perspectives with which to approach HIV/AIDS prevention and outreach efforts. While changing individual risk factors is indeed an important target for reducing the spread of HIV, these efforts will fail if not matched with efforts to address the social, political, and cultural factors that make HIV/AIDS an ongoing health threat.

Case Example

Alicia Treadwell was both anxious and excited about her new assignment. She had only been working at Rosedale AIDS Program for seven months, and she had just been assigned to the new Primary Prevention and Outreach program. Her task was to work with two colleagues to design outreach programs that were culturally sensitive and to network well with existing services, especially within a predominately African-American area of the Rosedale community where there had been a noticeable spike in new HIV/AIDS cases.

Alicia's Background. Alicia is an Anglo-American female from Akron, Ohio. She grew up in an area where the majority of her neighbors and classmates in high school were White, middle class, and valued educational and professional achievement. Her family was not wealthy by any means, but both of her parents worked and their combined income was enough for them to live comfortably. While Alicia was growing up, her family regularly attended a local Presbyterian church. Alicia excelled in school, and received a scholarship to attend a state university, where she began studying art history. During her first semester, an inspiring professor recommended Alicia read a series of essays written by a feminist author. After reading the essays, Alicia was struck by how powerfully they moved her. She began reflecting on her own life and the struggles she had faced as a woman. As she continued to study more works by feminist scholars, Alicia decided to do a double major and get a second degree in women's studies.

In both her art history and women's studies classes, Alicia became aware of social injustices based on other factors besides gender. For example, in one women's studies course, she wrote a research paper in which she examined scholarly articles criticizing the women's movement for generalizing White, middle-class women's experiences as normative, while disregarding the complex overlapping factors of race and class.

When Alicia was not in class she spent much of her time volunteering in her community. In fact, she was an active member with the Student Volunteer Alliance, an official university-sponsored club whose goal was to connect students to a number of volunteer opportunities. Through her activities with the Alliance, she gained leadership skills, recognized the value of volunteerism, and had the chance to work with a variety of social service agencies. She also volunteered with the homeless population.

After graduating with her two bachelor's degrees, Alicia still did not know exactly in which direction she would begin her career. She considered both her education and volunteer experience, then decided that she wanted to do something to make a difference in the world around her. She applied to her university's school of social work, and enrolled in a master of social work program the fall after she finished her undergraduate work.

Alicia's Social Work Experiences. The school of social work that Alicia attended was practicum based, meaning students had two field placements to fully immerse them in the social work practice experience. Her first field experience was as an intern at a domestic violence shelter. She was placed there because of her continued interest in women-related issues. While working at the clinic, she realized that several of the clients were African-American and Latina women. One of the clients that Alicia was assigned to work with at the shelter as a case manager was a fifty-four-year-old African-American woman named Diana who disclosed her HIV-positive status. At first, Alicia was uncomfortable. She felt as though she shouldn't react that way, but she was learning about the self-reflective process in her program, and knew she needed to be honest with herself and acknowledge any biases she may have. Alicia had never knowingly interacted with anyone who was HIV positive before. In addition, she felt awkward that she came from a place of such privilege in regards to her good health and being a member of the majority racial group in the United States. She was relatively young and new to the field of social work, however, and was afraid her client would think she wasn't qualified to work with her. Even more important, Alicia thought she would not be able to relate to her client, leading her to anticipate difficulty in building a healthy working relationship.

After personal reflection and seeking guidance from her supervisor, Alicia determined that she would address the potential barriers head on: she would tell Diana that in social work practice the client is the expert rather than the practitioner. Only Diana could know what was best for her own life. Alicia was there to collaborate in the process, offer information and resources, and advocate for what was in Diana's best interest. Alicia did not pretend she was more culturally competent than she was. She asked questions that helped her better understand Diana's background experiences, values and beliefs, and health condition.

After three months of case management with Diana, Alicia was amazed at the progress they had made together. Moreover, she learned the powerful lesson of empowerment and the wonders it can do to building a trusting relationship. She also found a new passion, as she had discovered that African Americans are disproportionately infected with and affected by HIV/AIDS. This prompted her to choose an ASO for her second field placement. Eventually, this placement led to the next step in her career at a similar organization in the neighborhood of Rosedale.

Rosedale

Rosedale is a primarily African-American neighborhood in the city of Midfield, a midsized city in the southern region of the United States. Midfield was established in 1860 with the development of a railroad system. It was a hub for business related to oil, cattle, and agriculture. By the turn of the twentieth century, the western part of the town had been settled primarily by African Americans. Although they suffered hardship during the Great Depression, the residents of Midfield survived to prosper in strength and spirit. Local businesses continued to thrive throughout the 1950s and 1960s, strengthening Midfield's status as a predominantly middle-class city based on entrepreneurship.

Today, the neighborhood of Rosedale comprises African Americans (72 percent), followed by Hispanics (21 percent), White Americans (5 percent), and other races (2 percent). Ten years ago, Rosedale built an African American Heritage Center; the Center has served as a landmark and meeting place that brings many of the members of the community and local families together. Even more central to the heart of the neighborhood are the Black churches: the Church of New Hope, Rosedale Missionary Church, and All Saints Ministerial Church. In addition to their spiritual and cultural heritage, Rosedale residents are proud of their locally owned restaurants and businesses and their high level of civic engagement.

Rosedale residents face many challenges when compared to the rest of the Midfield. The average household income is lower for Rosedale than for the rest of the city, and the poverty rate is higher. Compared to other schools in the Midfield Independent School District, the elementary, middle, and high schools in Rosedale receive the least funds, have typically lower test scores on statewide achievement tests, and have higher drop-out rates. Another challenge that residents of Rosedale face is home ownership: fewer than half of the residents own their own homes. Additionally, Rosedale, like most communities, has been impacted by an economic downturn. To date the unemployment rate runs close to 11 percent, higher than it has been since the 1970s.

Rosedale and HIV/AIDS. According to data from the state, 21 percent of the residents of Rosedale took an HIV test within the previous year, and 40 percent reported ever being tested. Of those who had been tested, the rate of testing HIV positive was 24.2 out of 100,000, almost twice that of the national average, which was 12.5 in 2007. This shows that although there is a relatively high testing rate in the town, there is still a growing AIDS epidemic, meaning that prevention efforts need be coupled with risk-reduction prevention interventions.

Rosedale AIDS Program

The Rosedale AIDS Program (RAP) originally emerged in the mid-1980s from grassroots efforts. As of present day most of the public had heard of the AIDS epidemic, but people primarily associated the disease with White, gay men. In fact, the executive director and a number of the first employees and board members of RAP fit this description, creating a feeling of uncertainty among the residents of Rosedale. As most of Rosedale was African American, the new AIDS program felt out of place: it was run by outsiders. How were these "experts" supposed to understand local problems of the neighborhood? The residents resonated with the general sentiment, "You mean you're going to come in here talking about sensitive topics such as sex and drugs when you don't even know us?" There was a level of distrust between Rosedale residents who were HIV positive and needed the services and the RAP service providers because of what appeared to be a cultural divide.

New Directions. In 2007, the executive director of RAP resigned for personal reasons, opening the position for a new leader, and, ultimately, creating the pathway for organizational change. With this resignation, RAP had an opportunity to develop a more relevant response to Rosedale's culture and the shift in the AIDS epidemic.

RAP's new executive director, Marcus Patterson, is an African-American man in his mid-thirties. He grew up in the Rosedale neighborhood and attended college at the local university in Midfield. He is well liked in the community, and many community members know him and his family. Marcus is focused, driven, and motivated to increase RAP's effectiveness. Because of this attitude, he often seems very serious and does not take the time out of his work day for fun. To some of the staff, his approach is intimidating. However, anyone who gets to know him knows that Marcus is a very kind and generous person. He has very strong spiritual beliefs and he values integrity. His top two priorities for RAP are to (1) increase the cultural competence of the agency, including hiring staff that are diverse, and (2) focus on outreach and prevention to reach the residents of Rosedale.

One year ago, Marcus, with agreement from the board, determined that it was time to make some structural changes in the agency. RAP laid off one of its middle managers. This created great turbulence in the agency, as this manager was well liked by some of his colleagues. With the departure of this manager, several other staff members decided they wanted to leave; this turnover created an opening for Alicia to start working at RAP after her graduation.

Organizational Culture. Between 2007 and 2010, RAP increased its proportion of employees who were African American and Latino. However, the upper management is still predominantly White. There seems to be a divide between the upper management and the front-line workers, where the front-line workers feel as though they are left out of the decision-making and information-sharing processes. Moreover, there are cliques in the agency based on role (counselors as opposed to case managers), education level (licensed social workers as opposed to peer workers), length of time at the agency (the old guard and the newcomers), and race. Despite these challenges, there is still a sense of shared passion for the work itself. Everyone at the agency is brought together with the common desire to help people living with HIV and AIDS and to prevent the spread of HIV.

With a new executive director and employees that better reflect Rosedale's racial composition, RAP is beginning to develop some rapport in the community. Because of this change, there is an influx of new community members volunteering, including joining the board. This is stimulating the development of new ideas and is ultimately resulting in better relationships with RAP clients.

Programs and Services. When RAP first opened its doors in 1995, they offered a variety of services, including

• Case management to help HIV-positive clients meet basic needs

• A crisis hotline, called the AIDS-Helpline

• Support groups for HIV-positive individuals and their family members and caregivers

• Street-based outreach and testing services

Now, RAP has expanded to twenty-two employees and has a variety of new programs:

- Financial assistance, along with budgeting and financial management services

- Employment services

- A food bank

- Dental care

- Primary prevention and outreach services

Work in Progress

The Team. At their first meeting, Alicia wanted to spend some time getting to know her two other team members, Mike Brookings and Rachael Thomas, so they spent some time learning about one another. Mike was one of the original founders of RAP. He was White, gay and, like Alicia, had his master degree in social work. Mike joined the AIDS movement as a street-based outreach worker in the 1980s because he had witnessed so much death and suffering related to AIDS among his closest friends. Because of their similar educational experiences and practice frameworks, Alicia and Mike hit it off well. Alicia also got along well with Rachael. Rachael was African American and a proud mother of two. Rachael had a bachelor's degree in public health and had become involved in AIDS work when her uncle was diagnosed with HIV seven years ago. Although Alicia got along well with both of her teammates, Rachael and Mike had very differing ideas about how to design a HIV-prevention strategy. While this seemed like a challenge in the beginning, it really helped to generate dialogue, discussion, and new ideas.

Developing a Collaborative Process. Together, the team came up with a collaborative approach to engage community members in the process of developing the HIV outreach and prevention campaigns. But first, before identifying partners in this project, they decided to host a community forum to gauge the range of local ideas and opinions on the topic of HIV/AIDS in Rosedale and what could be done about it.

For two weeks, the outreach and prevention team contacted local church leaders, business leaders, and neighborhood task force representatives. They hung flyers in all of the public locations where it was permissible to advertise that RAP was hosting a community forum on HIV/AIDS in Rosedale. They made sure that they had arranged for accommodations such as child care in order to limit any barriers to people being able to attend.

Twenty-seven Rosedale residents attended the public forum. Of those who attended, it was apparent that most knew the basics about HIV/AIDS: that there was no cure, that it was transmitted through bodily fluids exchanged during sex, and blood, and that the best ways to protect themselves from it were to not share needles, and to use condoms or be abstinent. However, there were still a lot of myths and misunderstandings about whether or not people could become infected through kissing, touching someone with AIDS, or using public restrooms. Additional beliefs that were shared among participants were the possibility of the AIDS conspiracy theory and distrust of medical workers. Most participants believed that some members of the community wanted to deny that HIV/AIDS was a problem or wanted to avoid the topic altogether.

There were two contrasting opinions voiced at the forum. The first was that HIV/AIDS was a disease that people contracted because of their immorality: sex outside of marriage, drug use, and homosexuality. People who voiced this opinion believed that an HIV-prevention effort was important, but that the primary message should be based on values of abstinence and sobriety. Prominent voices in this group were Mrs. Larkin (a concerned elder and well-known member of the Rosedale Missionary Church), Matthew Wellington (owner of a local restaurant), and Paula Parker (owner of a local beauty salon).

The second primary opinion was that HIV/AIDS was a human disease that puts all people at risk. Although they definitely supported people's decisions to abstain and to be sober, they believed outreach efforts should focus on using condoms and clean needles. Supporters of this argument were Reverend Raymond Watson of the Church of New Hope, Jenny Oliver from Pathways Substance Abuse and Chemical Dependency Center, and Abigail Collins of the Rosedale Community Health Clinic.

Inviting the Stakeholders. The prevention team decided to ask the prominent voices to the table to work on finding a common solution. Alicia set up individual, personal meetings with Mrs. Larkin, Mathew Wellington, Paula Parker, Reverend Watson, Jenny Oliver, and Abigail Collins. In each meeting, Alicia told these participants that she appreciated what they had shared at the forum and that she would value their participation in the project. She told them why she thought they would be a good fit. All but Mrs. Larkin agreed to participate.

Creative Brainstorm. Before tackling the major points of contention, Alicia encouraged the group of collaborators to find common ground. After the group had set ground rules, they asked themselves a few questions. What do we agree upon in regards to HIV/AIDS in Rosedale? What is the scope of the problem? Why is this problem important to me? Why do I think this problem is important to the community? What are shared values and beliefs that can be helpful in HIV-prevention efforts?

By going through this activity, the collaborators realized that they had much in common. They agreed that HIV/AIDS is a significant and growing health concern and that they had to do something about it. They realized that they all valued Rosedale and were proud to be a part of the community. They all shared the vision of a healthy community. They recognized overlapping health concerns of poverty, drug use, low-performing schools, and discrimination that were related to HIV/AIDS, and wanted to take a holistic approach to addressing the AIDS epidemic. They also recognized the strengths of the community: the cultural pride, hard work, family focus, and spirituality.

Alicia facilitated the group discussion, and, at the end, all of the participants were glad to be a part of this effort and knew that they had something unique to add and something to share with their collaborators.

Getting to Know Mrs. Larkin. In the meantime, Alicia had determined that she needed to get to know Mrs. Larkin and understand why she did not want to participate in the collaboration. She called Mrs. Larkin and asked her if it would be okay for them to meet over lunch and get to know each other better. Alicia reflected back to when she was working with Diana at the women's health clinic, about the importance of rapport and trust. Alicia knew that because she was a newcomer to the Rosedale neighborhood she would have to gain the respect of longtime residents. She would have to build trust with Mrs. Larkin. After their first successful meeting, Alicia and Mrs. Larkin began having lunch together frequently. Alicia shared her personal story, her journey to the field of HIV/AIDS and why she wanted to be in Rosedale. Mrs. Larkin was reserved at first, but began opening up to Alicia after a few meetings. She eventually shared that a dear friend's husband had cheated on her, and, in doing so, infected her friend with HIV. That was why she was so passionate about HIV/AIDS being a moral issue: if her husband had been faithful, her friend would have her full health.

Alicia didn't try to change Mrs. Larkin's mind; that was not her job. She only wanted to let her know that her voice and opinions were important to the group. She would add much depth and richness if she was willing to participate. Mrs. Larkin said that she would think about it, but that she was still not ready. HIV/AIDS-related health concerns were important to her, but she was not fully convinced that her perspective would be heard. Alicia respected Mrs. Larkin's decision, and the two of them continued to meet periodically.

An Afrocentric Worldview. Alicia had studied the Afrocentric worldview in her social work studies and thought it would be important to use this information to shape any type of outreach messages targeting Rosedale. She printed out materials about Afrocentrism and took them to the next prevention team meeting with Mike and Rachael. Mike thought the information was useful and began studying it from the point of view of his personal knowledge. Rachael came up with an idea: "Why don't we let the collaborators come up with their own principles and values of what Afrocentrism means to them? That way it is more practical and tangible rather than theoretical." Mike and Alicia liked Rachael's idea, and together the team decided that Rachael would lead the discussion on Afrocentrism, letting the collaborators determine their own principles and values that shape their worldview. In the large meeting, participants identified the following themes:

- Emphasis on collective experience ("We're all in this together.")

- Devotion to family and community.

- Pride of being African American.

- The importance of strong African-American leaders.

- Spirituality.

- Holistic health that incorporates body, mind, and spirit.

Once group members had identified these themes, participants actually had fun creating HIV-prevention and outreach initiatives. In fact, whether or not the messages should target abstinence and sobriety or condom use and clean needles became a moot point; instead they focused on their cultural identity and how that could be used to inspire people to make healthier, safer choices.

The Final Products

Status Sure: Safe for Me, My Family, and My Community. The first outreach program the group developed was a community-wide testing campaign. This campaign, Status Sure: Safe for Me, My Family, and My Community, is based largely on advertisement to get the word out about why testing and knowing one's HIV status is important. The first component of the campaign was media driven, primarily using billboards, posters, and radio ads. The bill-boards and posters portrayed a young, adult, African-American woman with the caption "I'm status sure. Are you? Get tested for HIV today to be sure of your status," with RAP contact information at the bottom. The radio advertise-ments are played on the two most popular radio stations—one that targets adolescents and one that targets young to middle-aged adults. The advertise-ments feature a poem in freestyle verse composed by a local artist. It covers how AIDS impacts African Americans and, like the visual advertisements, dis-cusses the importance of HIV testing and being status sure.

The second component of the campaign, a community awareness event to be held at the Rosedale African-American Heritage Center, is to be initiated after the media campaign has been in effect for about a month so that com-munity members will be more likely to recognize the phrase "status sure" as referring to knowing one's HIV status. This campaign component highlights the importance of being a leader in the African-American community, cou-pled with the idea that a responsible leader will know his or her HIV status. At this event, several leaders in the Rosedale community have already agreed to be tested for HIV, including Reverend Raymond Watson, Mayor Marissa Clai-borne, School Superintendent Robyn Marlow, and Sheriff Joseph Cardin. Each of these leaders will make a public service announcement via the local media stating, "I'm proud to be a leader and proud to be status sure."

Third, in addition to well-known leaders, other community members who play a vital role in the life of the community (but may not be well known) have agreed to participate. They include mothers, fathers, grandparents, teachers, neighbors, nurses, doctors, police officers, and firefighters. These community members will film a public service announcement with each saying some-thing along the lines of, "My name is Emma Wright. I'm proud to be a grand-mother and proud to be status sure. Do you know your HIV status?"

Overall, this campaign used the collaborative groups ideas of devotion to family and community, pride of being African American, and the importance of strong, African-American leaders.

Beautify Your Life with Sexual Health. In Rosedale, the beauty salon and barber shop offer safe communal places where people gather and share information, knowledge, and stories about themselves and the community while taking care of their physical appearance. The collaboration developed a campaign called Beautify Your Life with Sexual Health. This is a sexual safety promotion campaign that encourages a host of safer sex behaviors, from choosing abstinence to choosing a safe, healthy, trustworthy sexual partner, and consistent condom use. This campaign will emphasize the importance of feeling beautiful on the outside and making decisions that make the community members feel safe, healthy, and beautiful on the inside. In this way, it incorporates the principles of the collective experience, pride in being African American, and holistic health that incorporates body, mind, and spirit. Steps the group identified for moving forward with this project include the following:

- Set up meetings to get to know owners of local beauty salons and barber shops and present them with information on the importance of the campaign, Beautify Your Life with Sexual Health.

- After owner approval, train barbers and beauticians in HIV knowledge, awareness, and prevention.

- Provide information materials (flyers and brochures) to shops and salons for them to display.

- Develop posters to display on location.

Healthy Body, Healthy Mind. The Rosedale AIDS Program has as a primary goal to be able to work with other social service organizations, including the Rosedale Community Health Clinic, Dimmick Mental Health Services, and Pathways Substance Use and Chemical Dependency Treatment Center, because these organizations address problems that co-occur with HIV infection. The group chose to reach these three organizations through an outreach effort entitled Healthy Body, Healthy Mind. The point of this outreach is to emphasize that sexual health is an important element that needs to be balanced with physical health and mental health. It is based on the values of pride in being African American and holistic health that incorporates body, mind, and spirit. As part of this effort, the collaboration tried to recruit African-American artists from the Rosedale neighborhood to design art work with the theme Health Body, Health Mind to display in the Rosedale Community Health Clinic, Dimmick Mental Health Services, and Pathways Substance Use and Chemical Dependency Treatment Center. Steps that members of the collaboration agreed to take include these:

- Set up contacts with organizational leaders.

- Meet organizational leaders and present them with information and importance of the outreach effort, Healthy Body, Healthy Mind.

- After approval, educate practitioners and social workers at these organizations about RAP services, HIV/AIDS and its impact among African Americans, and the importance of sexual health so they may relay this information to patients and clients.

- Distribute informational materials for patients and clients.

- Develop posters and flyers to hang at the agencies with information on upcoming STD and HIV classes offered at RAP, on testing, and on other RAP services.

Engaging the Rosedale Inter-Faith Alliance. Finally, the group determined that involving spiritual leaders was important to decreasing stigma of HIV/AIDS in Rosedale. This, they were concerned, would be a challenge. How do you market a message of HIV prevention that is culturally sensitive to the spiritual beliefs of church members when topics such as sex and drug use are often taboo? Fortunately, they already had Reverend Watson on the collaboration, and he was a member of the Rosedale Inter-Faith Alliance. Below are creative ideas generated to begin involving spiritual leaders in the HIV/AIDS efforts within the community.

- Begin building relationships with church pastors, leaders, and members by meeting with them individually and sharing with them why they are passionate about this issue.

- Host a focus group with members from the churches to find out where they stand on the issue and engage them in a similar collaborative process.

- Set up a meeting between these spiritual stakeholders and the community collaboration to reach a common agreement about what may be feasible in an outreach effort for the churches.

- Develop an agreed-upon plan of action and a timeline with which to launch the efforts.

As a primary part of this effort, the collaboration realized that they needed to reach out to Mrs. Larkin. She was a strong voice in Rosedale Missionary Church, and they knew that without her help her church would never participate in the collaborative process. Paula called Mrs. Larkin, because Mrs. Larkin was one of her clients at Paula's Beauty Salon and they already had an amiable relationship. Mrs. Larkin told Paula that she would think about it and that she might come to the next meeting to observe.

At the next meeting, Alicia was surprised to see Mrs. Larkin. Mrs. Larkin walked up to Alicia, took her hand and said, "Thank you." She then proceeded to take a seat in a chair that had remained empty and to fill her spot as a collaborator.

Critical Inquiry Questions

1. How did Alicia's own reflective processes prepare her for outreach work in Rosedale?

2. What challenges did the outreach and prevention team face, and how did they anticipate or seek to address those challenges?

3. How do you think the changing culture of RAP influenced the work of the outreach and prevention team in the community?

4. What specific actions did Alicia take to build rapport with the community?

5. Moving forward, what additional challenges do you think the collaboration will face? What ideas do you have to address them?

References

Bauman, K. J., & Graf, N. L. (2003). *Educational attainment: 2000.* U.S. Census Bureau. Retrieved from www.census.gov/prod/2003pubs/c2kbr-24.pdf

Brooks, R. A., Etzel, M. A., Hinojos, E., Henry, C. L., & Perez, M. (2005). Preventing HIV among Latino and African American gay and bisexual men in context of HIV-related stigma, discrimination, and homophobia: Perspectives of providers. *AIDS Patient Care STDS, 19*(11), 737–744.

Bureau of Justice Statistics. (2009). *Prison statistics.* U.S. Department of Justice, Office of Justice Programs. Retrieved from http://www.ojp.usdoj.gov/bjs/prisons.htm

Centers for Disease Control and Prevention (CDC). (2009a). Fighting HIV among African Americans. *The Body Pro: The HIV Resource for Health Professionals.* Retrieved from http://www.thebodypro.com/content/whatis/art50362.html

Centers for Disease Control and Prevention (CDC). (2009b). *HIV/AIDS Surveillance Report, 2007. Vol. 19.* Atlanta: U.S. Department of Health and Human Services (DHHS), CDC: 2009.

Crosby, R., DiClemente, R. J., Charnigo, R., Snow, G., & Troutman, A. (2009). A brief, clinic-based, safer sex intervention for heterosexual African American men newly diagnosed with an STD: A randomized controlled trial. *American Journal of Public Health, 99,* S96–S103.

DiClemente, R. J., Wingood, G. M., Rose, E. S., Sales, J. M., Lang, D. L., Caliendo, A.M., . . . , Crosby, R. (2009). Efficacy of STD/HIV sexual risk-reduction intervention for African American adolescent females seeking sexual health services: A randomized controlled trial. *Archives of Pediatrics & Adolescent Medicine, 163*(12), 1112–1121.

DiClemente, R. J., Wingood, G. M., Harrington, K. F., Lang, D., Davies, S., Hook, E., . . . , Robillard, A. (2004). Efficacy of an HIV prevention intervention for African American adolescent girls: A randomized controlled trial. *Journal of the American Medical Association, 292,* 171–179.

Ferguson, Y. O., Quinn, S. C., Eng, E., & Sandelowski, M. (2006). The gender ratio imbalance and its relationship to risk of HIV/AIDS among African American women at historically Black colleges and universities. *AIDS Care, 18*(4), 323–331.

Freimuth, V. S., Quinn, S. C., Thomas, S. B., Cole, G., Zook, E., & Duncan, T. (2001). African American views on research and the Tuskegee syphilis study. *Social Science and Medicine, 52*(5), 797–808.

Fullilove, R. E. (2006, November 16). *African Americans, health disparities, and HIV/AIDS: Recommendations for confronting the epidemic in Black America.* Washington, DC: National Minority AIDS Council.

Galbraith, J., Ricardo, I., Stanton, B., Black, M., & Feigelman, S. (1996). Challenges and rewards of involving community in research: An overview of the "Focus on Kids" HIV risk reduction program. *Health Education Quarterly, 23,* 383–394.

Gilbert, D. J., & Goddard, L. (2006). HIV prevention targeting African American women: Theory, objectives, outcomes from an African-centered behavior change perspective. *Family Community Health, Supplement 1, 30*(1), S109–S111.

Gullette, D. L., Rooker, J. L., & Kennedy, R. L. (2009). Factors associated with sexually transmitted infections in men and women. *Journal of Community Health Nursing, 26*(3), 121–130.

Hatter, D. Y., & Ottens, A. J. (1998) Afrocentric world view and Black students' adjustment to a predominantly White university: Does worldview matter? *College Student Journal, 32*(3), 472–480.

Henry J. Kaiser Family Foundation, The. (2009). *Views and experiences with HIV testing among African Americans in the U.S.* Retrieved from http://www.kff.org/hivaids/upload/7927.pdf

Herek, G. M. (2009). *Fight AIDS, not people with AIDS!* Retrieved from http://psychology.ucdavis.edu/rainbow/HTML/aids.html

Herek, G. M., & Capitanio, J. P. (1999). AIDS stigma and sexual prejudice. *American Behavioral Scientist, 42*(7), 1130–1147.

Hill, R. B. (1971). *The strength of Black families.* New York: Emerson-Hall.

Hill, R. B. (1999). *The strengths of African American families: Twenty-five years later.* New York: University Press of America.

Jemmott, J. B. III, Jemmott, L. S., & Fong, G. T. (1992). Reductions in HIV risk-associated sexual behaviors among Black male adolescents: Effects of an AIDS prevention intervention. *American Journal of Public Health, 82,* 372–377.

Jemmott, J.B. III, & Jemmott, L.S. (1996). Strategies to reduce the risk of HIV infection, sexually transmitted diseases, and pregnancy among African American adolescents. In Resnick, R. J. & Rozensky, R. H. (Eds.), *Health psychology through the life span: Practice and research opportunities* (pp. 395–422). Washington DC: American Psychological Association.

Jemmott, L. S., Jemmott, J. B. III, & O'Leary, A. (2007). Effects on sexual risk behavior and STD rate of brief HIV/STD prevention interventions for African American women in primary care settings. *American Journal of Public Health, 97,* 1034–1040.

Krueger, L. E., Wood, R. W., Diehr, P. H., & Maxwell, P. W. (1990). Poverty and HIV seropositivity: The poor are more likely to be infected. *AIDS, 4*(8), 811–814.

Li, X., Stanton, B., Feigelman, S., & Galbraith, J. (2002). Unprotected sex among African-American adolescents: A three-year study. *Journal of the National Medical Association, 94,* 789–796.

Maman, S., Abler, L., Parker, L., Lane, T., Chirowadza, A., Ntogwisangu, J., & Fritz, K. (2009). A comparison of HIV stigma and discrimination in five international sites: The influence of care and treatment resources in high prevalence settings. *Social Science and Medicine, 68*(12), 2271–2278.

Minton, T. D., & Sabol, W. J. (2009). *Jail inmates at midyear 2008: Statistical tables.* Bureau of Justice Statistics, U.S. Department of Justice, Office of Justice Programs. Retrieved from http://www.ojp.usdoj.gov/newsroom/pressreleases/2009/BJS090331.htm

National Institute on Drug Abuse (2006). *Young African American adults at high risk for HIV, STDs even in absence of high-risk behavior.* National Institutes of Health, U.S. Department of Health and Human Services (DHHS). Retrieved from http://www.nih.gov/news/pr/dec2006/nida-05.htm

Rountree, M. A., Chen, L., Brown, A., & Pomeroy, E. C. (2009). HIV testing rates and testing locations among Whites, African Americans, and Hispanics in the United States: Data from the Behavioral Risk Factor Surveillance System, 2005. *Health and Social Work, 34*(4), 247–255.

Sandfort, T.G., & Dodge, B. (2008). "And then there was the Down Low": Introduction to Black and Latino Male Bisexualities. *Archives of Sexual Behavior, 37*(5), 675-682.

Shoptaw, S., Weiss, R. E., Munjas, B., Hucks-Ortiz, C., Young, S. D., Larkins, . . . , Gorbach, P. M. (2009). Homonegativity, substance use, sexual risk behaviors, and HIV status in poor and ethnic men who have sex with men. *Journal of Urban Health: Bulletin of the New York Academy of Medicine, 86*(1), S77–S91.

St. Lawrence, J. S., Brasfield, T. L., Jefferson, K. W., Alleyne, E., O'Bannon, R. E., & Shirley, A. (1995). Cognitive-behavioral intervention to reduce African American adolescents' risk for HIV infection. *Journal of Consulting and Clinical Psychology, 63,* 221–237.

Stanton, B., Fang, X., Li, X., Feigelman, S., Galbraith, J., & Ricardo, I. (1997). Evolution of risk behaviors over 2 years among a cohort of urban African American adolescents. *Archives of Pediatrics & Adolescent Medicine, 151,* 398–406.

Stanton, B. F., Li, X., Ricardo, I., Galbraith, J., Feigelman, S., & Kaljee, L. (1996). A randomized, controlled effectiveness trial of an AIDS prevention program for low-income African-American youths. *Archives of Pediatrics & Adolescent Medicine, 150*, 363–372.

Sterk, C. E., Theall, K. P., & Elifson, K. W. (2003). Effectiveness of a risk reduction intervention among African American women who use crack cocaine. *AIDS Education and Prevention, 15*(1), 15–32.

Stolberg, S. A. (2008, January 5). In global battle on AIDS, Bush creates legacy. *The New York Times.* Retrieved from http://www.nytimes.com/2008/01/05/washington/05aids.html?_r=2&ref=world&oref=slogin

Substance Abuse and Mental Health Services Administration (SAMHSA). (2009). *Results from the 2008 National Survey on Drug Use and Health: National findings.* Office of Applied Studies, NSDUH Series H-36, HHS Publication No. SMA 09-4434. Rockville, MD.

U.S. Census Bureau. (2008). Table 3: Annual estimates of the population by sex, race and Hispanic or Latino origin for the United States: April 1, 2000 to July 1, 2007 (NC-EST2007-03). Population Division, U.S. Census Bureau, Washington, DC.

U.S. Department of Justice—Federal Bureau of Investigation. (2008). *Hate crime statistics: Table 1, Incidents, offenses, victims, and known offenders.* Retrieved from http://www2.fbi.gov/ucr/hc2007/incidents.htm

Waites, C. (2009). Building on strengths: Intergenerational practice with African American families. *Social Work, 54*(3), 278–287.

Wilton, L., Herbst, J. H., Coury-Doniger, P., Painter, T. M., English, G., Alvarez, M. E., . . . , Carey, J. (2009). Efficacy of an HIV/STI prevention intervention for Black men who have sex with men: Findings from the Many Men, Many Voices (3MV) Project. *AIDS and Behavior, 13*, 532–544.

Wingood, G. M., DiClemente, R. J., Mikhail, I., Lang, D., Hubbard McCree, D., Davies, S., . . . , Saag, M. (2004). A randomized controlled trial to reduce HIV transmission risk behaviors and sexually transmitted diseases among women living with HIV: The WiLLOW program. *Journal of Acquired Immune Deficiency Syndromes, 37*, S58–S67.

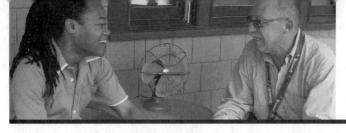

5

Culturally Competent Social Work Practice with Latinos with HIV

Diana Rowan

> From the depth of need and despair, people can work together, can organize themselves to solve their own problems and fill their own needs with dignity and strength.
>
> **—César Chàvez**

Introduction

Latinos are the largest, fastest-growing, and youngest minority group in the United States, and bear a disproportionate burden of HIV and AIDS. This disparity in the prevalence of HIV in Latinos is important to both social work practitioners and policy makers. This chapter examines the multiple vulnerabilities of Latinos with HIV and presents strategies for social work interventions that are culturally tailored. Case examples are used to illustrate various practice-related concepts throughout the chapter.

In 2010, Latinos accounted for 16 percent of the U.S. population, or 50.5 million people (U.S. Census Bureau, 2011), but 20 percent of the new cases of HIV and 17 percent of people living with HIV/AIDS. The AIDS diagnosis rate is three times that of non-Hispanic Whites, but one-third that of Blacks. Several factors contribute to these high rates. They include obstacles to prevention efforts for Latinos and the fact that HIV diagnoses usually come later in the disease progression than they do in non-Hispanic Whites, as is the case with the Black population. Furthermore, Latinos are slower to receive medical care for HIV disease than any other group. Also, many Latinos with HIV or AIDS do not receive adequate medical care. One study found that about 50 percent of Latinos with HIV were eligible for Medicaid (compared to 32 percent of Whites), and that 24 percent were uninsured (compared to 17 percent for Whites).

Note: Portions of this chapter were previously published in Rowan, Furman, Jones, and Edwards (2008).

Social workers must tailor services for HIV and AIDS prevention and care for Latino populations in order to meet their needs in a culturally appropriate manner. Structural risk factors are complex and interlocking, and they heighten Latinos' vulnerability to HIV infection. They include homophobia within the Latino culture, religious objections to condom use, restrictive immigration laws, discrimination, economic underdevelopment, xenophobia (fear of foreigners), and unequal access to power due to widespread poverty. Individual risk factors (Guilamo-Ramos, Bouris, & Gallego, 2010) include problem drinking and drug use, risky sexual behaviors, lack of mental health care, low self-efficacy (or confidence), incarceration, unemployment, undocumented immigration status, housing instability, social isolation from family supports in home country, and language barriers. Also, Latinos are overrepresented in the criminal justice system, and a higher percentage of Latino inmates compared with White inmates are HIV infected (Guilamo-Ramos et al., 2010). Latinas (Latino women) have even poorer health than Latinos (Latino men), use fewer health services, and suffer from higher rates of disease, disability, and early death (Cianelli, 2010). The fact that Latino and Latina vulnerabilities occur at both structural and individual levels requires social workers to consider multiple levels of intervention to effectively reduce the risk of HIV infection and increase access to care for those living with HIV or AIDS.

Latinos, HIV/AIDS, and Social Work

Social workers must develop unique skills, values, and knowledge for working with any specific population (Furman et al., 2009; Leigh, 1985). The following section briefly addresses issues in working with Latinos with HIV and AIDS.

Knowledge

Social work practice with Latinos is as diverse and complex as the group itself (Furman & Negi, 2007). The term "Latino," sometimes used interchangeably with the term "Hispanic," refers to people whose ancestry can be traced to the countries of Latin America and the Caribbean. However, many Latinos are native born and are not immigrants. For example, the ancestors of many Latinos did not come to the United States, but were Mexican nationals whose ancestral territories were annexed by the United States as part of the Treaty of Guadalupe Hidalgo at the end of the Mexican-American War. Similarly, Puerto Ricans living on mainland Puerto Rico have been citizens of the United States for nearly a century.

For many Latinos, the term itself is a social construction that is less important to their identity than are other factors (Furman & Negi, 2007). Most Latinos, for instance, identify primarily by their nation of origin. For instance, Guatemalan descendents of the Maya identify primarily by their ethnic group (Little, 2004). However, in spite of the diversity in the Latino population, thinking of Latinos as a group is useful for several reasons. First, with the exception of Brazilians, who speak Portuguese, and those who primarily speak indigenous languages, Latinos are bound by the historical use of Spanish. Second, many Latinos have come to view themselves as an increasingly powerful political entity whose unity is a considerable source of power (Gregory, Steinberg, & Sousa, 2003). National and local elections in the United States are increasingly influenced by Latino votes, and recent legislative initiatives concerning immigration have been slowed, in part, by politicians' concern about the impact of legislation on Latinos as a voting block. Finally, Latinos share many values that are rooted in postcolonial Latin America. The centrality and importance of these values often conflict with those of the dominant U.S. society, and set Latinos apart as a distinct and evolving group.

Values and Their Translation into Skills

Respect for culturally imbedded values is extremely important to social work practice with Latinos. The values presented here are only a partial list, but they form a core that binds Latinos and will help social workers who provide services to this population, especially those who are unfamiliar with Latino culture. All of these values have important practice implications for working with Latinos with HIV and AIDS. In general, these values are extensions of the overall collectivist values that many Latinos hold, which differ from the more individualistic values of the dominant American culture. These collectivist values have been shown to be adaptive, in that they have historically led to group cohesion during times of social disruption and distress (Cabrera & Padilla, 2004), and have served as protective factors against some types of psychosocial problems, such as substance abuse (Sale et al., 2005).

Familismo

Social workers and other professionals in the United States who are new to working with Latinos often misinterpret the importance of family and its centrality in how Latinos view identity and existence (Lugo Steidel & Contreras, 2003; Valenzuela & Dornbusch, 1994). White Americans view the individual as the essential unit of analysis; they tend to think of people as individuals who live in the context of environments and groups (Williams, 2003). Social work is largely a reflection of this individualistic focus. For instance, one of the central organizing principles of social work practice is "person in the environment" (Ashford, LeCroy, & Lortie, 2001). Viewed from this perspective, the individual is located in various levels of systems that form its social context and create its reality. However, implicit within this perspective is the centrality of the individual to practice. This perspective breaks down for work with Latinos, who view themselves as inextricably connected to family life in ways that White Americans cannot understand (Garcia & Zuniga, 2007). Some social workers are confused by Latinas' willingness to sacrifice their well-being for their families and may diagnose them as having poor boundaries or insufficient individuation. Social workers may then seek to help women develop individual goals and more ego strength. However, these concepts are inconsistent with Latinos' culture, in which such concepts sound selfish (Cauce & Domenech Rodríguez, 2002). Thus, when working with Latinos, social workers need to suspend their negative assumptions about how clients relate to their family members and adopt a strengths-based orientation.

Personalismo

Personalism, or *personalismo*, refers to the Latino preference for warm, personal, and engaged relationships (González-Ramos, Zayas, & Cohen, 1998). Cold, impersonal, highly structured, and bureaucratic services often make Latinos feel unwelcome. Although respecting professional roles and expertise is extremely important in the Latino culture, this respect is not expressed in a detached and distant manner. Professionals are expected to be engaging, warm, kind, and empathic. It is valuable for social workers to share some personal information about themselves, particularly about their families. Self-disclosure of this nature is an important practice skill. Often, this helps Latinos feel a sense of trust: their social workers are then viewed as authentic and caring people. This is especially important when providing services to Latinos, such as newly immigrated or undocumented residents, who may have good reason to mistrust mainstream institutions.

Orgullo and Respeto

Orgullo, or pride, is an extremely important value in Latino communities. *Orgullo* is manifested as pride for one's cultural identity, pride about one's skills and capacities, and pride for the ability to maintain one's family. *Orgullo* at times may make it difficult for Latinos to seek and receive help, because they often perceive a need for help as harming their sense of self (Delgado & Humm-Delgado, 1982). *Respeto*, or respect, is a key value in Latino communities. Because treating individuals with dignity and respect is a core social work value, social workers should find adhering to *respeto* congruent with their practice. However, what constitutes respect can differ greatly between Latinos from different countries of origin, and between individuals within groups. It is therefore important for social workers to ask their clients about their own understanding of respect, and to ask what he or she can do to make the client feel respected. As a general guideline, social workers can demonstrate respect by valuing the cultural and personal worth of all of their clients. It is also important that social workers spend time establishing a quality helping relationship before intervening in a manner that could make a Latino feel judged or criticized. Workers from other cultural contexts should use analysis and clinical interpretations of Latinos judiciously, especially early in treatment. Over time, Latinos develop *confianza* (confidence) with their social worker, but this confidence can be lost through too much critical analysis, which Latinos can view as disrespectful: tact and delicacy are important cultural means of expressing respect.

Machismo

In Latino society, machismo is a constellation of ideal male characteristics that include physical power, social domination, and a discounting of feminine characteristics. The roots of machismo have been traced to the influence of Catholicism on indigenous peoples and the reaction of indigenous men to their own subjugation at the hands of Spanish conquistadors (Hardin, 2002). Too often, only the negative aspects of machismo have been highlighted. Taylor and Behnke (2005) however, suggest that a central component of machismo is the role of Latino fathers, their capacity to provide for the family, and the lengths to which they will go to do so. Latino men who, for socioeconomic reasons, are unable to engage in this prosocial aspect of machismo, may engage in other, less positive ways of proving their worth and masculinity. Thus, when working with Latinos, it is important to recognize that machismo can often be a double-edged sword. Many Latino men believe they can handle problems on their own and therefore neglect to seek services, yet workers can help Latino men to tap into the more positive aspects of machismo— their responsibility to family and community—as a motivation for seeking help and resources.

Connected to machismo is the expectation that men will be dominant in sexual relationships, and that sexual activity promotes their masculinity and sense of virility. Consequently, in some Latino homes, men who have extramarital relations believe they are not violating social rules as long as they continue to serve as protectors and providers for their family (Cianelli, 2010). Men are expected to have had multiple sex partners before marriage. This expectation, along with extramarital sex, increases the risk of HIV transmission for both men and women. Furthermore, because Latino men view conceiving children, even outside of their primary relationship, as enhancing their machismo, they may not be receptive to the use of condoms (Cianelli, 2010). With regard to HIV prevention, social workers can leverage the value of machismo by pointing out to Latino men that safe sex practices are in line with their goal of protecting their families (Alvarez et al., 2009).

Marianismo

The other side of machismo is *Marianismo*, a word derived from the Virgin Mary of Catholicism. In *Marianismo*, women are expected to be subservient and obedient to the men in their families (Sherraden & Barrera, 1997) and docile, pious, and caring mothers. This has important implications in terms of safe sex and sexual choice. Because *Marianismo* calls for women to be pure and to acquiesce to their partners' sexual desires (Alvarez et al., 2009), it is often difficult for a Latina to ask her partner to use a condom. Some research (Sanchez, Rice, Stein, Milburn, & Rotheram-Borus, 2010) has also suggested that religious norms and fear of domestic violence prevent Latinas from attempting to negotiate condom use in relationships that their male partners represent as monogamous. The hierarchical relationship structure in Latino couples "often supports discrimination, harassment, and economic manipulation of women, thus placing them at greater risk for contracting HIV" and other sexually transmitted infections (STIs) (Cianelli, 2010, p. 59). *Marianismo* and *familismo* explain why Latinas routinely prioritize the care and safety of their husbands and children over their own safety and health needs.

Simpatía

Another value tied to gender-based social roles is *simpatía*. *Simpatía* calls for conformity, harmony, and pleasant social relations, and it emphasizes the importance of nonconfrontational relationships (Alvarez et al., 2009). *Simpatía* and *Marianismo* present significant challenges for HIV-prevention workers. Social workers must approach Latinas with lessons on condom negotiation in a sensitive manner that acknowledges culture-bound obstacles. One suggestion social workers might make is that Latinas leverage their man's machismo-related desire to be the protector of the family to encourage condom use.

Service Delivery Considerations for Latinos with HIV/AIDS

As noted above, culturally sensitive practice with Latinos with HIV and AIDS must reflect understanding of the large degree of within-group variation. The information presented must be based on assessment of the needs of clients and their systems. There is great heterogeneity among Latinos in the United States, whose countries of origin are diverse. The majority of Latinos in this country are of Mexican origin, but many other locations are represented, including Puerto Rico, El Salvador, Cuba, and others. The cultural backgrounds of these subgroups are diverse, though they all use Spanish as a primary language, except for Brazilians, who speak Portuguese. Also, within the Spanish language, there are variations in diction, speech patterns, vocabulary, and vernacular usage unique to the region of origin (Furman et al., 2009). Social workers should understand that while there are commonalities among Latino cultures, there are also differences. With regard to social work practice with HIV, it is important to understand that one's nation of origin may affect both the level of and mode of risk of infection. For example, the highest rates of newly diagnosed cases of HIV infection are in the counties along the United States–Mexico border (Alvarez et al., 2009). Latino men born in Puerto Rico are more likely to acquire HIV as a result of injection drug use or high-risk sexual contact with women than from sexual contact with men. Latino men born in Central America, South America, Cuba, Mexico, or the United States are more likely to contract HIV through sexual contact with other infected men than from sexual contact with women or injection drug use. Latinas, regardless of country of origin, acquire HIV by having sex with infected men or through injection drug use (Alvarez et al., 2009, p. 8). Since different regions have varied behavioral risk factors and rates of HIV prevalence, social workers should inquire about the client's region of origin rather than assuming homogeneity of risks.

Cultural Relevance

Following are suggestions for delivery of effective, culturally relevant social work interventions to Latinos with HIV and AIDS.

Spanish-Speaking Service Providers for Less-Acculturated Clients. There are various degrees of acculturation in the U.S. Latino population. For clients who are less acculturated and who speak mostly Spanish, social workers should provide services in Spanish to reduce misinformation and miscommunication (Aronstein, 1998; Deren, Shedlin, & Beardsley, 1996; Guilino, 1998). For example, the details about antiretroviral (ARV) medication regimens may be complex and difficult to understand even without a language barrier, so social workers should remove the potential for miscommunication whenever possible. Furthermore, social workers should give medical terminology regarding AIDS symptomatology and pharmacology to clients in easy-to-understand, jargon-free language.

To provide culturally competent social work to Latinos, it is not enough to simply translate into Spanish materials and programming that were designed for a mainstream American audience. Sanchez et al. (2010, p. 409) recommend "HIV interventions for Latinos be developed not only with language in mind, but with a language infused of idioms, ideas and examples" that reflect the cultural norms of Latinos along the acculturation continuum. Social workers should place Spanish HIV-prevention literature and information on HIV/AIDS testing and services in areas frequented by many Latinos, such as bodegas, neighborhood laundromats, and churches.

Services for less-acculturated Latinos should be located in neighborhoods where these populations are found. Access to health-care and social services should be facilitated in a manner that goes beyond a superficial policy of having "translation services available upon request." A recent report prepared by the Latino Commission on AIDS (2010) found a critical shortage of bilingual and bicultural health professionals in the South, constraining service delivery in a part of the United States where HIV infection rates are high. Affordable, conveniently located clinics and agencies should have evening hours (Hirsh, Higgins, Bentley, & Nathanson, 2002) and should be staffed with interpreters. Ideally, services should be provided by members of the health-care team who speak Spanish, thus eliminating the need for a third person. Also, programs for HIV care and prevention should be constructed by social workers who are literate with Latino culture, regardless of whether they speak Spanish. Focus groups of members of the HIV-positive Latino community can help inform development of culturally tailored services.

Culture-Bound Illnesses and Folk Healing in Medical Care. A patient's ailments are often a subject of discussion with the social worker working with patients with HIV. Culturally sensitive practice requires awareness of culture-bound illnesses such as *empacho*, which is a stomach ailment; *embrujado*, which is erratic behavior thought to be caused by bewitchment (Koss-Chioini & Canive, 1993); and *ataque de nervios*, a panic reaction following a time of grief (Guarnaccia, DeLaCanceela, &

Carillo, 1989). Awareness of these conditions in Latin culture can help the practitioner determine what is a culture-bound syndrome and what may indicate a need for medical or psychiatric intervention.

In evaluating culture-bound syndromes in Latinos, the social work practitioner must be aware of the role of folk healers, priests, and other non-allopathic medical personnel who treat such illnesses. In immigrant populations coming from Mexico and Central America, the *curandero*, or folk healer, would treat such illnesses. A potential problem is that *curanderos* sometimes claim that they can cure HIV (Bowden, Rhodes, Wilkin, & Jolly, 2006) and numerous other culture-bound illnesses through traditional interventions such as the use of herbs (Land, 2000), teas purchased at a *botanica* (botanical shop) (Delgado & Santiago, 1998), and intercession and healing services. These can reduce clients' efforts to avoid infection or participate in conventional allopathic medical treatments. Social workers should advise clients to use alternative herbal therapies only with physician approval, because they can interfere with the mechanisms of some ARV medications.

Sometimes culture-bound traditions impede care or place an individual at risk. For example, some Latino immigrants have been known to wear amulets (available at local *tiendas*) around their wrists to protect them from sexually transmitted diseases (STDs) (Bowden et al., 2006). Social workers should address myths such as this one with facts, in order to save lives.

Recognition of the Importance of Traditional Religion. Reciting prayers, blessing oneself with holy water, wearing holy artifacts (Land, 2000), and lighting religious candles are all important elements of the Latino practice of Catholicism. Prayers to the Our Lady of Guadalupe or other representations of the Virgin Mary are common, especially during times of crises. Acknowledgement that these are important practices to Latino clients may be helpful in establishing a bond with clients and building *respeto*.

Sexuality and Latino Culture. One Latina service provider interviewed in a study by Bowden and colleagues (2006, p. 553) reported, "The Catholic influence that sex is for procreation and not for pure enjoyment, combined with the idea that talking about sex encourages more sexual activity, poses barriers to educating the Hispanic population about HIV/AIDS." The silence surrounding sexuality in Latino culture affects different Latino subgroups in varying ways and poses different challenges to social workers.

HIV-Positive Lesbian, Gay, Bisexual, Transgender (LGBT) and Latino Men Who Have Sex with Men (MSM). Diaz (1998) noted that open discussion of sexuality is often taboo in Latino culture. When this sexuality taboo and the concept of machismo collide, many gay Latinos feel alienated from their own culture. Hunter and Hickerson (2003, p. 24) noted, "The primary allegiance for Latino lesbian and gay persons usually remains with their ethnic identity, their community, and most prominently, their family." Disclosing both their HIV status and their same-sex sexuality can cost these individuals their family support (Hunter & Hickerson, 2003). To complicate matters, some men identify as heterosexual yet engage in risky (unprotected) sexual behavior with other men, without informing their female partners (Wolitski, Jones, Wasserman, & Smith, 2006). Fear of social repercussions about their sexual orientation can lead Latino men to identify as heterosexual, while secretly engaging in sex with men (Brooks, Etzel, Hinojos, Henry, & Perez, 2005). Fernandez et al. (2005) found that 43 percent of Latino MSM were having unprotected sex, and 22.5 percent of those men were HIV positive.

There is a religious component to the stigma and judgment associated with being homosexual in the Latino community. In one sample of U.S. Latinos, 60 percent identified as being Catholic (Jayson, 2010). The messages of "sometimes virulent homophobia" coming from some churches (Brooks et al., 2005, p. 738) not only impact the self-esteem of Latino MSM, but also affect HIV prevention by driving risky sex practices underground. Furthermore, the Catholic church's "condemnation of homosexuality, ban on the use of condoms, and insistence on abstinence has made it impossible for the Catholic Church to work effectively to suppress the spread of HIV, particularly among Catholic Latino populations" (Brooks et al., 2005, p. 740).

Social workers working with HIV-positive lesbian, gay, bisexual, transgender (LGBT), and Latino MSM must maintain constant awareness of the role that their culture plays in expressions of their sexuality. They bear triple minority status (HIV positive, LGBT/MSM, and Latino) in the mainstream culture and are at high risk for stigmatization in their own culture.

Gender Roles of Latinas. Women of color have a history of disenfranchisement, oppression, and marginalization in both the U.S. and global communities. This oppression is expressed in a myriad of ways. One method of controlling women's sexuality is to control their access to reproductive health information and services.

Latinas have suffered this kind of oppression and as a result are reluctant to push for condom use because they "fear verbal and physical abuse and because condoms are associated with prostitution, poor hygiene, and contraception" (Land, 2000, p. 90). Social workers can help confront the oppression in Latinas' primary relationships by making referrals to culturally sensitive physicians and other medical professionals who can educate them about issues surrounding their reproductive health. Social workers can also provide assertiveness training to Latina clients to help facilitate more equality in their relationships.

The value that Latinos place on the importance of the extended family has been well documented. Latino families provide both tangible as well as intangible support to their members. However, Latinas are often the main caregivers in the home; when they are HIV positive, they must carry the burden of caring for themselves as well as for the other people in the household. Often they ignore their own needs for rest and reduced stress (Remor, Penedo, Shen, & Schneiderman, 2007). In addition to the numerous household responsibilities of HIV-positive Latinas, pervasive cultural attitudes mandate that caretaking of household members be done solely by the immediate family, perhaps even prohibiting the hiring of cleaning and caregiving services. Social workers should educate caregivers about burnout and provide linkages to organizations offering respite care in order to help clients deal with the stress of caregiving.

Circular Migration. Social work with immigrants from Latin countries necessitates an understanding of risk factors for HIV infection associated with traditional migration and transmigration patterns. Many Latinos migrate to the United States to pursue educational or employment opportunities. Traditional labor migrants eventually settle in one region, attracted by better economic, political, and environmental conditions. They encounter a wide range of threats, including low wages, unstable housing conditions, lack of access to health-care and social services, long work hours, low literacy, lack of English-speaking proficiency, and widespread anti-immigrant sentiment. Those who have immigrated without documents also fear deportation. Some view immigration to the United States as a temporary relocation rather than a permanent move, and therefore leave family members behind, causing them stress and loss of support (Guilamo-Ramos et al., 2010). Transmigrants continually move to different places, countries, and cultures (Furman et al., 2009), driven by economic and social reasons. They encounter high levels of poverty, increased social isolation, and high stress, which combine to take a high psychological and physical toll.

Latino migrant and transmigrant farm workers are generally young men who are far from home for long periods. This situation frequently leads them to have a high number of sex partners, sex with commercial sex workers, and sex with other men, all of which are high-risk behaviors for HIV infection (Denner, Organista, Dupree, & Thrush, 2005). When these men return home to their families, they may unknowingly infect their wives.

In 2010, the United States lifted a twenty-two-year immigration ban that had stopped anyone with HIV/AIDS from entering the country. While this is a victory for social justice and human rights advocates, it does not eliminate all discrimination with regard to immigration. Social work advocacy is needed for a fair immigration policy for all Latinos.

Box 5.1. The List of Ten Messages

When conducting individual or group-level interventions with Latinos living with HIV, part of the social work role is to provide education and raise awareness. Below is a list of ten messages that can be shared with Latino clients who have recently learned of their HIV-positive status (adapted from Merck Sharp & Dohme Corporation, 2010):

1. Embrace your spirituality with a positive mindset. (*Adopta tu espiritualidad de manera positiva.*) Your spirituality can be an effective source of support. You can use prayer and meditation to find a calmer place.

2. Build a trusting relationship with your doctor and other health-care providers. (*Crea confianza en tu relación con tu doctor.*) Even though it may be embarrassing to discuss private issues with your doctor, you need to be honest and tell them about health problems, drug and alcohol use, and your sex life. Also, tell them about issues that affect your home life.

3. Make sure someone on your health-care team speaks Spanish. (*Asegúrate de que alguien en tu equipo médico hable español.*) You may be able to express symptoms, feelings, or fears more easily in Spanish. If needed, a bilingual health-care provider can also help translate lab results and other important communications that are written in English.

4. Set goals and stick to them. (*Fíjate metas y cúmplelas.*) Plan for the future. Decide with your health-care provider when you need to start medications. Use a calendar to remind you of check-ups. Keep track of your lab results (CD4 count, viral load, cholesterol, and glucose levels). Make sure you report uncomfortable side effects of medications. It may be possible to make adjustments.

5. Don't replace your doctor-prescribed medication with herbal remedies. (*No sustituyas los medicamentos quete recetó tu doctor con plantas medicinales.*) Your family and friends might recommend the use of herbal remedies. Traditional remedies can be good for you but only if you use them correctly. You must tell your doctor what other drugs and herbs you are taking, because some remedies can interact with your HIV medications.

6. If you move often, don't interrupt your treatment. (*Si te mudas a menudo, no interrumpas tu tratamiento.*) There are a lot of reasons why you might move often: to find good sources of income, to be closer to family members, or because of immigration issues. If there is a need to move, be sure to keep getting medical attention. Take your lab reports and medications with you. Your current church can help refer you to another supportive community of faith in your new area.

7. Take advantage of the rights to which you are entitled. (*Tienes derechos. ¡Reclámalos!*) There are many resources available, but use the ones that are right for you. Social workers can offer advice and put you in touch with medical professionals who will understand your situation. Don't let your financial situation, gender, sexual orientation, or immigration status get in the way of your health and well-being.

8. You should tell your sex partners your status. (*Sin embargo, todos tus compañeros sexuales tienen que estar enterados de tu estatus.*) Your HIV status is very personal and you might not be ready to tell everyone. That is okay, but sex partners should know of any risks. Give some thought to how you will handle

this conversation. Consider telling your close friends and family. You may be surprised at how supportive your loved ones can be. Still, who you choose to tell, and when, is up to you.

9. Practice safer sex. (*Practica sexo más seguro.*) STIs are a concern for everyone. If you have recently learned of your HIV-positive status, you may not currently be thinking about an intimate relationship, but the time will come when you are ready to have a physical relationship and you will need to be smart about being safe. Use a condom. It doesn't just protect your partner, but also protects you from any STIs.

10. Take care of yourself so you can take care of your family. (*Cuídate para que puedas cuidar a tu familia.*) You probably put your family first and you should be proud of that. When you take care of your own health you may feel selfish. You must take HIV care seriously. Make sure you go to medical check-ups, listen to the advice of your health-care team, and follow your treatment plan. When you make the right choices for yourself, you will be doing the right thing for the people you love.

Latino Support Group Case Example

A common method of service delivery in AIDS service organizations (ASOs) targeted at subgroups of the HIV and AIDS population is the use of culture-specific or age-specific support groups. At a local ASO in a city in the southeastern United States, targeted support groups for Latinos with HIV are offered. Based on group dynamics seen at the ASO, the following is a composite case example of a Latina social worker facilitating a support group for Latinos infected or affected by HIV. Note the following Latino-related themes: the worker establishes personal contacts with the clients, views the group as an extended family, sees the need for Spanish-speaking practitioners and culturally sensitive agency procedures, recognizes the machismo tendency to see females as caregivers, and acknowledges the importance of spiritual beliefs and practices. The following AIDS-related themes are illustrated: the need for support at times of crisis such as hospitalization, the fact that many persons living with HIV and AIDS are without support due to isolation or death of a partner, judgments about the mode of one's transmission, the presence of debilitating symptoms such as forgetfulness due to AIDS-related dementia, and the questions of if, when, or how to disclose one's sero-positive status to family members. The support group is led in Spanish, but the dialogue is presented in English for the reader.

Case Example

Isabel heads down the hall of her workplace, an urban ASO located on the outskirts of a Latino community. She is on her way to lead a support group offered once a month for Latino clients. She knows who will be at the group meeting because she conscientiously calls or text-messages each of the members the day before to remind them of the meeting time and to find out if they will attend. She knows this is much more effective than mailings, flyers, or email messages. Her group responds well to her personal contacts. (Isabel has thus effectively used *personalismo* to reach her clients and encourage attendance for the support group.)

As she enters the group room, an older Latina named Rosa is talking with other members about their visit to see María in the hospital earlier in the week. María, a group member, has had revolving door hospitalizations for kidney failure, as a consequence of her AIDS.

"Who will visit María tomorrow?" Rosa asks.

"I will. Do you want me to pick you up, also?" responds José, a young man who contracted HIV through an injection drug habit. (José is offering tangible support to María and providing others the opportunity to participate by offering transportation to the hospital. He views the group as an extended family.)

"Yes, I would. She needs visitors. We're all she has.…I don't have anyone to visit me since my dear husband died of respiratory failure from his AIDS so I'll be there for María," says Rosa. (Rosa shows compassion for María and provides support since she is aware of the hardships associated with dealing with illness without a partner.)

After a few minutes of group discussion about María and the importance of feeling connected to a group of supportive people at times of crisis, the door to the group room opens.

"Sorry we're late," says a young couple, in unison. "We had trouble finding the place."

"Did the receptionist lady give you directions? Because I got lost my first time, too. I couldn't follow all those crazy street names. Look, just remember to turn left at the fire station, then left at the bright pink daycare center, and you're here," explains Chico. (Chico fills in a gap in agency procedures by providing directions with landmarks so that the couple can more easily find the meeting location.)

Isabel smiles because she has noticed that her clients respond well to directions using landmarks. She's learned to use that method to help get them to their numerous medical and resource appointments around the city. She knows it is the young couple's first meeting, but she doesn't want to lose an opportunity to point out the importance of promptness.

"Try to be on time, because it's important to get in that habit. What happens if you're late with a dosage of medications or you're late for your new doctor or late for your appointment for emergency rent help?" Isabel asks.

"They skip over you. Yep, they do," confirms Rosa.

"Remember, if anyone needs a calendar, I have some free ones from drug companies to share with you. It's very important to keep your appointments written down so you won't miss them if you have memory difficulties," explains Isabel.

"I've been having a hard time with forgetting things the last couple of months," confides José. "I found something that helps. I have Chico call me the morning of my appointments to make sure I remember and I do the same thing for him." (Notice how the group members find supportive solutions to dealing with symptoms like AIDS-related dementia by calling each other on the day of their appointments.)

"Yeah, when he remembers ... which is rarely!" chides Chico, with a laugh.

"I don't need anyone to call me. Lupe tells me what I need to do. She keeps it all straight," says Julio. Julio and his wife, Lupe, are regular attendees, but rarely participate in the group discussions.

"Does she make your appointments, too?" asks Isabel, the group facilitator.

"Of course! What's a wife for?" laughs Julio.

The group members look puzzled and concerned.

José asks Lupe, "Why are you taking all the responsibility for your husband's care?"

Lupe shrugs her shoulders and looks to Julio in a subordinate manner.

Chico, a gay man who contracted the virus from a partner who did not disclose his own positive status, says, "Honey, your man needs to take care of his own stuff . . . and Mister, you need to take responsibility for your own treatment." (The group notices the cultural values of machismo and confronts both Lupe and José with their responsibility for themselves and the way the disease is affecting each of them.)

Julio seems threatened and volleys back, "What do you know about marriage anyway, you [Spanish gay slur]!" (Julio demonstrates prejudice and bias in regard to Chico's sexuality by insulting him.)

José chimes in with, "Hey, we're all family in here. We don't put each other down. It doesn't matter how you got it, now you have to deal with it."

Isabel intervenes, interjecting the importance of personal responsibility and taking ownership for care. "Mr. Sullivan may extend you more grace in your case management meetings," says Isabel, making reference to the fact that Mr. Sullivan, a non-Latino practitioner, may be overcompensating in an effort to be culturally sensitive. "I will not allow group family members to be disrespectful in this place," adds Isabel.

"That is the truth," adds Rosa.

"Julio, you may not understand this now, but from now on if you need something from me, I'd like you to make the call, not Lupe," explains Isabel. She feels that Julio's disengagement from the coordination of his care is part of his denial of being HIV positive and shows that he doesn't want to deal with it.

The group discussion continues, with various members drawing out the new couple and learning their story. They have both recently been diagnosed, and are struggling with the decision of whether to tell their families back in Guadalajara. (Lupe and Julio also struggle with whether to reveal their HIV status to their families, which is a major decision that could result in reduced support from their families.)

"I'd like to close the meeting with a prayer to Our Mother Mary, asking for help for María in the hospital," says Rosa, gathering up the hands of those on each side of her. (By closing the meeting with a prayer to a Catholic saint, group members sense that the social worker values and respects their religious beliefs.) The group closes in prayer for one of their "family" members.

This case example demonstrates how both values and skills are involved in providing services to Latinos with HIV and AIDS. The case also points out the complexities of providing culturally competent services. Developing cultural competence is a lengthy process, and while we have explored some key issues in working with HIV-positive Latinos, social workers should view the development of cultural competence as a life-long journey. This is especially true when working with a population as diverse as the Latino population. Working with Latinos with HIV and AIDS challenges social workers to understand the confluence of complex psychosocial factors. These are two groups who have been the recipients of tremendous discrimination: Latinos and HIV-positive individuals.

Community-Level Interventions

In addition to direct practice interventions, social workers need to engage in advocacy on organizational and community levels to ensure that competent services are developed. Two recent initiatives aimed at HIV prevention and care for the Latino community have been developed at the federal level. In 2007, the CDC's Division of HIV/AIDS Prevention created "the Hispanic/Latino Executive Committee, to ensure coordination, support, and success of cross-cutting HIV prevention activities targeting Hispanics/Latinos in the U.S. and Puerto Rico" (Alvarez et al., 2009, p. 10). The Obama Administration announced in 2009 a five-year communications campaign, entitled Act Against AIDS (Actúa contra el SIDA), to refocus attention on HIV/AIDS in the United States in order to reduce complacency. The campaign features messages targeted at specific high-risk communities, including the Latino community (Dean, 2009).

Conclusion

Social workers are well positioned to address many of the systemic and individual variables that place Latinos at high risk for HIV infection and lack of access to care (Guilamo-Ramos et al., 2010). Our strengths perspective and systems thinking equip us to deliver culturally appropriate, values-sensitive, evidence-based prevention and care programs that are critical to mitigation of the effects of HIV and AIDS on Latinos in the United States. Nevertheless, the profession needs to continue on the journey to culturally competent care for these Latinos.

Questions for Reflection

1. What is your ethnicity? How would you explain it to a person unfamiliar with anyone who is a member of your ethnic group? How might a social worker tailor HIV-prevention messages to members of your ethnicity?

2. What has been your level of interaction with members of the Latino culture? What might be some personal obstacles for you to working effectively with this population group?

3. What is your position on U.S. immigration policy? How might your position affect your ability to work with this population?

4. Imagine that you are working with a person who you discover is in the United States without documentation. Your agency has a policy to not report this to authorities. Would you have a moral problem working with this person?

5. Do you believe that the goal for all people arriving in the United States should be to acculturate as quickly as possible toward a mainstream American lifestyle? Why or why not?

6. Which is a more strengths-based term: illegal alien, illegal immigrant, or undocumented worker?

7. A homosexual/MSM Latino man with HIV is said to be triple minority. Which of these three minority statuses do you feel carries the greatest stigma for him?

8. Role-play with an imaginary Latina client how she could negotiate for condom use with her husband, whom she suspects of having sex outside of their relationship.

Web Resources

National Latino AIDS Awareness Day (NLAAD) (October 15): http://www.nlaad.org/

Latino Commission on AIDS: http://www.latinoaids.org/

AIDSinfo (NIH): www.aidsinfo.nih.gov

The Body: www.thebody.com/espanol.html

Gay Men's Health Crisis AIDS Hotline: http://www.gmhc.org/en-espanol

TuSalud—The Latino Wellness Magazine: www.tusaludmag.com

National Latino AIDS Action Network: http://www.latinoaidsagenda.org/

References

Alvarez, M., Jakhmola, P., Painter, T., Tailepierre, J. D., Romaguera, R. A., Herbst, J. H., & Wolitski, R. (2009). Summary of comments and recommendations from the CDC consultation on the HIV/AIDS epidemic and prevention in the Hispanic/Latino community. *AIDS Education and Prevention, 21*(Supplement B), 7–18.

Aronstein, D. (1998). Organizing support groups for people affected by HIV. In D. Aronstein & B. Thompson (Eds.), *HIV and social work: A practitioner's guide* (pp. 293–302). Binghamton, NY: Harrington Park Press.

Ashford, J. B., LeCroy, C. W., & Lortie, K. L. (2001). *Human behavior in the social environment: Multidimensional perspective.* Belmont, CA: Wadsworth/ Thomson Learning.

Bowden, W. P., Rhodes, S., Wilkin, A., & Jolly, C. (2006). Sociocultural determinants of HIV/AIDS risk and service use among immigrant Latinos in North Carolina. *Hispanic Journal of Behavioral Sciences, 28*, 546–562.

Brooks, R., Etzel, M., Hinojos, E., Henry, C., & Perez, M. (2005). Preventing HIV among Latino and African American gay and bisexual men in a context of HIV-related stigma, discrimination, and homophobia: Perspectives of providers. *AIDS Patient Care and STDs, 19*(11), 737–744.

Cabrera, N. L., & Padilla, A. M. (2004). Entering and succeeding in the 'culture of college': The story of two Mexican heritage students. *Hispanic Journal of Behavioral Sciences, 26*(2), 152–170.

Cauce, A. M., & Domenech Rodríguez, M. (2002). Latino families: Myths and realities. In J. Contreras, A. Neal-Barnett, & K. Kerns (Eds.), *Latino children and families in the United States: Current research and future directions* (pp. 3–25). Westport, CT: Praeger.

Cianelli, R. (2010). Editorial—HIV: A health-related disparity among older Hispanic women. *Hispanic Health Care International, 8*(2), 58–64.

Dean, H. (2009). Foreword: HIV/AIDS prevention in the Hispanic/Latino community. *AIDS Education and Prevention, 21*(Suppl. B), 1–2.

Delgado, M., & Humm-Delgado, D. (1982). Natural support systems: Source of strength in Hispanic communities. *Social Work, 27*(1), 83–89.

Delgado, M., & Santiago, J. (1998). HIV/AIDS in a Puerto Rican/Dominican community: A collaborative project with a botanical shop. *Social Work, 43(2)*, 183–186.

Denner, J., Organista, K., Dupree, J. D., & Thrush, G. (2005). Predictors of HIV transmission amongst migrant and marginally housed Latinos. *AIDS and Behavior, 9*(2), 201–210.

Deren, S., Shedlin, M., & Beardsley, M. (1996). HIV-related concerns and behaviors among Hispanic women. *AIDS Education and Prevention, 8*(4), 335–342.

Diaz, R. M. (1998). *Latino gay men and HIV: Culture, sexuality, and risk behavior.* New York: Routledge.

Fernandez, M. I., Perrino, T., Bowen, G. S., Hernandez, N., Cardenas, S., Marsh, D., & Rehbein, A. (2005). Club drug use, sexual behavior, and HIV risk among community and internet samples of Hispanic MSM: Implications for clinicians. *Journal of Social Work Practice in the Addictions, 5*(4), 81–100.

Furman, R., & Negi, N. (2007). Social work practice with transnational Latino populations. *International Social Work, 50*(1), 107–112.

Furman, R., Negi, N., Iwamoto, D., Rowan, D., Shukraft, A., & Gragg, J. (2009). Social work practice with Latinos: Key issues for social workers. *Social Work, 54*(2), 167–174.

Garcia, B., & Zuniga, M. A. (2007). Cultural competence with Latino Americans. In D. Lum (Ed.), *Culturally competent practice: A framework for understanding diverse groups and justice issues* (3rd ed.) (pp. 299–327). Belmont, CA: Thompson Higher Education.

González-Ramos, G., Zayas, L. H., & Cohen, E. V. (1998). Child-rearing values of low income, urban Puerto Rican mothers of preschool children. *Professional Psychology: Research and Practice, 29*, 377–382.

Gregory, P. G., Steinberg, Y. J., & Sousa, C. M. (2003). *Voluntary community involvement of Latinos: A literature review.* Unpublished manuscript. Retrieved from http://www.ucce.ucdavis.edu/files/filelibrary/5433/8114.pdf

Guarnaccia, P., DeLaCanceela, V., & Carillo, E. (1989). The multiple meanings of Ataque deNervios in the Latino community. *Medical Anthropology, 11,* 47–62.

Guilamo-Ramos, V., Bouris, A., & Gallego, S. (2010). Latinos and HIV: A framework to develop evidence-based strategies. In C. A. Poindexter (Ed.), *Handbook of HIV and social work: Principles, practice, and populations* (pp. 291–309). Hoboken, NJ: John Wiley & Sons.

Guilino, P. U. (1998). Individual clinical issues. In D. Aronstein & B. Thompson (Eds.), *HIV and social work: A practitioner's guide* (pp. 165–182). Binghamton, NY: Harrington Park Press.

Hardin, M. (2002). Altering masculinities: The Spanish conquest and the evolution of the Latin American machismo. *International Journal of Sexuality and Gender Studies, 7*(1), 1–22.

Hirsh, J., Higgins, J., Bentley, M., & Nathanson, C. (2002). The social constructions of sexuality: Marital infidelity and sexually transmitted disease—HIV risk in a Mexican migrant community. *American Journal of Public Health, 92*(8), 1227–1237.

Hunter, S., & Hickerson, J. (2003). *Affirmative practice: Understanding and working with lesbian, gay, bisexual, and transgender persons.* Washington, DC: NASW Press.

Jayson, S. (2010, March 16). Catholic Church, and religion in general, losing Latinos in USA. *USA Today.* Retrieved from http://www.usatoday.com/news/religion/2010-03-16-latinoreligion16_ST_N.htm

Koss-Chioini, J. D., & Canive, J. (1993). The interaction of popular and clinical diagnostic labeling: The case of embrujado. *Medical Anthropology, 15,* 171–188.

Land, H. (2000). AIDS and women of color. In V. Lynch (Ed.), *HIV/AIDS at year 2000* (pp. 79–96). Needham Heights, MA: Allyn and Bacon.

Latino Commission on AIDS. (2010). *Shaping the new response: HIV/AIDS and Latinos in the Deep South.* The Deep South Project. Retrieved from http://www.latinoaids.org/downloads/deepsouthreport.pdf

Leigh, J. W. Jr. (1985). The ethnically competent social worker. In J. Laird & A. Hartman (Eds.), *A handbook of child welfare: Context, knowledge, and practice* (pp. 449–459). New York: Free Press.

Little, W. E. (2004). *Mayas in the marketplace*. Austin, TX: University of Texas Press.

Lugo Steidel, A., & Contreras, J. M. (2003). A new familism scale for use with Latino populations. *Hispanic Journal of Behavioral Sciences, 25*, 312–330.

Merck Sharp & Dohme Corporation. (2010). *10 Tips for Latinos to live well with HIV*. Author.

Remor, E., Penedo, F., Shen, B., & Schneiderman, N. (2007). Perceived stress is associated with CD4+ cell decline in men and women living with HIV/AIDS in Spain. *AIDS Care, 19*(2), 215–219.

Rowan, D., Furman, R., Jones, A., & Edwards, K. (2008). Social work practice with Latinos living with HIV/AIDS. *Advances in Social Work, 9*(2), 142–156.

Sale, E., Sambrano, S., Springer, J. F., Pena, C., Pan, W., & Kasim, R. (2005). Family protection and prevention of alcohol use among Hispanic youth at high risk. *American Journal of Community Psychology, 36*(3–4), 195–205.

Sanchez, M., Rice, E., Stein, J., Milburn, N., & Rotheram-Borus, M. J. (2010). Acculturation, coping styles, and health risk behaviors among HIV positive Latinas. *AIDS and Behavior, 14*, 401–409.

Sherraden, M. S., & Barrera, R. E. (1997). Culturally protective health practices: Everyday pregnancy care among Mexican immigrants. *Journal of Multicultural Social Work, 6*(1/2), 93–115.

Taylor, B. A., & Behnke, A. (2005). Fathering across the border: Latino fathers in Mexico and the U.S. *Fathering: A Journal of Theory, Research, & Practice about Men as Fathers, 3*(2), 99–120.

U.S. Census Bureau. (2011). *Overview of race and Hispanic origin: 2010. Census briefs*. Retrieved from http://www.census.gov/prod/cen2010/briefs/c2010br-02.pdf

Valenzuela, A., & Dornbusch, S. M. (1994). Familism and social capital in the academic achievement of Mexican origin and Anglo adolescents. *Social Science Quarterly, 75*, 18–36.

Williams, B. (2003). The worldview of dimensions of individualism and collectivism: Implications for counseling. *Journal of Counseling and Development, 81*, 370–374.

Wolitski, R. J., Jones, K. T., Wasserman, J. L., & Smith, J. C. (2006). Self-identification as "down low" among men who have sex with men (MSM) from 12 U.S. cities. *AIDS and Behavior, 10*, 519–529.

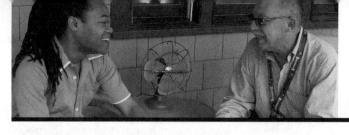

6

HIV/AIDS: Introduction to Prevention for Men Who Have Sex with Men
Jeff Driskell

There's this illusion that homosexuals have sex and heterosexuals fall in love. That's completely untrue. Everybody wants to be loved.

—Boy George

Introduction

The first cases of AIDS (acquired immune deficiency syndrome) were identified in 1981 by physicians providing care to gay and bisexual men living in urban communities. These men were diagnosed with rare opportunistic infections typically not seen in people with healthy immune systems. The two most commonly diagnosed opportunistic infections were Kaposi's sarcoma (KS) and pneumocystis carinii pneumonia (PCP). Medical providers were unable to explain why gay and bisexual men were experiencing these rare infections. The initial name given to the disease by public health officials and the media was GRID (gay-related immunodeficiency syndrome), or gay cancer. Shortly after the beginning of the epidemic, scientists discovered that these rare infections had no boundaries and that all people, including injection drug users, hemophiliacs, babies, and heterosexuals, were susceptible to HIV (human immunodeficiency virus) infection. To be more inclusive of all those impacted with and by this disease, GRID became known as AIDS, which today is considered the final stage of the disease process.

One of the greatest pieces of knowledge that was discovered early in the epidemic is that HIV is transmitted through specific behaviors such as sharing of needles and unprotected sexual activities. Historically, HIV was transmitted via blood transfusion. Federal policies and procedures have been put in place to eradicate this mode of transmission. This information regarding modes of transmission was vital, providing a foundation for prevention efforts that targeted specific risk behaviors.

Men Who Have Sex with Men

Before proceeding further, it is important to define and clarify the concept of men who have sex with men (MSM). The term MSM is often used in HIV/AIDS–related care and prevention, indicating that although some men engage in sexual behaviors with other men, they may not self-identify as gay or bisexual. We must not assume that because men engage in sexual practices with other men that they define themselves as gay or bisexual. This is especially significant when working with other cultural groups who do not use gay or bisexual vernacular. Other examples would be men who engage in sex with men only when women are not available (such as during incarceration or when working in isolated locations) or when they perform the behaviors for purposes of survival (i.e., for money, drugs, or housing). Thus, the focus in HIV prevention work is often on the behavior and not on the group with which the client identifies. MSM can be a hidden population, making it difficult to recruit and provide outreach for prevention interventions. Throughout this chapter, when referencing MSM (men who have sex with men), the reader should understand it to mean that these men may identify as gay men, bisexual men, or heterosexual men who have sex with men.

In addition to clarifying the concept of MSM, this chapter will provide a context of HIV/AIDS and its impact on the MSM population. HIV infection in the United States continues to disproportionately affect MSM. Although there has been an overall decline in HIV infection rates in the United States since the inception of the disease, MSM remain the only group in which there has not been a steady decline. For example, in 2006 MSM accounted for more than half (53 percent) of all new HIV infections in the United States (Centers for Disease Control and Prevention [CDC], 2008). Between 2005 and 2008 alone there was an estimated 17 percent increase in HIV infections among MSM (CDC, 2008). In 2006, White MSM accounted for almost 46 percent of new HIV infections, African-American MSM between the ages of thirteen and twenty-nine accounted for more than half (52 percent) of new HIV infections, and Latino MSM between thirteen and twenty-nine represented about 43 percent of all new infections. Within the MSM community alone, young African-American MSM have the highest rates of HIV infection as compared to other racial groups of MSM. A more recent study conducted by the CDC (2008) suggests that one in five MSM in twenty-one cities is infected with HIV, and nearly half are unaware of their status. These disturbing statistics point to the need for effective prevention efforts and additional government funding targeted to the unique prevention needs of MSM.

As a result of these alarming statistics, recent federal governmental policy initiatives (i.e., Health Resources Service Administration [HRSA]) and behavioral research recommendations (Kelly et al., 1997; Koester et al., 2007; Morin et al., 2004) have emphasized a need to integrate HIV prevention with HIV primary care in order to have effective and acceptable HIV-prevention programs, particularly for higher-risk individuals. In order for such interventions to have a public health impact, it is critical that social workers provide MSM with acceptable and tailored prevention services to help them maintain safer sexual and drug use behaviors.

This chapter will introduce the various theoretical models used to develop effective HIV-prevention interventions for MSM. In addition, readers will learn about elements associated with the successfulness of interventions as they relate to reducing high-risk sexual and drug use behaviors. It is important to note that although this chapter focuses on various theories to help guide the development and implementation of prevention efforts, change and action must also occur at other systemic levels (i.e., structural barriers, policy initiatives, and funding) if we are to curb the rates of HIV infection over an extended period.

Factors Related to HIV Infection

When MSM become infected with HIV, it often means that they have engaged in behaviors that put them at risk, such as unprotected or risky sex, or sharing of needles. However, to understand HIV-related risk in a larger context, it is important to conduct a holistic assessment from an ecological perspective. At the most basic level, it is important for social workers to address the following components when conducting comprehensive risk assessments with MSM, which include biological, psychological, demographic, sociocultural, and behavioral factors.

(1) **Biological.** HIV-negative MSM who have a diagnosable STI (sexually transmitted infection) are at increased risk of contracting HIV if they engage in risky sexual behavior. Why? As a result of the STI, the body's immune system is compromised, and thus is more susceptible to infection. Furthermore, HIV-positive MSM who have an STI are at a greater risk of exposing sexual partners to HIV through

the shedding of blood or pus through open sores. The greater the amount of virus in an HIV-positive MSM's system, the more infectious the fluids. The amount of virus (viral load) is typically higher during the initial acute phase of infection when the person is likely unaware of the infection. HIV-negative or unknown-status MSM are at increased risk of infection if they engage in receptive anal sex with an HIV-infected sex partner(s). It is known that unprotected receptive anal sex is the highest sexual risk activity for contracting HIV as there can be trauma (tearing of tissue) to the anus, creating an opportunity for fluid to enter the bloodstream. Finally, research has indicated that men who are uncircumcised are at a greater risk of contracting, as well as transmitting, HIV. This vulnerability is a result of the large number of cells within the foreskin that are often targeted by HIV in addition to the potential trauma (i.e., tearing) of the foreskin during sex.

(2) Psychological. When referring to psychological aspects related to risk, we are talking about the MSM's personality factors in addition to how they think and feel, which ultimately have an impact on their behavior. For example, an HIV-negative young MSM who feels he is at little risk of infection may choose to engage in unprotected, receptive anal sex. This belief may be based on the fact that he believes HIV/AIDS is a manageable disease and not debilitating or life threatening. Furthermore, MSM who have low self-esteem or who feel isolated may engage in potentially risky behaviors as a way of coping with these unsettling feelings. Other psychological states include individuals with compulsive behaviors, depression, and anxiety.

(3) Demographic. There are a number of demographic factors that impact risk, including age, sexual orientation, and geographical location. For example, MSM have the highest rates of infection in the United States. Among ethnic minority groups, African Americans are disproportionately impacted by HIV/AIDS in that they have higher rates of AIDS diagnoses. This is in part due to poverty and unequal access to health care, prevention services, or programs.

(4) Sociocultural. This component refers to gender and power differences, social attitudes, cultural beliefs around health or illness, cultural beliefs around condom use, and the impact of stigma associated with specific drug use, sexual behaviors, sexual orientation, and HIV status. When referring to stigma, it is the process of being continually devalued based on an individual's sexual orientation, sexual practices or drug use behaviors. Other factors include lack of adequate access to health care, which often promotes prevention opportunities; economic factors such as living in poverty; racism; complacency, prevention fatigue, or burnout; religion norms; and both externalized homophobia and internalized homophobia.

(5) **Behavioral.** Certain risk behaviors can increase any individual's chances of HIV infection, including both sexual and drug use behaviors. As stated above under the Biological category, HIV can be transmitted through unprotected receptive and insertive anal sex. MSM who inject drugs (e.g., methamphetamine) or share works (i.e., needles, bleach, cotton) are also at increased risk of HIV infection or transmission. The combination of unprotected sex and drug use is particularly dangerous, which leads to increased probability.

Prevention

MSM continue to be one of the highest at-risk groups for HIV infection, which makes them a priority for prevention efforts. At the onset of the HIV/AIDS epidemic, prevention efforts for MSM targeted those who were HIV negative, as well as those who were unaware of their HIV status. The focus of prevention has typically been geared toward behavioral elements such as communicating or negotiating sexual safety, reducing the number of sexual partners, and increasing condom use. As new treatments have improved the quality and longevity of life for those living with HIV/AIDS, it is clear that there is an increase in need to address the unique aspects of prevention. Although only a small percentage of government funding supports HIV/AIDS prevention, funding is slowly increasing. The goal associated with this new direction is to assist those living with HIV/AIDS in adopting and maintaining safer sexual and drug use behaviors. Neglecting the prevention needs of HIV-positive MSM could potentially lead to the acquisition of other STIs or the acquisition of other strains of HIV (Crepaz et al., 2006). Furthermore, there is the possibility of spreading HIV/AIDS to HIV-negative and unknown-status sexual or drug-using partners.

In order to support MSM and their unique prevention needs, social workers must develop, implement, and evaluate appropriate and effective prevention interventions. Specifically, interventions that influence health behaviors are most effective when guided by health promotion theory. The remainder of this chapter will highlight elements associated with effective interventions as well as some of the various theories that impact behavior change.

Levels of Prevention

When developing HIV-related prevention interventions, it is important to indicate the level at which the prevention program will take place. There are three standard public health levels from which to choose: primary, secondary, and tertiary.

Primary prevention focuses on preventing disease, harm, or injury. This involves engaging in actions to prevent the initial occurrence by focusing on or identifying risk factors and risk conditions. For example, one would classify development of a prevention program geared toward HIV-negative or unknown-status MSM who have been identified as engaging in high-risk sexual or drug use behaviors as primary prevention.

Secondary prevention has a goal of stopping or slowing down the progression of harm or disease, or both, as soon as possible. In this case, social workers would target prevention efforts toward MSM who have already been diagnosed with HIV and who are at risk of HIV transmission to sexual or drug-using partners. In addition, secondary prevention with HIV-positive MSM has a goal of eliminating exposure to other diseases or infections that could complicate their current health status.

Tertiary prevention can be thought of as treatment. The goal would be to reduce the occurrence of relapse of a chronic disorder or disease. For example, if you were working with HIV-positive MSM who were being medically treated for HIV, it would be important to discuss and support medication adherence. Non-adherence to HIV medications can potentially lead to medication resistance. Drug resistance can result in limited medication treatment options as well as an increase in viral load, which affects the immune system.

Along with selecting the appropriate level of prevention, one also must decide at which level you will implement your intervention. Interventions can take place at the individual, group, or community levels. An intervention can be defined as a specific activity (or activities) with the goal of bringing about behavior change or risk-reduction practices. See table 6.1 as it illustrates the various prevention intervention levels that are used to guide prevention efforts for MSM.

Table 6.1. Various Prevention Intervention Levels

Intervention Level	Example
Individual	Counseling, Testing, and Referral. The goal is to encourage routine HIV testing for MSM who may be at risk of HIV infection. It is beneficial because it promotes early access to care for those diagnosed with HIV. In addition, it is an opportunity for risk reduction or prevention counseling (CDC, 2001).
Group	Many Men, Many Voices (3MV). This is a seven-session small-group intervention targeting Black men who do not identify as gay or bisexual. The goal is to reduce rates of STIs (Wilton et al., 2009).
Community	d-up: Defend Yourself! This is a community-level intervention targeting Black MSM. The primary goal is to address social norms around condom use (Jones et al., 2008).

Characteristics of Effective Prevention Interventions

There is a science behind developing and implementing effective prevention interventions to target sexual and drug use risk behaviors. Effective interventions contain a number of characteristics. See table 6.2 as it provides an overview of these characteristics.

Behavioral Theories and Models

Theory can be thought of as a way to predict, understand, or analyze such things as behavior. In such cases, the prediction of behaviors and attitudes is not uncommon. Theories are made up of a series of assumptions and concepts; the concepts are typically targeted in prevention interventions. For example, one concept that is often assessed and targeted is self-efficacy. This term is defined as having the confidence in oneself to implement a desired behavior within a specific context. Taking it further, you may want to assess your clients' level of condom use self-efficacy (their belief that they can use condoms) the next time they are at a sex party.

Typically, HIV transmission and acquisition are based on people's behaviors and are often shaped by personal and environmental influences. On an intrapersonal level, attitudes, beliefs, knowledge, motivation, behavioral skills, and past experiences can shape behavior. At the interpersonal level, advice, opinions and beliefs of others, and behaviors of friends and family can influence decision making. Finally, at the community or group level, innovations adopted by popular community leaders, new policies, and a change in community norms all can affect behavior. It

Table 6.2. Characteristics of Effective Prevention Interventions

Concept	Definition
Comprehensive	Intervention that addresses multiple domains (e.g., family, peer, norms, resources, and community) and influences the development and perpetuation of behaviors to be prevented.
Varied Teaching Methods	Interventions involve diverse teaching methods that focus on increasing awareness and understanding the problem behavior and on acquiring or enhancing skills (e.g., role-play, workbook).
Sufficient Dosage	Programs provide enough intervention to produce desired effects and provide follow-ups as necessary to maintain effects.
Theory Driven	Programs have a theoretical justification, are based on accurate information, and are supported by empirical research (e.g., Social Cognitive Theory).
Positive Relationships	Programs provide exposure to adults and peers in a way that promotes strong relationships and supports positive outcomes.
Socioculturally Relevant	Programs are tailored to the community and cultural norms of the participants and make an effort to include the target group in the program development and implementation.
Evaluation	Programs have clear goals and objectives and make an effort to systematically document results relative to their goals (e.g., process evaluation, outcome evaluation).
Well-Trained Staff	Program staff supports the program and are provided with training regarding the implementation of the intervention (e.g., they are trained in the use of motivational interviewing).
Appropriately Timed	Programs are initiated early enough to have an impact on the development of the problem behavior, and are sensitive to the developmental needs of the participants.

Source: Nation et al. (2003).

is important to note that although theories are used to predict behaviors and to guide prevention interventions, social workers also can use the various concepts and core elements associated with theories related to conducting assessments on individuals, groups, and communities.

A number of theories and core elements have been used as frameworks in the development of HIV-related prevention interventions for MSM. Many of these theories have been tested and supported as effective interventions. In table 6.3 there are a few examples of prevention interventions that have been supported by evidence in reducing HIV transmission or acquisition. Table 6.3 presents three Diffusion of Effective Behavioral Interventions (DEBI) recommended by the CDC. View additional interventions at the website for The Diffusion of Effective Behavioral Interventions Project (DEBI) at http://www.effectiveinterventions.org/en/AboutDebi.aspxTable

Many of these theories contain concepts that reflect the personal and environmental influences discussed above. Keep in mind that it is common for many prevention interventions to include more than one theory, thus using and targeting multiple concepts. This allows for the intervention to address a number of critical elements that have an impact on change. In a meta-analysis of studies that address behavior change, Fishbein and colleagues (2001) identified eight elements that are critical for positive behavior change. These elements are all relevant to MSM prevention interventions. Fishbein and colleagues also suggested that interventions are more likely to reduce rates of HIV transmission or acquisition if they contain these elements. This is why many prevention efforts use more than one theory to guide the intervention.

1. There are no environmental barriers to make the behavior change impossible.

2. The person has developed positive intentions to perform the new behavior.

3. The person has the skills necessary to perform the behavior.

4. The person has a positive attitude toward the behavior.

Table 6.3. Selected Diffusion of Effective Behavioral Intervention Approaches (DEBIs) Related to Prevention of HIV in MSM

Intervention	Target Population	Sample Core Elements
Many Men, Many Voices (3MV)	Young, Black MSM Group-level interventions	Build self-esteem, increase self-efficacy, learn risk-reduction skills
MPowerment	Young gay and bisexual MSM Community-level intervention	Development of a core group, formal outreach in the community, social marketing and publicity campaigns
Personalized Cognitive Counseling	MSM of all racial groups and ages	One-to-one behavioral risk-reeducation counseling, behavior risk assessment, and use of cognitive behavioral techniques to address thoughts, attitudes, and beliefs

5. The social pressures to perform the new behavior outweigh the pressure to not perform the new behavior.

6. The person perceives the behavior to be more consistent than inconsistent with his or her self-image.

7. The person's emotional response to implementing and performing the new behavior is more positive than negative.

8. The person believes that he or she can perform the behavior (self-efficacy).

The next section introduces theories used in HIV prevention. Using theory to guide prevention interventions is critical to supporting the likelihood that the intervention will be successful. Based on the assumptions and concepts associated with each theory, you will see the link associated with the elements of positive behavior change identified by Fishbein and colleagues (2001) above. The theories are separated into three main categories: (1) intrapersonal or individual, (2) interpersonal, and (3) community or group.

Intrapersonal-Level or Individual-Level Theories
Health Belief Model (Rosenstock, 1974; Rosenstock, Strecher, & Becker, 1994)

Originally, Rosenstock (1974) developed the Health Belief Model as a systematic method to help explain and predict health behavior by focusing on attitudes and belief systems. Over the years the model has been modified and used to guide intervention development. In general, the Health Belief Model assumes that if behavior change is going to occur, behavioral researchers need to address a number of areas. There are two main concepts associated with this model: (1) perceived threat (perceived susceptibility, severity), and (2) outcome expectations (perceived barriers, perceived benefits, self-efficacy level, and cues to action, such as media, personal influence, and reminders). Although Rosenstock does not list them as specific concepts, this model also takes into account sociodemographics (age, gender, ethnicity, socioeconomics, personality) as having an influence on the model as it relates to behavior change. See table 6.4 for concepts and definitions.

In conducting risk assessments of MSM, social workers should strive to incorporate the above concepts as a way to assess and understand their client's perceptions of engaging in risk behavior as well as perceptions of their avoidance of safety

Table 6.4. Health Belief Model: Concepts and Definitions

Concept	Definition
Perceived Susceptibility	A belief about the likelihood of getting a disease or condition.
Perceived Severity	A belief about how serious a condition and what its clinical and social consequences may be.
Perceived Benefits	A belief about the benefits associated with adopting a new behavior.
Perceived Barriers	A belief about the negative aspects associated with adopting a new behavior.
Cues to Action	Strategies used to activate readiness to adopt a new behavior. A strategy to raise awareness.
Self-efficacy	Confidence in a person's ability to take action.

Source: Rosenstock (1974); Rosenstock et al. (1994)

measures such as condoms. In order to understand these perceptions, you may want to ask questions related to the concepts associated with the Health Belief Model. For example, workers can ask the following questions:

1. How likely is it that you believe you could contract HIV?

2. In what ways would your life be impacted if you were to become infected with HIV?

3. What would be the benefits if you decided to use condoms while engaging in anal sex?

4. What things get in the way of you being safer when it comes to sex with other men?

5. How confident are you that you could use condoms the next time you have sex?

Transtheoretical Model (Prochaska & DiClemente, 1983).

This is commonly referred to as the "stages of change" model. It postulates that people move through various stages related to behavior and behavior change. There are six primary stages: precontemplation, contemplation, preparation, action, maintenance, and relapse. See table 6.5 for stages and definitions. As people progress through each stage, their progress indicates a higher level of commitment and motivation to change the specific risk behavior. It is important to note that movement through the stages can vary. Some people may progress, others may regress, and some may stay stagnant.

Table 6.5. Transtheoretical Model: Stages and Definitions

Stage	Definition
Precontemplation	Does not intend to take action within the next six months.
Contemplation	Intends to take action within the next six months.
Preparation	Intends to take action within the next thirty days and has taken some behavioral steps in this direction.
Action	Changed overt behavior for less than six months.
Maintenance	Changed overt behavior for more than six months.
Relapse	Retreats to old behaviors and patterns.

Source: Prochaska & DiClemente (1983).

In order to assess and prepare for intervention, social workers can use the Transtheoretical Model to help identify the stage in which an MSM may be, in terms of behavior change and motivation for change. For example, if an MSM is in denial about his drug use or the seriousness of his risky sexual behaviors, then developing a behavioral plan for change would be premature. This individual is clearly in the precontemplative stage based on the fact he or she does not see a problem with engaging in unprotected anal sex. The social worker would have to begin at the precontemplation phase and assist in creating an argument for change. For example, when a client is in denial, the social worker's role is to help raise awareness and conduct a risk-benefit analysis. Again, the goal is to help the client move from a place of being "stuck" and in denial to ownership of his behavior, thus fostering motivation for change.

Below are a set of example questions to assess at which stage a client may be at in terms of their behavior(s).

1. What do your friends think about the impact your drug use is having on your life?

2. How does your drug use fit with your personal value of being as healthy as possible?

3. What benefits do you gain from having unprotected anal sex with your partners?

4. What are the costs to you for having unprotected anal sex with your partners?

5. What needs to happen in order for you to move forward with a plan that would support you in reducing or stopping drug use?

Theory of Reasoned Action (Ajzen, 1991; Fishbein & Ajzen, 1975)

The theory of reasoned action was originally developed to better understand behavior change based on the causal connection between beliefs, attitudes, norms, and intentions. Thus, intentions to avoid a risk behavior are determined by a person's beliefs, attitudes, and norms (see table 6.6). When assessing beliefs, it is

Table 6.6. Theory of Reasoned Action: Concepts and Definitions

Concept	Definition
Behavioral Belief	An individual's belief about consequences of particular behavior. The concept is based on the subjective probability that the behavior will produce a given outcome.
Attitude toward the Behavior	An individual's positive or negative evaluation of self-performance of the particular behavior. The concept is the degree to which an individual positively or negatively values performance of the behavior. The individual's attitude is determined by the total set of accessible behavioral beliefs linking the behavior to various outcomes and other attributes.
Normative Belief	An individual's perception about the particular behavior, which is influenced by the judgment of significant others (e.g., parents, spouse, friends, teachers).
Subjective Norm	An individual's perception of social normative pressures, or relevant others' beliefs that he or she should or should not perform such behavior.
Perceived Behavioral Control	An individual's perceived ease or difficulty of performing the particular behavior. We assume that perceived behavioral control is determined by the total set of accessible control beliefs.
Control Beliefs	An individual's beliefs about the presence of factors that may facilitate or impede performance of the behavior. The concept of perceived behavioral control is conceptually related to self-efficacy.
Behavioral Intention	An indication of an individual's readiness to perform a given behavior. We assume that intention is an immediate antecedent of behavior. The behavioral intention is based on attitude toward the behavior, subjective norm, and perceived behavioral control, with each predictor weighted for its importance in relation to the behavior and population of interest.
Behavior	An individual's observable response in a given situation with respect to a given target. Behavior is a function of compatible intentions and perceptions of behavioral control in that perceived behavioral control is expected to moderate the effect of intention on behavior, such that a favorable intention produces the behavior only when perceived behavioral control is strong.

Sources: Ajzen (1991); Fishbein & Ajzen (1975).

important for a social worker to assess people's view of potential consequences of a risky behavior (e.g., consequences of unprotected anal sex), as well as their beliefs about the opinions of their significant others (friends, family, romantic partners) of the risky behavior. Belief consequences are what form a person's attitude toward the risky behavior. Furthermore, opinions from significant others and the desire to conform to those opinions assist in forming subjective norms. As a result, if a person's attitude and subjective norms disagree with the risky behavior, his or her intentions to change the behavior increase. Accordingly, intentions are the most important determinant of actual behavior change. Importantly, theories tend to be modified over time and, as a result, Ajzen (1991) expanded the theory of reasoned action to the theory of planned behavior by adding the concept of perceived behavioral control (control beliefs and perceived power) to the causal model (table 6.6). For example, if an MSM client has not had much success using condoms with sex partners, he has demonstrated poor behavioral control. The client may have strong intentions to use condoms but, based on history, may not be able to consistently implement condom use. Following are sample assessment questions that can be used to gain a better understanding of a person's beliefs, norms, attitudes, and intentions as they relate to sexual practices.

1. How might your friends feel if they were to find out you were having unprotected sex?

2. What are your thoughts about using condoms for anal or vaginal sex?

3. What do you think may be the possible outcome(s) if you choose not to use condoms?

4. What are some of the things that may get in the way of you using condoms?

5. What are your intentions to use a condom the next time you have sex?

Interpersonal-Level Theories
Social Cognitive Theory (Bandura, 1977, 1986, 1994)

Social Cognitive Theory is another theory that is an extension of an existing theory. Social Cognitive Theory was originally coined Social Learning Theory (Bandura, 1977). Albert Bandura (1977, 1986) created a triadic framework that identifies three influences on behavior: (1) personal factors, (2) environmental factors, and (3) behavioral factors. Bandura later defined the interaction among these concepts as reciprocal determinism. In summary, these influencing factors become the guide that reinforces and shapes the beliefs that determine behaviors. Thus, a change in any one of these three domains will have an influence on the others. Research using Social Cognitive Theory's conceptual focus on transactions between personal factors, behavior, and environment has shown that focus to be effective in reducing the rates of HIV infection among high-risk populations. Personal characteristics include cognitions, beliefs, and expectations associated with their ability to change their behavior and their attitude toward the behavior itself. Two constructs embedded in this theory suggest that behavior change and maintenance of that behavior are a function of expectations about one's ability to perform a certain behavior (self-efficacy), in addition to the expectations regarding the outcome resulting from performing that behavior (outcome expectations). These tend to be the concepts more widely used in HIV prevention with MSM. See table 6.7 for additional concepts associated with Social Cognitive Theory.

For example, an HIV-infected MSM who has high self-efficacy for disclosure, regardless of the situation, is more likely to disclose his HIV status to his sex partners. In contrast, an HIV-infected MSM who has low self-efficacy for disclosure and is in aversive situations may be less motivated to disclose and, as a result, may internalize negative experiences (Bandura, 1994). In relation to HIV disclosure, HIV-infected MSM who have a pattern of not disclosing to sex partners and who have low self-efficacy for doing so may be more likely to avoid disclosure altogether. Following are example questions to assess the concepts associated with social cognitive theory.

Table 6.7. Social Cognitive Theory: Concepts and Definitions

Concept	Definition
Reciprocal Determinism	Behavior changes that result from interaction between a person and the environment
Outcome Expectations	Beliefs about the likelihood and value of the consequences of behavioral choices
Self-efficacy	Beliefs about one's ability to perform certain actions in various situations; also a concept wherein individuals gain control over their own behaviors rather than being passive acceptors of their environment
Observational Learning Reinforcement	Learning to perform new behaviors by exposure to interpersonal or media means, particularly via peer modeling

Source: Bandura (1977, 1986, 1994).

1. On a scale of 1 to 7, how important is it that you disclose your HIV status the next time you have sex with another man? (1 = not important at all, 7 = extremely important).

   a. If the client responds by saying 5, you may want to ask what it would take to move from a 5 to a 6.

2. On a scale of 1 to 7, how confident are you that you will use condoms the next time you have sex with another man? (1 = not confident at all, 7 = extremely confident).

   a. If the client responds by saying 3, you may want to ask what it would take to move from a 3 to a 4. This information helps guide the prevention plan by identifying target strategies in order for change to occur.

   b. You can also assess strengths by asking, "I noticed you said a 3 and not 2. Can you help me understand that?"

3. What do you believe might happen if you were to disclose your HIV status to your next potential sex partner?

Community-Level or Group-Level Theories

Diffusion of Innovations theory (Oldenburg & Parcel, 2002; Rogers, 2002) is a macro-level approach to prevention because it has a community focus. The purpose of this theory is to help explain how a new idea, behavior, or object (innovation) spreads (diffuses) among individuals within a specific community (Rogers, 1983). In order for effective diffusion, the approach must not be of focus solely on individuals, but rather on community or large groups, through communication channels and social systems (networks with members, norms, and social structures). Diffusion of Innovations Theory posits that people are most likely to adopt new behaviors (e.g., use condoms) based on favorable evaluations of the innovation conveyed to them by similar others whom they respect (see table 6.8). For example, the Mpowerment Project is a community-level intervention that targets young MSM. This project uses the power of peer influence to have an impact on the perceptions of norms surrounding sexual risk taking. Community change, therefore, comes about through a process of informal communication and modeling by peers within personal networks. The goal is to change young MSM's perceptions and behaviors around sexual risk-taking norms and condom use (Kegeles,

Table 6.8. Diffusion of Innovations Theory: Concepts and Definitions

Concept	Definition
Diffusion	Overall spread of the innovation, the process by which the innovation is communicated through certain channels over time by members of a social system
Dissemination	The planned, systematic efforts designed to make a program or innovation more widely available
Innovation	An idea, practice, or object that is perceived as new by an individual or group
Communication Channels	Means by which messages are spread, including mass media, interpersonal channels, and electronic communication
Social System	Interrelated units that are engaged in joint problem solving to accomplish a common goal, having structure, including norms and leadership
Innovation Development	All decision and activities (and their impacts) that occur from the early stage of an idea to its development and production
Adoption	Uptake of the program or innovation by the target audience
Implementation	Active, planned efforts to implement an innovation within a defined setting
Maintenance	Ongoing use of an innovation over time
Sustainability	The degree to which an innovation or program of change continues over time
Institutionalization	Incorporation of the program into the routines of an organization or broader policy or legislation

Sources: Oldenburg & Parcel (2002); Rogers (2002).

Hays, & Coates, 1996). One of the strategies that Rogers (1983) encourages is the use of an opinion leader in bringing about changes in MSM's perceptions and behaviors. Popular opinion leaders are influential in spreading information about an innovation (e.g., condom use). For example, in the Black MSM community, opinion leaders may include clergy. How might you collaborate with clergy to spread (disseminate) ideas (innovation) about safer sexual practices?

In preparing to develop a community-level intervention program for MSM using the DOI model, social workers must ask several questions in terms of assessment. Consider the following questions:

1. Which innovation(s) would reduce sexual risk taking by targeting the MSM community (e.g., regular HIV testing, condom use, disclosure of HIV status)?

2. How likely is it for the target MSM community to adopt the innovation?

3. What people in the community are seen as opinion leaders (popular men within the gay community, clergy, business people)?

4. By which means (communication channels) would the innovations best be spread (e.g., word of mouth, use of opinion leaders to spread the message, social events)?

5. Once the innovation(s) has been adopted, what strategies might be used to sustain the adoption (e.g., social marketing campaigns, follow-up social events)?

HIV-Prevention Intervention Example: The Milestone Project

The integration of both care and prevention services for HIV-positive MSM is critical for prevention efforts. The following prevention intervention is a case that illustrates the key elements associated with positive behavior change, which is discussed above, this chapter.

Case Example I

> The Milestone Project is a prevention project tailored to meet the prevention and care needs of HIV-positive MSM. The intervention takes a holistic approach with a special emphasis on sexual health. The goals associated with this project are to (1) reduce unsafe sexual practices or behaviors among high-risk HIV-positive MSM, (2) reduce the possible transmission of HIV/AIDS, as well as other STIs, to HIV-negative and unknown-status sex partners, and (3) avoid the acquisition reinfection with other STIs or other strains of HIV. The approach involves one-on-one counseling sessions between the client and the prevention case manager (PCM) and medical social worker. The intervention is conveniently located within a health center that traditionally provides medical care to the MSM community.

> The Milestone Project model is comprehensive in that it addresses both HIV-related care and HIV prevention. For example, the PCM not only provides prevention counseling (i.e., HIV disclosure strategies, negotiated safety), but also assists the client with case management needs (i.e., health insurance,

medication adherence support). In addition, the project includes an educational element that involves the use of a workbook. This workbook contains a number of topics related to the prevention needs of MSM. For example, some of the topics include HIV disclosure, sexual boundaries, and achieving the relationships the clients want. In addition, the Milestone Project uses role-play scenarios to practice various skills. For example, HIV disclosure to sex partners can be challenging for HIV-positive MSM. There are risks involved in disclosing one's HIV status. For example, the loss of a sexual experience, stigma, fear of rejection, or losing face by sharing one's HIV status with other members within the gay, bisexual, or transgender community. That being said, should HIV-positive MSM always disclose their status to sex partners? Under which circumstances should HIV-positive MSM disclose their HIV status? Questions like these can be useful for HIV-positive MSM to consider as these may be situations they may encounter. In general, the use of role-play helps build self-efficacy (confidence).

It is known that single-session interventions tend to be ineffective at behavior change among populations at risk for HIV (e.g., Kamb et al., 1998). Individuals who participate in the Milestone Project are encouraged to commit for one year. The intervention begins with an initial comprehensive intake. Following the intake are four primary counseling sessions, guided by the use of the workbook. The initial sessions typically take place within the first two months of the intervention. Clients then participate in booster sessions at three, six, nine, and twelve months. In between sessions, prevention case managers provide case management assistance on an as-needed basis.

The project integrates concepts associated with Social Cognitive Theory, the Health Belief Model, the Transtheoretical Model, and the IMB Model (information, motivation, behavioral skills). For example, the concept of self-efficacy is linked to one's confidence in using condoms within various situations or contexts, as well as confidence in disclosing one's HIV status to potential sex partners. In relation to the Health Belief Model, counseling sessions address the perceived benefits and barriers associated with condom use for anal sex.

The design of the Milestone Project was based on a preliminary needs assessment of the MSM community, as well as on previous research. It was important to include the target population in the development of this intervention. As a result, the project staff developed a community advisory board that consisted of HIV-positive MSM. The role of that board was critical in designing a culturally appropriate and relevant intervention. The community advisory board provided feedback on the workbook content and strategies on how to market the project, including the use of appropriate language, images, community norms, and recruitment.

One of the strategies used in bringing about behavior change with this population is the use of motivational interviewing. All PCMs and medical social workers receive motivational interviewing training, as well as both individual and group supervision. All PCMs are licensed social workers and are required to stay current on continuing education.

The types of evaluation exemplified in this project include formative, process, and outcome evaluations. The formative aspect incorporated a needs assessment of the MSM community and review of the literature. The literature provided the purpose and rationale for this intervention for HIV-positive MSM. Furthermore, the needs assessment assisted in providing additional rationale to justify the goals of the project. During the implementation phase, an external evaluation team conducted a process evaluation to ensure the project staff was implementing the project as outlined. This evaluation included key informant interviews (clients, project staff, and directors). At the onset of the project, clients completed a baseline assessment. In addition, they completed assessments at six and twelve months. These assessments helped capture outcome data in terms of any behavior changes that took place during their time in the Milestone Project.

Case Example II

Michael is a forty-two-year-old HIV-positive White gay male who came to the clinic for health-care related needs. During an initial comprehensive assessment, workers identified that Michael not only had care-related needs, but also sexual health and prevention needs. As a result, a prevention case manager (PCM) told Michael about the PCM program known as the Milestone Project. Michael was initially apprehensive about participating, but later agreed. An initial meeting was scheduled between Michael and the PCM in order for him to learn more about the program. After about four sessions, the PCM identified a trend in Michael's behavior. It was apparent that he was engaging in unprotected anal sex with anonymous men, and that he was struggling with disclosing his HIV status to his sex partners. The PCM was able to identify and name these patterns of behavior, leading to the development of a more concrete prevention treatment plan that would address his individual prevention needs. However, before implementing such a plan, it was important for the PCM to identify and establish mutual goals with the client. For example, if Michael was not ready to change his sexual and HIV-disclosure practices, then a plan for him to use condoms and increase disclosure to sex partners would have been premature. The PCM first had to assess Michael's readiness to change. Before proceeding, take a minute to reflect on the following questions:

- If you were the PCM working with Michael, what theory or model might you use to help guide you in assessing his readiness to change?

- What specific question(s) might you ask to assess his readiness for change both in terms of condom use and HIV disclosure? Provide at least two sample questions.

An additional area of struggle for Michael involves disclosure of his HIV status to sex partners. Keep in mind that just because he does not disclose his HIV status does not mean that he is engaging in risky sexual behavior. The PCM discussed with Michael his disclosure patterns in relation to his sexual practices. Michael expressed that he does not disclose his status in every sexual encounter that he engages in and only in some situations does he use condoms. Before proceeding, reflect on the following questions:

- If you were the PCM working with Michael, what theory or model might you use as a framework to help understand and predict his condom use behaviors? For example, you may want him to think about his intentions to use condoms or heighten his awareness of his risks associated with unprotected sex.

- What theory or model can you use as a framework to better understand and predict his disclosure behaviors? For example, you may want to assess his confidence in disclosing his HIV status in certain situations.

- What question(s) might you ask to assess Michael's beliefs around his condom use patterns? How are these questions linked to the theory(s) you previously identified to understand his condom use behaviors?

- What questions might you ask to assess Michael's beliefs around disclosing his HIV status to his sex partners? How are these questions linked to the theory(s) you previously identified to understand his disclosure behavior?

- What theory or model might you use as a framework to fortify Michael's belief in his ability to change his behaviors? Hint: Think in terms of self-efficacy.

Once the PCM was able to assess Michael's needs and readiness for change, he used a workbook-based approach to guide their sessions. Two of the topics in the workbook were HIV disclosure and sexual risk limits. These topics were the foundation for the next series of sessions with Michael. Again, continuous assessment is essential in prevention interventions.

Questions for Reflection

1. Identify and differentiate the three levels of prevention.

2. Based on the case scenario involving Michael, at what level did the intervention take place (primary, secondary, or tertiary)? What evidence do you have to support your conclusion?

3. Based on the prevention illustration, the Milestone Project, identify and give an example for each of the characteristics of effective prevention programs used in the program.

4. Name the theory best associated with each statement:

   a. heightening clients' perceptions of own risk

   b. strengthening clients' intention to change risk behaviors

   c. fortifying clients' belief in ability to change behavior

   d. increasing clients' readiness to change behavior

   e. spreading new ideas and behaviors through a social network

5. Locate a peer-reviewed research article that addresses an HIV-prevention intervention for MSM. Identify the level of prevention and the theory(s) used to guide the intervention Remember, the theory may not be explicitly stated in the article, but rather various theoretical concepts of a theory may be addressed. Were you able to identify more than one of the theories presented in this chapter in the intervention?

6. Using the Diffusion of Effective Behavioral Interventions Project website, identify an effective intervention that targets MSM. What is the target population? Be as specific as possible. At which level of prevention does the intervention take place? What theory(s) is used to guide the intervention? What are the core elements associated with the intervention? What are the target behaviors? (http://www.effectiveinterventions.org/en/AboutDebi.aspx).

References

Ajzen, I. (1991). The theory of planned behavior. *Organizational Behavior and Human Decision Processes, 50,* 179–211.

Bandura, A. (1977). *Social learning theory.* Englewood Cliffs, NJ: Prentice Hall.

Bandura, A. (1986). *Social foundations of thought and action: A social cognitive theory.* Englewood Cliffs, NJ: Prentice Hall.

Bandura, A. (1994). Social cognitive theory and exercises of control over HIV infection. In R. J. DiClemente & J. L. Peterson (Eds.), *Preventing AIDS. Theories and methods of behavioral interventions* (pp. 25–59). New York: Plenum.

Centers for Disease Control and Prevention (CDC). (2001). Revised guidelines for HIV counseling, testing and referral and revised recommendations for HIV screening of pregnant women. *Morbidity and Mortality Weekly Report, 50*(RR19), 1–58.

Centers for Disease Control and Prevention (CDC). (2008). Men who have sex with men–STD surveillance 2006. Retrieved from http://www.cdc.gov/STD/STATS/msm.htm

Crepaz, N., Lyles, C. M., Wolitski, R. J., Passin, W. F., Rama, S. M., Herbst, J. H., . . . , Stall, R. (2006). Do prevention interventions reduce HIV risk behaviors among people living with HIV? A meta-analytic review of controlled trials. *AIDS, 20*(2), 143–157.

Fishbein, M., & Ajzen, I. (1975). *Belief, attitude, intention and behavior: An introduction to theory and research.* Reading, MA: Addison-Wesley.

Fishbein, M., Triandis, H. C., Kanfer, F. H., Becker, M., Middlestadt, S. E., & Eichler, A. (2001). Factors influencing behavior and behavior change. In A. Baum, T. A. Revenson, & J. E. Singer (Eds.), *Handbook of health psychology* (pp. 3–17). Mahwah, NJ: Lawrence Erlbaum Associates.

Jones, K. T., Gray, P., Whiteside, O., Wang, T., Bost, D., Dunbar, . . . , Johnson, W. (2008). Evaluation of an HIV prevention intervention adapted for Black men who have sex with men. *American Journal of Public Health, 98*(6), 1043–1050.

Kamb, M. L., Fishbein, M., Douglas, J. M., Rhodes, F., Rogers, J., Bolan, G., . . . , Peterman, T. A. (1998). Efficacy of risk-reduction counseling to prevent human immunodeficiency virus and sexually transmitted diseases: A randomized controlled trial. *Journal of the American Medical Association, 280,* 1161–1167.

Kegeles, S. M., Hays, R. B., & Coates, T. J. (1996). The Mpowerment Project: A community level intervention for young gay men. *American Journal of Public Health, 86*(8), 1129–1136.

Kelly, J. A., Murphy, D. A., Sikkema, K. J., McAuliffe, R. L., Roffman, R. A., Solomon, L. J., . . . , Kalichman, S. C. (1997). Randomized, controlled, community-level HIV-prevention intervention for sexual risk behavior among homosexual men in US cities. Community HIV Prevention Research Collaborative. *Lancet, 350*(9090), 1500–1505.

Koester, K., Maiorna, A., Vernon, K., Myers, J., Dawson-Rose, C., & Morin, S. (2007). Implementation of HIV prevention interventions with people living with HIV/AIDS in clinical settings: Challenges and lessons learned [Electronic Version]. *AIDS and Behavior, 11*(5S), S17–29. DOI: 10.1007/s10461-0079233-8.

Morin, S. F., Koester, K, A., Steward, W. T., Maiorana, A., McLaughlin, M., Myers, J. J., . . . , Chesney, M. A. (2004). Missed opportunities: Prevention with HIV-infected patients in clinical care. *Journal of Acquired Immune Deficiency Syndromes, 36*(4), 960–966.

Nation, M., Crusto, C., Wandersman, A., Kumpfer, K. L., Seybolt, D., Morrissey-Kane, E., & Davino, K. (2003). What works in prevention? Principles of effective prevention programs. *American Psychologist, 58*(6/7), 449–456.

Oldenburg, B., & Parcel, G. (2002). Diffusion of health promotion and health education innovations. In K. Glanz, B. K. Rimer, & F. M. Lewis (Eds.), *Health behavior and health education: Theory, research, and practice* (3rd ed.). San Francisco: Jossey-Bass.

Prochaska, J. O., & DiClemente, C. C. (1983). Stages and process of self-change of smoking; Toward an integrative model of change. *Journal of Consulting and Clinical Psychology, 51,* 390–395.

Rogers, E. M. (1983). *Diffusion of innovations* (3rd ed.). London: Free Press.

Rogers, E. M. (2002). Diffusion of preventive interventions. *Addictive Behaviors, 27*(6), 989-993.

Rosenstock, I. M. (1974). Historical origins of the health belief model. *Health Education Monographs, 2*, 328–335.

Rosenstock, I. M., Strecher, V. J., & Becker, M. H. (1994). The health belief model and HIV risk behavior change. In R. J. DiClemente & J. L. Peterson (Eds.), *Preventing AIDS: Theories and methods of behavioral interventions* (pp. 5–24). New York: Plenum.

Wilton, L., Herbst, J. H., Coury-Doniger, P., Painter, T. M., English, G., Alvarez, M. E., . . . , Carey, J. W. (2009). Efficacy of an HIV/STI prevention intervention for Black men who have sex with men: Findings from the Many Men, Many Voices (3MV) Project. *AIDS and Behavior, 13*(3), 532–544.

7

Social Work with At-Risk Adolescents and Young Adults: HIV Prevention and Care

Diana Rowan and Rebecca Stamler

We have a powerful potential in our youth, and we must have the courage to change old ideas and practices so that we may direct their power toward good ends.

—Mary McLeod Bethune, Civil Rights Leader and Educator

The Disproportionate Impact of HIV on Young People

In the United States, young people aged thirteen to twenty-nine accounted for 39 percent of all new HIV (human immunodeficiency virus) infections in 2009. For comparison, young people of these ages made up only 21 percent of the U.S. population. Those aged twenty to twenty-four had the highest number and rate of HIV diagnoses of any age group.

Data from 2007 show that most HIV transmission in youth aged thirteen to twenty-four occurred via sexual exposure. The specific routes of transmission are as follows (Futterman, Lewis, Stafford, & Johnson, 2007):

- HIV transmission among young males

  - Sexual contact with other males: 76 percent

  - High-risk heterosexual contact: 11.5 percent

  - Injection drug use: 7.5 percent

  - Sexual contact with other males during drug use: 4.5 percent

  - Other (including perinatal infection): 0.5 percent

- HIV transmission among young females

  - High-risk heterosexual contact: 85 percent

  - Injection drug use: 14 percent

  - Other (including perinatal infection): 1 percent

Rates of HIV infection disproportionately affect specific minority population groups, including racial and ethnic minorities and sexual minorities. In 2009, African Americans accounted for 55 percent of all HIV infections reported in youth. Young males who have sex with males (young MSM) accounted for 27 percent of all new infections in the United States and 69 percent of new infections among persons aged thirteen to twenty-nine. Among young African-American men who have sex with men (MSM), new infections increased 48 percent from 2006 through 2009 (CDC, 2011). Of those youth aged thirteen to nineteen who were living with HIV, 70 percent were African American, 15 percent were White non-Hispanic, 13 percent were Hispanic, and fewer than 2 percent were Asian American or Pacific Islander and American Indian or Alaska Native. More than 60 percent of the cases in males were reported to have involved male-to-male sexual contact. These alarming trends justify the need for increased emphasis on prevention of HIV infection in all young people, especially in minority youth.

Why Are Young People at High Risk for HIV Infection?

Adolescents are prone to engaging in risk-taking behaviors. Many adolescents engage in sexual intercourse with multiple partners. In addition, particular groups of adolescents, including MSM, injection drug users, and youth who exchange sex for money, drugs, or goods, engage in greater risk-taking behaviors, placing them at risk for infection with HIV and other sexually transmitted diseases (STDs). Among the sexually experienced, adolescents aged fifteen to eighteen years have the highest rates of reported STDs.

Teens in the United States are not unique. In many parts of the world, STDs and unplanned pregnancies have always occurred among adolescents. However, over the past few decades the onset of puberty and initiation of sexual intercourse have occurred at earlier ages, while the age for marriage has risen. Many adolescents begin sexual intercourse by age fifteen, with inconsistent protection and with multiple partners, which facilitates infection of HIV and other STDs (HIV InSite, 2011).

In addition to risk-taking behaviors, there are several biological reasons for heightened HIV infection rates in young women. Before puberty, the exocervix of the uterus is lined with only a single layer of columnar cells, which leaves young women more vulnerable to infection with HIV, chlamydia, and gonorrhea. During puberty, these cells are progressively replaced by multilayer squamous cells, which are less susceptible to infections. Furthermore, HIV and STDs are transmitted with greater efficiency from males to females because of the greater amount of surface area of the female genital tract. Also, women are more likely to remain asymptomatic, and hence HIV/STD infections go unnoticed and untreated for longer periods in women than in men (HIV InSite, 2011).

Tens of thousands of teens in the United States have lost a parent to acquired immune deficiency syndrome (AIDS). More youth are living with a parent or parents who have HIV or AIDS. In addition to the emotional devastation that life with HIV can bring, parental illness may raise youths' vulnerability to HIV risk behaviors. Children of parents living with HIV frequently live in the same high-prevalence communities as their parents, which increases their risk of acquiring HIV. A study in the Bronx showed that, of eighty-one youth who contracted HIV due to risky sexual behaviors, 21 percent reported having at least one parent who was also HIV positive (Chabon, Futterman, & Hoffman, 2001).

Adolescent Psychosocial Development

Erik Erikson's theory of psychosocial development is one of the best-known models for understanding identity development, and it is especially useful for understanding the common conflicts of adolescent development. Erikson describes eight stages through which each healthily developing human should pass, from infancy to late adulthood. In each stage, the person confronts, and hopefully masters, new challenges. Furthermore, each stage builds on the successful completion of the earlier stages. If the individual does not successfully master challenges at each stage, the theory suggests those challenges will reappear as problems in the future. The eight stages, the major psychosocial crisis to be resolved in each, and the typical age range when each is experienced are presented below.

The Eight Stages of Psychosocial Development

1. Hope: Trust vs. Mistrust (Infants, 0 to 1 year)

2. Will: Autonomy vs. Shame and Doubt (Toddlers, 2 to 3 years)

3. Purpose: Initiative vs. Guilt (Preschool, 4 to 6 years)

4. Competence: Industry vs. Inferiority (Childhood, 7 to 12 years)

5. Fidelity: Identity vs. Role Confusion (Adolescents, 13 to 19 years)

6. Love: Intimacy vs. Isolation (Young Adults, 20 to 34 years)

7. Care: Generativity vs. Stagnation (Middle Adulthood, 35 to 65 years)

8. Wisdom: Ego Integrity vs. Despair (Seniors, 65 years onward)

According to this model, the major developmental challenge faced by each youth is to consolidate his or her own identity. During the typical adolescent developmental stage of "identity vs. role confusion," youth are working toward mastery of a number of tasks, such as:

• Maintenance of a constant self-esteem

• Development of inner regulatory controls

• Control of mood stability

• Comfort in one's body

• Establishment of direction in life

• Confidence about approval from significant peers and family members

Developmental Traits of Adolescence

The common challenges of psychosocial development in adolescence help a social worker better understand how youth view taking risks and why prevention approaches designed for adults are not as effective with adolescents. In short, youth are not simply adults with less life experience. They view their own vulnerability, regulate their self-esteem, and experiment with different identities in ways that are not commonly seen in adults. Thus, social workers cannot expect youth to respond to HIV-prevention education in the same way as adults. Four developmental traits of adolescence are discussed with respect to HIV-prevention education: invulnerability, low or unregulated self-esteem, identity formation, and the search for autonomy.

Invulnerablity. Developmentally, adolescents have a tendency toward experimentation and risk taking. They have less ability than adults to understand the potentially tragic consequences of dangerous behaviors and sometimes feel immortal or invulnerable to life-threatening events. Adolescent invulnerability can explain why some teens do not change unsafe sexual practices in response to educational efforts alone.

One method for countering this outlook is to present concrete instances in which young people who are similar in age and looks reveal their HIV-positive status, talk about the impact of HIV on their lives, and urge other teens to modify their behaviors. This approach is similar to the method used by Mothers Against Drunk Driving (MADD), in which young people convicted of drunk driving with a fatality and victims' families speak about the impacts of the choice to drink and drive.

Low Self-Esteem or Unregulated Self-Esteem. Self-esteem is one's evaluation of oneself, which can vary over time. In some individuals, it is based less on self-evaluation than it is on the perception of how others see them. Adolescence is a life stage when both low self-esteem and unregulated self-esteem (in which the evaluation of oneself fluctuates from positive to negative) are common.

It is essential for social workers to frequently assess for levels of self-esteem when working with adolescents, since it can change often throughout the day. (The related concepts of self-concept and self-worth are more durable and less likely to fluctuate quickly.) The level of young people's self-esteem is often related to how motivated they will be to take care of themselves and to preserve their choices for the future. Furthermore, the ability to be emotionally and sexually intimate, to seek mutual sexual fulfillment, and to discuss sexuality and safe sex methods are impeded if an adolescent has low self-esteem. Adolescents (and many adults) often regulate their self-esteem through external sources, such as:

• Drug experimentation

• Excessive alcohol use

• Risky sex

• Reckless behaviors

Low self-esteem can cause a person to bypass careful decision making. Social workers can help youth process criteria for choosing to have a sexual experience with someone (including when, who, with what, protection options, and what behaviors). Social workers can help role play how to counteract "ploys" for sex.

Some especially vulnerable clients may have such low self-esteem, be depressed, be addicted to substances or destructive behaviors, or be from such a chaotic family situation that it might be a challenge to convince them that life is worth living. In these cases, referral for intensive clinical mental health counseling and psychiatric evaluation is appropriate.

Box 7.1. Sample Activity

Here is a sample activity to use with young people in an individual or group setting, which teaches about self-efficacy, empowerment, and decision making.

Ask the youth this question:"What causes a girl to go against her personal commitment and go along with her boyfriend's insistence to not use a condom?"

Possible answers could be peer pressure, lack of education, short-term decision making, or low self-esteem, among others. Ask the youth which of these reasons might be potential areas of vulnerability. Follow up by asking the client if he or she has ever felt like the girl in this example.

Other questions to pose with sexually active youth are, "What are your personal criteria for selecting partners for various sex acts? How might drug or alcohol use impact your ability to stick to your list? What do you do if a person you are with pressures you to participate in sexual activity, but that person does not meet your criteria?"

If these and other questions are hypothetically posed in a group setting, even youth who are not comfortable enough to verbally participate can benefit through active listening.

Identity Formation. Finding new identifications, loyalties, and interests outside of one's family setting is a central step in adolescent development. Belonging to a group, whether it is social, virtual, or descriptive, is often of great importance during adolescence and young adulthood. The high school years in particular can be dominated by obsession about a clique membership. Sometimes youth decide for themselves which group best suits them, and other times it is decided for them, causing identity confusion. A quick survey of current high school clique blogs revealed the following common associations: jocks, band geeks, emos, goths, gangstas, trouble makers, hot chicks, prep, nerds, cheerleaders, overachievers, gamers, freaks, skaters, ghetto wannabees, repeat graders, sluts, popular kids, rich kids, poor kids, stoners, loners, and drop-outs. Studies of the psychology behind gang membership show that the value of membership and belonging is powerful enough to impact young people's values. Online social media provide virtual gathering sites for youth and adults, and widen the options for expression. Online communication and virtual gathering places make it even easier for teens to try on new identities and practice various expressions of identity. The internet widens the opportunities for affiliations. Thus, it is not uncommon for an adolescent gamer to identify his or her closest social group as fellow gamers in other parts of the world, people with whom they may have never met or spoken. Social workers who understand that experimentation with identity expression is normal for this developmental stage will be more successful in building rapport and developing common respect with adolescent and young adult clients.

A large part of identity consolidation (figuring out who we are) involves developing one's sexual orientation and gender identity, which will be discussed in detail later in the chapter. Other aspects of sexual identity and expression are

- Multiple partners versus monogamy

- What sex behaviors are acceptable

- How closeness and intimacy are related to sex

- Understanding safe sex versus safer sex

- Anonymous hook-ups versus long relationships

Search for Autonomy. The achievement of autonomous functioning involves the disengagement from family ties and engagement with the world of peers and social institutions. Many social work interventions are with adolescents who, for various reasons, prematurely disengage from family. The desire for autonomy can lead adolescents into an intense, sometimes frantic search for relationships outside of their family, where they can feel safe and as if they belong. When these relationships involve risky sexual behaviors, injection drug use, or drug and alcohol use that lowers inhibitions, they become very relevant to considerations about HIV transmission.

HIV/AIDS Education for Adolescents and Young Adults

Research shows that most people in the United States, including adolescents, understand that HIV is transmitted sexually, yet many people continue to be infected. This means that prevention specialists must make efforts to combat the "it can't happen to me" fallacy. AIDS education service providers need to deliver appropriate information to adolescents while keeping in mind that the target audience is not developmentally skilled at

- Delaying gratification

- Containing impulse control

- Self-soothing

- Changing habits

- Combating peer pressure

One way to neutralize these factors is to appeal to youths' interest in

- Respecting themselves

- Taking care of their partners

- Being in control of their future

HIV prevention and general safe sex strategies need to be presented to this population with a nonjudgmental attitude. Adolescents are quick to respond negatively to being told what they need to do or to being made to feel that they do not have choices. When working with adolescents on any issue, social workers should avoid portraying behavior choices as right or wrong; this stance elicits either oppositional behavior or superficial compliance. Instead, workers should present factual information in a nonthreatening manner to allow young people to feel empowered to make choices by listening to their own inner voices.

Because peer pressure has a very strong impact on both behavioral choices and self-esteem in young people, providing education in a group setting can be effective. Group dynamics can be a powerful tool in teaching and discussing new concepts. As informal leaders in a peer group begin to listen and express agreement with statements about safe sex and protecting oneself against HIV and STDs, the rest of the group will often follow more willingly.

Interventions that lay out factual pros and cons of safe sex are a good match for adolescents, who are more literal and less abstract in their cognitive development than adults. Group discussions are effective, as are skill rehearsal activities. An example is role-play of how to ask a partner to use a condom. (More details on condom negotiation skills are presented in Chapter 12.)

It is not essential that an HIV/AIDS educator who works with young people be young in age. Sometimes it can be helpful in social work interventions to try to match ages and other characteristics, such as race, ethnicity, or religious background of the worker and the client or client system. However, more important than matching characteristics is that the worker conveys a nonjudgmental attitude and a desire to understand the reality of the young people's lives. A culturally competent approach is not only essential, but the degree to which the worker is invested in culturally sensitive practice is a good predictor of success. (Chapters 1, 3, and 5 discuss strategies for culturally competent practice in more detail.)

Impacts of Drugs and Alcohol on HIV Prevention

Use and abuse of alcohol and drugs can lower inhibitions and impair judgment and may lead adolescents (and adults) to engage in risky sexual behaviors. (Chapter 12 presents a thorough discussion of sexual behaviors and drug use with respect to HIV prevention and transmission.) The following are high-risk behaviors that are often seen in adolescents and young adults:

• Failure to use condoms correctly or consistently

• Sexual intercourse or other sexual behaviors while under the influence of drugs or alcohol, or both

• High-risk sexual behaviors for extended periods

• Injection drug use, especially when sharing dirty needles

• Participation in exchange sex, for money, drugs, or other goods

• Exposure to date rape or club drugs that increase risks for HIV infection

  • Rohypnol (Roofies)

  • Xanax

  • Clonipin

  • Gamma hydroxybutyrate (GHB)

  • Ketamine (Special K)

- Use of club drugs to heighten sexual performance, which is especially prevalent among young MSM, gay, bisexual, and transgender youth to increase sexual pleasure and endurance.

Social workers should take straightforward approaches with clients about how substance use impairs making decisions. Even with information and support, some adolescents will refuse to stop drug use and will continue risky sexual practices. Social workers in this situation have to accept their own limitations and set healthy boundaries.

Assessment with Adolescents and Young Adults

Social workers are trained to conduct thorough assessments prior to engaging in interventions with clients, based on the foundational principle that social work practice is best when it meets the clients where they are. An important point to remember when conducting assessments with adolescents and young adults is that we cannot judge maturity or development level based on how an individual looks. Data need to be gathered that help the social worker assess the following:

- Developmental level (not just chronological age)

- Cognitive ability (not just educational grade level)

- Amount of knowledge about sex and HIV/AIDS

- Relationship status

- Sexual orientation or questioning issues

- Gender identity issues

- Sexual history (including sexual abuse)

- History of drug and alcohol use

Each of these areas may be addressed in a standard psychosocial assessment, but special efforts should be made to ask age-appropriate questions about sexual knowledge and experience. The worker should not wait for an adolescent client to bring up the topic of sex. Adolescents may have been conditioned to not discuss sex with adults, may fear judgments or a scolding, or may be waiting for the worker to raise the issue. When speaking with adolescents, it is important to remember the following guidelines (AIDS Education and Training Centers, 2007):

1. Youth don't always ask the questions to which they want answers.

2. Youth responses may vary greatly in terms of being very comfortable talking about everything to being extremely guarded.

3. Youth are more likely to be concrete thinkers than abstract thinkers.

4. Youth may hold values and beliefs that influence their behavior or limit the information they provide you (e.g., they might think it is not proper to discuss private matters outside of the home).

The HEADSS Assessment Model

The AIDS Education and Training Centers (2007) modified an approach for conducting a psychosocial assessment of adolescents. The approach has been modified further here, to be more strengths-focused. Social workers will benefit from asking youth the following questions, ideally without the parent(s) or guardian present. If the accompanying adult is present for any part of the interview, the worker should allow the youth to introduce the adults to the worker but should direct the questions to the youth. Ideally, the interview should be conducted in the first language of the youth, to maximize his or her ability to understand the questions and to communicate clearly. Certain questions should be phrased as open ended when possible, which means they must be answered with answers longer than "yes," "no," or simple phrases; these questions also increase the likelihood of gaining more information during an assessment or interview.

H-HOME

- Where do you live?

- Who do you live with?

- Do you have brothers or sisters? What are they like?

- Are there any new people living in your home?

- How much time do you spend at home?

- What are the rules like there?

- What are the arguments about at home?

- If you have a problem, do you discuss it with anyone? Who?

- Have you ever run away from home?

- What would you like to change about your home?

Question to avoid: "Tell me about mom and dad." This phrasing does not allow for the youth to discuss the separation or divorce of parents, being raised in a single-parent home, being raised by another guardian, being in foster care, being emancipated, or without a permanent place to stay.

E-EDUCATION

- What is the last school that you attended?

- What grade was that? (If the client responds with answers that indicate he or she is still in school, proceed with the questions. If not, ask about what led the client to leave school.)

- What do you like best and least about school?

- How important are your grades to you? Have they changed lately?

- Have you ever failed any classes or repeated any grades?

- Do you ever cut classes?

- How much school have you missed in the last . . . (year, month)?

- How do you get along with the other kids in your classes?

- Have you ever been teased, bullied, or attacked at school?

- Do you work after school or on weekends?

- About how much time do you spend on homework in a week?

- Have you been in any afterschool activities or sports?

- How do you get along with teachers or employers?

- What are your career or vocational goals?

Question to avoid: Don't lead with "How are you doing in school?" The youths may not be enrolled in school. And if they are and their academic performance is not strong, this phrasing does not give them an opportunity to discuss strengths.

A-ACTIVITIES

- What do you do with your free time?

- Do you watch TV? If so, how often do you watch TV? Which shows are your favorites?

- How important is music to you? What kind? Why?

- Do you read or write for fun? How so?

- What activities do you do during and after school?

- Are you active in sports? Do you exercise?

- What are you good at? What do you wish you were good at?

- Describe the last time you would say that you had fun. When was it? Who were you with?

- Do you like to hang out mostly with people your age or people of a different age?

- Do you spend the most time with people of your gender? Another gender?

- How important to you are your friends?

- Are you the type to have one or two friends or a lot of friends?

- Do you have a car?

- What do you do on weekends? Evenings? Do you go to parties?

- Have you ever been involved with the police?

Question to avoid: Don't lead with, "What do you do with your friends?" The youth may not identify as having friends and this question can lead to them feeling judged or not understood.

D-DRUGS

With younger teens, it is best to begin by asking about their friends' and family's drug use. Depersonalization increases the chances of gathering honest answers.

- Do any of your family members drink or use drugs? If so, how do you feel about it? Is it a problem for you?

- If you go out with friends or to a party, do any of the people there drink or do drugs?

- Do you smoke cigarettes? Have you ever smoked one?

- Have you ever tried alcohol? When? What kind and how often?

- Do any of your friends drink or use drugs?

- Do you or your friends drink or use drugs and then drive?

- Have you been in a car accident lately? Did it involve drugs or alcohol?

- What drugs have you tried? Have you ever injected steroids or drugs? If so, when did you first try drugs or inject steroids or drugs? How often do you use steroids or drugs?

- How do you get money to pay for drugs?

- Are drugs used or available in places where you hang out?

Question to avoid: Don't lead with the question, "Do you use drugs?"

S-SEXUAL ACTIVITY/IDENTITY

Note that if the youth reports having had no sexual partners, the social worker may need to exclude some of these questions. This disclaimer is qualified, however, with mentioning that adolescent clients may not admit to sexual activity when first asked, and continuing a conversation about sex and relationships for a few minutes may lead to them disclosing the truth about their past sexual history.

- Are you now or have you ever been in a relationship? When? How was it? How long did it last?

- What is or was that experience like for you?

- How do you define "sexual activity"?

- Do you consider yourself ready for sex? Did you have any sexual activity in current or prior relationships? How comfortable are you with sexual activity?

- Have you ever had sex outside of relationships?

- How many sexual partners have you had?

- How old were you when you first had sex? How old was your partner?

- Do you have sexual activities with men? Women? Both?

- Do you most identify as straight, gay, or do you not discriminate? How do you know which is right for you?

- Do you think you need to have sex to find out if you're lesbian, gay, or bisexual?

- (For females) Do you want to become pregnant? Have you ever been pregnant? (For males) Do you want to get someone pregnant? Have you ever gotten someone pregnant?

- Have you ever had an infection as a result of having sex? If so, what did you do about it?

- Do you use condoms or another form of contraception for STD and HIV prevention? If so, what type of birth control do you use? How much of the time? (10 percent, 50 percent, 99 percent, or 100 percent of the time?)

- Have you ever felt disrespected or uncomfortable with something someone did to you during sex?

- If someone were to sexually abuse or rape you, what would you do?

- Have you ever had sex unwillingly?

- Have you ever had sex in exchange for money, drugs, clothes, or a place to stay?

- Have you ever been tested for HIV? Do you think you need to be tested? If not, what type of person should get tested? (This question helps to evaluate the individual's knowledge of HIV risks.)

- (For females) Do you menstruate regularly? Have you ever had a pelvic examination? Has anyone told you about breast self-examinations? (For males) Have you had a testicular examination? (For males and females) Have you been examined for STDs?

Questions to avoid: Don't ask a male youth, "Do you have a girlfriend?" and don't ask a female youth, "Do you have a boyfriend?" These questions imply heterosexuality and close the door on the youth feeling comfortable to discuss feelings aligned with identification as lesbian, gay, bisexual, transgender (LGBT), or questioning. Furthermore, don't lead with questions like "Have you ever had sex?" or "Are you gay?" This is too much, too fast. Also, allow room for the youth the express an identity outside the binary model of "male or female."

S-SUICIDE/DEPRESSION

- How do you feel today, on a scale of 0 to 10 (0 = very sad, 10 = very happy)?

- Have you ever felt less than a 5? How long did that feeling last?

- What made you feel that way? What made it get better?

- What is the biggest problem where you live right now? On a scale of 1 to 10, how bad is it? Are there other problems at home?

- On the same scale, how happy are you at school? Is this number higher or lower than it used to be?

- On the same scale, how happy are you with your friendships and relationships? Is this number higher or lower than it used to be?

- (If the youth previously reported being bullied) With regard to being bullied, on the same scale, how severe was the bullying?

- How are your sleeping habits? Are you sleeping a lot more than you used to? Are you having trouble sleeping? (Sleep disturbances can be an indicator of depression.)

- How are your eating habits? Do you have a good appetite? (Frequent fad dieting, crash diets, anorexic or bulimic behavior, and obesity with significant overeating or bingeing are all indicators of significant psychological distress. Enquiring about a youth's body image perceptions and whether or not she or he pursues thinness, fears being fat, or has poor dietary or abnormal eating habits provides insight on whether the individual needs a referral for an evaluation for an eating disorder.)

- (If the youth previously expressed feelings of being a sexual minority, such as LGBT or questioning) How does being a sexual minority impact the number you rated for how you feel today?

- Have you ever or do you ever think about hurting yourself or think that life isn't worth living, or hope that when you go to sleep you won't wake up?

- Do you think about death often? Do you ever think about your own death?

If the youth admits to suicidal ideation, assess for whether the individual has a plan on how he or she would attempt suicide. If they have a plan, further assess for access to the method, such as a gun, a car to drive off a cliff, and so on. Immediately refer anyone expressing suicidal or homicidal thoughts to a mental health professional for expert evaluation and treatment. The mental health professional will conduct a suicide risk depression screening, including the following:

Suicide Risk/Depression Screening

1. Sleep disorders (problems falling asleep, early or frequent waking, or greatly increased sleep and complaints of increasing fatigue)

2. Appetite or eating behavior change

3. Feelings of boredom

4. Emotional outbursts and highly impulsive behavior

5. History of withdrawal or isolation

6. Hopeless or helpless feelings, both of which are significant predictors of depression and suicide risk

7. History of past suicide attempts, depression, or psychological counseling

8. History of past suicide attempts or depression in the family

9. History of drug or alcohol abuse, acting out or crime, recent change in school performance

10. History of recurrent serious "accidents," which may actually be intentional attempts to harm self

11. Psychosomatic symptomatology

12. Significant current and past losses, such as deaths of family or friends, or loss of important relationships

13. Suicidal ideation

14. Self-injurious behaviors (such as cutting)

15. Decreased affect on interview, avoidance of eye contact, or depression posturing

16. Preoccupation with death (clothing, music, media, art)

17. History of psychosocial or emotional trauma

18. If LGBT, negative impact of discrimination and marginalization due to identity of being LGBT

Suggestions for Ending Interviews with Adolescents

• Ask the client to sum up their life in one word or to give the overall "weather report" for their life (sunny with a few clouds, very sunny with highs all the time, cloudy with rain likely, thunderstorm predicted, etc.).

• Ask the youth to tell you what he or she sees in the mirror each day. Specifically, look for youth who tell you that they are "bored." Boredom in adolescents may indicate depression.

• Ask the youth to tell you with whom they can trust and confide if there are problems in their lives, and why they trust that person. This is especially important if you have not already identified a trusted adult in their family system. Encourage them to explore other trustworthy adults that can help with problems and answer questions. Let them know you are interested in them and that you are someone who wants to help.

• Give the adolescents an opportunity to express any concerns you have not covered, and ask for feedback about the interview. If they later remember anything they have forgotten to tell you, remind them that they are welcome to call or text at any time, or to come back to talk about it.

• For adolescents who demonstrate significant risk factors, relate your concerns. Ask if they are willing to change their lives or are interested in learning more about ways to deal with their problems. This question can lead to a discussion of potential follow-up and therapeutic interventions.

• If the adolescent's life is going well, say so. If he or she is unable to identify strengths, the worker should identify strengths to help provide encouragement. Strengths can never be restated too often.

• Ask if there is any information you can provide on any of the topics you have discussed, especially health promotion in the areas of sexuality and substance use. Try to provide whatever educational materials in which young people are interested.

• Discuss perspectives and experiences about topics that are important to him or her in order to build rapport and trust.

Adolescent Sexual Minorities

Being an adolescent can be difficult enough without being judged about one's authentic identity. Sexual minorities face additional issues in their identity development whenever they begin to address their sexual orientation or gender identity. As the data presented earlier in the chapter show, young sexual minorities, specifically MSM, experience higher levels of HIV incidence.

Who Are Sexual Minorities?

Sexual minorities are a population that has come to include sexual orientation and gender identity; MSM, women who have sex with women (WSW), and LGBT individuals are among those who do not fit in the heterosexual majority. Sexual orientation describes the expression of emotional, sexual, or romantic attraction to another person, whether same-sex, other sex, both sexes, or none at all. Gender identity is more focused on a person's self-image or belief about being male or female. Transgender (TG) is an umbrella term to describe different ways of expressing authentic gender identity (e.g., transsexual, cross-dresser, gender queer, intersex, gender variant, or gender nonconforming). Adolescents may go through periods when they question their gender identity or sexual orientation, or both, which may remain fluid until they discover and accept their identity. Some young people remain fluid and identify as gender queer or gender nonconforming to refute binary groupings such as heterosexual or homosexual and male or female. Research that claims to focus on LGBT issues often concentrates on lesbian and gay populations, barely mentioning transgender concerns.

Gender Identity Development for Sexual Minorities

Adolescents focus much attention on building their authentic identity. Experimentation, exploration, and risk taking can lead to commitment to certain aspects of personal identity, including values, interests, career choices, social interactions, self-expression, gender identity, intimacy, and sexuality. Sexual minorities face additional issues in their identity development whenever they begin to address their sexual orientation or gender identity. LGBT adolescents are more likely to experience role confusion when they have inadequate support, few role models, and limited outlets for self-expression. Youth may postpone their exploration of authentic identity until they feel safe, whether due to lack of self-acceptance, lack of support from family and friends, or stigmatization from society at large, which may include systematic discrimination due to public policy.

Many sexual minority adolescents address their sense of self through the coming-out process. Several models of gay and lesbian identity development concentrate on stages of coming out. For example, the Cass Model (Barrett & Logan, 2002; Cass 1979) suggests six stages:

1. Identity confusion can be a painful and turbulent time. This stage involves the beginning awareness of same-sex attractions. Ignoring or suppressing feelings of being different from heterosexual peers can lead to shame, distress, self-judgment, and fear of repercussions.

2. Identity comparison is a step toward self-exploration. This stage involves acceptance of the possibility of being gay or lesbian, in addition to rationalizing why same-sex attraction may be happening. "This is just a phase," or "I'm just in love with this specific woman/man," might be typical self-talk.

3. Identity tolerance increases the commitment to being gay or lesbian. This stage involves a compelling need to connect to other people who are gay or lesbian, along with the sense of separation from the heterosexual majority. A good connection with the gay community can lead to a stronger sense of gay or lesbian identity.

4. Identity acceptance is a step toward self-acceptance and a commitment to one's identity. This stage involves more interactive involvement with gay and lesbian people, and disclosure of authentic identity, or "coming out," to significant heterosexual individuals.

5. Identity pride increases awareness of a connection to the gay community and the separation from heterosexism. There can be an "us versus them" attitude toward heterosexuals. This stage involves increased disclosure of authentic identity and possible involvement in political and social activism.

6. Identity synthesis is a stage of integration. This stage involves incorporation of gay or lesbian identity as a component of the whole sense of self.

Although these stages are sequential, it is not uncommon for people to revisit stages at different points in their lives. Typically, adolescent sexual minorities will be at earlier points in the stages and may need support to work through the challenges of each stage. Some people may remain stuck in a stage or two without advancing to identity synthesis.

There are fewer identity development models about gender identity, which can be even more complex than for sexual orientation. Parents and peers can add pressure to questioning adolescents to conform to the conventional binary definitions of gender and sexuality while adolescents tend to be more fluid in expression and development. Ethnic or racial cultural expectations also direct creation or reduction of barriers of personal adjustment.

Increased Stressors of Sexual Minority Adolescents

The risk of disclosure for LGBT teens can become a very challenging experience when they are faced with rejection, marginalization, discrimination, victimization, inequity, and harassment. Sexual minority youth are sometimes isolated or rejected by family and friends when they come out to them. If rejected from the family unit, many young people become homeless or dependent on unstable housing, vulnerable to predators and street survival-sex. Many youth may not be prepared for this new-found independence, which may lead to financial instability, unpredictable access to food, dropping out of school, employment problems, substance abuse, legal issues, and poor access to health care.

Risk of HIV is not included in the context of sexual identity development models, as most models are generally concerned with self-acceptance of authentic identity, informing others about their sexual orientation (coming out), and living an authentic identity. However, homophobia and transphobia can contribute to self-defeating attitudes and risky behaviors, including risk for HIV infection. Skilled professionals will need to be prepared to help a client work through acceptance of HIV status and the synthesis of this information.

Sexual Behavior Experimentation among Adolescents

There is a natural curiosity about sex in our increasingly provocative society. Sexual behavior is highly visible in mass media, especially on television, in movies, and on the internet. Adolescents' developing personalities are highly influenced by their environment and a certain level of risk taking in unconventional behaviors. Release of certain hormones throughout the body launches a new phase of life, which becomes a sexual awakening for some young people. It can be a confusing time for many sexual minority youth. Sexual risk taking can lead to increased stigmatization, and to STDs including HIV. High-risk behaviors include

• Unprotected oral sex

• Unprotected anal intercourse, insertive or receptive

• Forced sex

• Sex under the influence of alcohol or drugs

• Sex in exchange for resources

• Numerous partners

Some adolescents may experiment in sexual activity in their efforts to express and receive love, affection, and acceptance. Others seek a general release of stress and tension. Young MSM often engage in riskier sexual behavior than their heterosexual-exclusive peers; there is an expectation of sexual expression among young males who have sex with men. Whatever personal needs are being fulfilled, mental health professionals must address the high risk for contracting HIV through creative educational programs and prevention counseling about topics such as safe-sex practices, regular testing, and use of drugs or alcohol during sex.

Sexual minority youth often have experienced being excluded from their families and being kicked out of their homes. In order to survive, some of them decide to participate in sex work in exchange for money, goods, and services. In fact, these young people may take part in riskier behaviors to increase their gain, also increasing their vulnerability to HIV infection. Survival sex work is highly stigmatized, which may create an environment of self-censorship instead of self-disclosure. There is a growing inevitability to address the needs of those who are at such high risk. Homeless sexual minority youth who turn to sex work for goods, services, and money make themselves highly vulnerable to receiving and transmitting HIV. Innovative and inclusive youth-friendly programs are available in some larger cities at HIV/AIDS service agencies and organizations, but for those who remain fearfully silent, the demand for services is growing. Many adolescents do not even get themselves tested for HIV for fear that others will find out that they have been tested, or that they are HIV positive. Layers of marginalization increase the challenges for this population, whether due to sexual orientation, gender identity, race, or ethnicity, in addition to being HIV positive.

Adolescence is a transitional time when people begin to mature physically and sexually. It is a time to investigate abstract concepts and to understand various roles in life in order to commit to ideal values, interests, interpersonal relationships, self-expression, gender identity, intimacy, and sexuality. Each layer of a young person's identity must be explored in order to understand and establish his or her authentic identity. When psychosocial standards stigmatize aspects of identity markers, the youth's ability to navigate the natural process of puberty is more problematic. It is more complicated for a youth to question existing sexual orientation or gender identity when he or she has a sense that it is not safe to talk to about it.

Mental health professionals should be aware that sexual minority youth are at a higher risk than other youth. Low self-esteem, depression, substance abuse, victimization, self-injury, suicidal ideation, lack of family support (which can lead to increased marginalization), and other life stressors are more likely to reduce identity fusion and increase role confusion. Therefore, it is essential for mental health providers to design effective interventions with sexual minority youth in mind.

Transgender-Specific Issues

A population group at very high risk for HIV infection is transgender youth. Transgender youth may face supplementary issues in their identity development when they begin to address their gender identity in a culture that does not understand them. A major objective for transgender individuals is to pass as the preferred gender in an attempt to live a genuine life. Another significant issue for transgender adolescents is disclosure of authentic identity to family, friends, and teachers. It might also be perplexing for transgender youth to address sexual orientation in conjunction with adjusting to a positive gender identity. These young people experience societal discrimination, sexual harassment, bullying, and physical violence due to preconceived expectations of who they should be under binary expectations of gender expression. American society has little tolerance for behaviors that appear to fall outside of the binary model of male or female. Pressure to have unprotected sex can be greater with male-to-female (known as MTF) individuals because they do not become pregnant, which may lead to rape, as well as physical, emotional, and sexual abuse.

The World Professional Association for Transgender Health has published suggested standards of care for transsexual, transgender, and gender-nonconforming individuals, which are more restrictive for those under the age of eighteen. Protocol suggests specific clinical guidelines with reversible interventions and minimal incremental changes for easier adjustment to gender dysphoria. Increasing numbers of adolescents are choosing to live in their authentic gender in high school and begin early levels of transition. The standards of care recommend that genital surgeries, however, not be performed until an individual reaches legal age in a given country, and the individual has lived their desired identity for twelve months (World Professional Association for Transgender Health, 2011).

Hormone therapy can lead to further emotionality for transgender individuals, especially while they attempt to adjust to the correct dosage. Parents may deny consent for their child to access hormones, leading to a possibility of hormone abuse (e.g., obtaining illegal or street hormones). Methods of delivery for some hormones and silicone require intravenous injection, which can lead to risky behaviors for HIV when individuals share or poorly sanitize needles and syringes. In some cities, harm-reduction programs offer needle exchange programs for intravenous syringes and needles. Furthermore, social workers and other mental health professionals should be aware that hormone therapy can cause heightened emotionality for transgender individuals, especially while attempting to adjust to the correct individual dosage. Insurance does not pay for hormones, therapy, or other desired levels of transition, which can be very costly for individuals, as well as for families.

HIV-Positive Adolescents

The high incidence rates of HIV in adolescents and young adults show that HIV-prevention efforts are not always successful. Social workers at AIDS service organizations (ASOs), medical clinics, and other community-based agencies have the opportunity to work with adolescents who were recently diagnosed as HIV positive and those that have been living with the virus for some time, such as those who contracted the virus at birth (perinatal transmission). Below are some social work practice tips for working with adolescents and young adults who are living with HIV. You may find that these suggestions are applicable with other HIV-positive adult clients as well.

- If the HIV transmission occurred recently, it is likely that antiretroviral (ARV) medications will not be necessary for a while. Social workers should educate clients that even if ARVs are not yet necessary, HIV still requires medical supervision.

- Social workers should be aware that

  - Confidentiality is mandatory

  - The social worker may be the first helping professional contacted after someone is initially diagnosed

  - After HIV diagnosis, the adolescents' emotional response can be

    - Denial

    - Fear

    - Uncertainty

    - Lack of response

    - Anger

    - Depression

  - A variety of behaviors can occur, such as

    - Lack of cooperation with medical and support services

    - Noncompliance with medications (adherence)

    - Unhealthy lifestyle

    - Disinterest in monitoring CD4 count and viral load

- Alcohol and drug use may cause interference with ARV adherence. Social workers are often in a position to educate youth about how missing multiple medication dosages can cause complications in treatment, including mutation of the virus and a new search for a protocol to fight it.

- If youths' HIV status is "outed," discrimination can occur at home, work, school, and in the adolescents' social circles, leading to possible stigmatization from others.

- In addition to dealing with HIV, these youth also are dealing with normal developmental challenges of adolescence.

- Social workers may observe a range of behaviors in HIV-positive youth:

  - Counter phobic stance—strong and brave, teaching others about HIV

  - Overtly debilitated—depressed, ashamed, hopeless

  - Angry—acting out, even sexually

  - More psychologically stable—mix of fear, anger, or loss, with accompanying ability to acknowledge their feelings and access supports

- Youth may need assistance working through issues with regard to disclosure—if, when, how, and who they should tell about their HIV status.

- In addition to the adolescent who is living with HIV, there are many other individuals in their social network who are affected, such as

  - Parents or guardians

  - Siblings

  - Intimate partners—past, present, and future

  - Extended family

  - Friends—past, present, future

  - Other significant people in their lives

Community-Level Interventions Targeted at Adolescent HIV Prevention

Given the high incidence rates of HIV in younger people and in certain minority groups, such as African-American youth, Latino youth, and sexual minority youth, a wide range of HIV-prevention initiatives are needed. Cultural competence calls for tailoring the content and mode of delivery of the messages to the target audience. To be culturally relevant, public information campaigns should include youth-oriented components and be delivered in Spanish in Latino areas. Content must be age and generation appropriate. Because of limits on what information can be distributed in schools, social workers can educate through

- Web-based advertising

- Social networking sites

- Text messages

- Street outreach

- Clinic-based education

- Counseling

- Testing centers

- Youth groups at civic centers

- Youth groups at churches

Adolescents with Extreme Vulnerability to HIV Infection

In addition to racial and ethnic minority youth, there are specific groups of adolescents who need targeted HIV-prevention education and support:

- Transgender or gender-questioning youth

- Male youth who are gay, bisexual, or questioning (whether closeted or out)

- Youth who have run away

- Youth who are being sexually trafficked

- Incarcerated youth and young adults (juvenile delinquency facilities and jails)

- Youth in migrant families

- Homeless youth, including transitionally homeless and couch-surfing youth

- Youth who are victims of dating violence

- Youth in high-risk neighborhoods

- Members of the house/ball community

What Is the House/Ball Community?

The house/ball community is a relatively clandestine sub-culture of young African-American and, to a lesser degree, Latino MSM and male-to-female (also known as MTF) transgender persons who affiliate within an organized social structure, based on acceptance and celebration of their sexual gender expression (Bailey, 2009). Members of the house/ball culture, sometimes called the ballroom community, organize themselves in "houses," which are family-like social structures that offer family bonds often lacking in members' families of origin (Phillips et al., 2011). Balls are elaborate social events where members of houses "walk the runway" in specialized dance and performance competitions. Balls first appeared as part of the Harlem Renaissance in the 1920s and 1930s, where wealthy White people would come to experience the flourishing and exotic nightlife of Harlem, which included drag shows with Black men dressed in women's clothes. The ball scene has significantly evolved since those early days and is now not about the spectators, but about the celebration of an underground culture, of predominantly lesbian, gay, bisexual, and transgender people of color.

A study of a sample of 504 house/ball members in New York City showed that eighty-four (17 percent) were HIV positive and sixty-one (73 percent) were unaware of their HIV status prior to the testing done in the study (Murrill et al., 2008). The house/ball community has to date been understudied with respect to how the house/ball environment encourages HIV prevention and testing in young MSM and male-to-female transgender persons of color that affiliate to varying degrees with the sub-culture. In regions of the United States where the house/ball culture is active, it is estimated that 2 to 10 percent of young MSM of color affiliate with the community in nearby urban centers (Rowan, Long, & Johnson, in review). Cities known to have large ballroom communities include New York, Chicago, Baltimore, Washington, Detroit, Los Angeles, Atlanta, Charlotte, Miami, and Houston.

Members of the house/ball community bear multiple minority statuses, which typically include being people of color, being MSM in a heterocentrist society, or being transgender, and being prone to exhibiting behaviors outside of the mainstream. Furthermore, they are typically at risk for poverty, employment instability, violence (as perpetrators and victims), as well as a variety of health threats (Rowan et al., in review). Because the house/ball culture includes young MSM of color, the population group with the highest rates of new HIV infections, houses and balls offer unique opportunities for integrating HIV prevention, testing, and early treatment messages. The social work profession's commitment to culturally competent practice calls for these messages to be culturally affirming.

Implications for Mental Health Professionals

Nonjudgmental care is essential for sexual minorities, especially confused or questioning youth who are struggling with understanding their gender identity and sexual orientation. Professionals may express bias and prejudice through verbal and nonverbal communications In order to build a relationship with any service recipient, professionals must use inclusive terminology, especially during assessment interviews. Professionals should be careful not to assume that someone is lesbian or gay when they might be transgender, or vice versa.

There have not always been positive role models for sexual minority youth. In the past, television and movies often illustrated LGBT characters as comic relief; in recent years, real life stories are depicted more often. Ellen DeGeneres jeopardized her career by coming out as lesbian on her television sit-com. Chaz Bono has courageously shared his journey as a trans-man (female-to-male) with the public. There are, however, so many more adult LGBT individuals who are hesitant about open disclosure, thus making themselves unavailable as role models. Living in larger urban cities such as New York, San Francisco, Los Angeles, Boston, and Chicago increases access to services, support groups, and larger LGBT populations. Emotionally secure people best serve as role models and supporters in the lives of sexual minority youth to improve their resilience as they work through self-acceptance and identity commitment.

Chrysalis was a school-based program to improve life skills and to prevent HIV infection in multicultural transgender youth on Oahu, Hawaii (Bopp, Juday, & Charters, 2004). The group started in 1992, yet struggled due to poor funding. Chrysalis was reestablished with positive results in 1997, through the Life Foundation, an AIDS service organization; it ended again several years later, however, due to poor funding. A postoperative transgender health educator facilitated weekly two-hour meetings that took place after school on a high school campus; the program's focus was HIV prevention and improvement of life skills. A transgender peer facilitator provided a role model who had already experienced many of the significant issues that group members wanted to discuss. The program's goal was to reduce harmful behaviors and encourage incremental positive changes with a nonjudgmental approach. The objectives of Chrysalis were to

- Motivate students to stay in school and succeed

- Improve feelings of safety and belonging in school, home, and community

- Help participants build self-esteem, self-efficacy, and aspirations to a satisfying, healthy, meaningful, and productive life as an adult

- Decrease participants' risk of HIV or STD infections (Bopp et al., 2004)

The opportunity to talk about personal issues with others in a nonjudgmental environment offers empowerment and direction to participants. Discussions at Chrysalis often focused on school participation, risky behaviors for STDs, anatomy, sex reassignment surgery, career goals, alcohol and drug use, family, physical safety, and self-esteem. Members reported that Chrysalis taught them to have healthier relationships, better knowledge about condoms, and safer sex. When compared with transgender youth who were not in such a support program, Chrysalis group members were more likely to attend school without truancy, graduate from high school, manage teasing and bullying more effectively, and become more comfortable with their authentic selves (Bopp et al., 2004). The Chrysalis group could serve as a model for working with other minority groups, as well.

Case Example

The following case example illustrates many themes discussed in this chapter, with respect to HIV prevention, adolescent identity development, issues pertaining to sexual minorities, and activities in the house/ball community. Readers are then offered questions to challenge their ability to apply the chapter material to the case situations.

Jaylen is a seventeen-year-old African-American male who has recently moved into the freshman dorms at Big City College. Big City College is located about an hour's drive away from the rural community of his hometown, Tinytown, where his mother, two brothers, and two sisters live. He misses them and hopes he will make some new friends soon. He was popular at Tinytown High School and misses the attention he received as the lead actor in the school's musicals during his junior and senior years.

Jaylen did some dating in high school and took a spectacular-looking girl to the prom. He most enjoyed helping her and her girlfriends pick out their dresses. Everyone at the school knew he had an eye for fashion, and they were not surprised when he decided to study fashion merchandising at Big City College. He has a photo of himself and his prom date with their cheeks pressed close together in a frame on his dorm room desk. He is using the photo, just as he used her, to provide a cover for the fact that he is 100 percent sure that he is gay. Tinytown High School had some kids who were openly gay, but they endured what looked to Jaylen as unbearable teasing and abuse. There was no way he would have ever considered acknowledging his sexual orientation to anyone—not anyone—not his brothers, sisters, mother, friends, or the gay couple who lived on the next street. Jaylen's mother is a faithfully religious woman who is very active in the CME church in Tinytown. She is a role model in the community and conducts a peer support group for middle-school-aged African-American girls in the church, to teach them about purity and waiting until marriage to have sex with their husbands. Jaylen knows there is no way his mother would ever understand that he is sexually attracted to some of his guy friends, and that the girls he brought home over the years were just part of relationships he constructed to hold any gay rumors about him at bay. Jaylen passed off these rumors to his mother as being due to the fact that he was so focused on his clothes and appearance, and that his smaller size made it impossible for him to fit in and look good in hip-hop fashion. Jaylen was still in elementary school when he realized he would never fit into the stereotypical mold of a masculinized African-American male.

Jaylen noticed a flyer posted on campus for tryouts for models for a fashion show to raise money to combat AIDS in Africa. He was used to being told he looked like a model, and he got over any stage fright he might have had during the high school musicals, so he decided to try out. The show organizers were professionals from the fashion scene in Big City. Jaylen knew these were people who could help his career, so he was thrilled when they showed special interest in him, offered him a job, and invited him to events outside of the show rehearsals. He found himself sexually attracted to some of the men involved with the show and experienced significant anxiety about what to do, if anything. In his past, he had ignored these thoughts and worked to cover them up. For what seemed like ages, Jaylen had focused on what he had believed that God wanted for him and had prayed that God would send him a woman whom he would find attractive in a way no other has. But he wasn't in Tinytown anymore. He was in Big City, away at college and away from people who would tell his mother what he was doing and who he was doing it with. How exciting, and how scary!

On the night of the fashion show fundraiser, there was a party for the models and crew at one of the organizer's homes in the city. Jaylen had so much fun and was thrilled when one of the men asked him if he'd like to stay overnight at his house rather than attempt to find a way back to campus. That night Jaylen engaged in his first sexual experiences with a man. He felt like he was high, but he knew he hadn't taken any drugs. He felt magnificent until the morning when the man told him to get out. Jaylen went back to campus and ran into a couple of girls he knew. They kept asking him what was bothering him. They said he was acting so strange and he wondered how he would ever cover up what happened the night before.

The next night, and every night for five nights straight, he found himself back at the man's house, these times engaging in sex with multiple men all night long. They appeared to have fun introducing him to all kinds of sex behaviors and encouraged him to try everything, multiple times. Jaylen missed all of his classes that week and by the next weekend he found himself in the campus health center. He lost track of drugs he had been given and blood was coming out of his anus to a degree where he thought he was about to die. He almost wished he would die because, as he saw it, he had two choices and he could live with neither of them. One choice was to come out as gay and continue to pursue sex with men, whom he now found so sexually attractive he wondered how he could stand it. But, this choice would mean losing the love of his mother, being cursed by God, and being shunned as an African-American male in his community. The other choice was to deny this part of who he is and go back to expressing his identity as a straight African-American male, but continue to enjoy the closeness of his family. What would he do....

The physician who treated him at the campus health center told him he had sustained some damage to the lining of his rectum from an excessive amount of anal sex. Jaylen was embarrassed and wondered what this older man thought of him. The physician asked him if he had practiced safe sex. Jaylen laughed, thinking the doctor was making a joke about needing to protect himself from getting pregnant. After a couple of seconds, Jaylen realized that the man was deadly serious and the protection he needed was from HIV and other STDs, not pregnancy. He admitted to the physician that he had not used condoms. Jaylen thought back and realized he had not seen a condom used in the whole week he was at that man's house. The physician ran an Ora-Quick HIV test and Jaylen was relieved to learn he was HIV negative, though he was told he would have to be retested in a month or so. The physician referred him to the campus social worker, saying, "You better go talk to this woman right away, because it appears you are participating in some pretty high-risk activities. You need to get a grip on yourself, son, or you'll screw up your schooling and wreck your life."

"Wow," thought Jaylen. He was sobered by being told he was wrecking his life. What did that mean? And what would a social worker do for him? There was a social worker at his high school, but she was an old lady who sat in an office where the poor kids seemed to hang out. He went to see the campus social worker right away and was disappointed to learn he needed an appointment. This social worker, he learned, did hour-long therapy sessions.

The next morning Jaylen felt better physically but worse psychologically. The social worker asked him a long list of very personal questions, a lot of them about sex and drugs. She seemed to know more about gay sex than he did before the week prior. He learned that he would need to make some changes if he wanted to avoid getting infected with HIV. Jaylen was in shock that he was having to face such topics as HIV and AIDS. That was something for people in Africa, and for drug addicts and gays. Oh, but what was he?

He decided to "screw it," and not worry about the future. He was having enough stress solving his current problems, like being behind in all of his classes and avoiding his mother's calls and sisters' texts. He was happy when Friday night rolled around again and he got a ride back to the infamous house to see who was there. On Sunday, Jaylen awoke to the reality that he had been drugged and sodomized. He had found a bloody rolling pin lying on the living room floor near where he awoke. He was silent during the taxi ride back to his dorm. He was grateful that the driver was willing to let him go to his room for the cash to pay for the ride, since someone had emptied his wallet of the little bit of money he had.

Jaylen became depressed. He started drinking wine coolers and enjoyed both the way they tasted and the way they helped him tune out the noise in his head. The thoughts racing through his mind about what to do sometimes kept him from falling asleep. When he realized how high in calories the wine coolers were, he cut way back to just one or two a week. It was essential to him that he look good in his prized wardrobe. He was relieved he was able to keep up with his schoolwork, but he felt as if his soul had been broken. He felt guilty, victimized, stupid, embarrassed, ashamed, and fearful that his mother and family and friends in Tinytown would find out what he was. Another part of him felt relieved and wise that he had finally proved to himself that he was indeed a gay man. There were other gay men in his marketing classes, but they were White and seemed so much more sure of themselves and their sexuality.

On the Friday before Halloween, Jaylen mustered the energy to wear a very creative costume he designed that was reminiscent of the graveyard ghouls in Michael Jackson's *Thriller* video. While walking through the student union he was approached by two young men also wearing costumes. They had masks on, but Jaylen could tell they were both African American. His gay-dar also gave him the vibe that they were definitely the type to have sex with men. Darius and Ginger, as they said were their names, praised his costume and engaged him in an interesting conversation about how he crafted it. They invited him to a party at one of their friends' apartments that night, and encouraged him to wear his creation. Jaylen was avoiding all social events, especially parties, since the weekend when "you-know-what" happened, as he called it in his mind. The next week he ran into two guys, one of them looking extremely fine, and they reintroduced themselves as Darius and Ginger. This time they invited him to a "mini-ball" to be held at a local community center. He asked what a mini-ball was, and the men just laughed and said, "You just stick with us and we will change your world." Jaylen sensed they were genuine, promised himself he would not drink from any cups that he was not 100 percent sure had not been drugged, and decided to go with them. At the last minute, he slipped one, then two, then three condoms in his pocket, "just in case." He had been picking them up off of the social worker's desk each time he had met with her, and in the past month he had seen her six or seven times. She didn't tell him what to do or have any miracle answers, but she was a good listener, asked interesting questions, and did not seem in the least bit repulsed by the behaviors he had been telling her about. For a White woman, she seemed to understand the Black condition fairly well, acknowledging that racism was indeed alive and well.

Darius and Ginger introduced Jaylen to the rather clandestine sub-culture of the house/ball community. There, he found a supportive network of African-American males who preferred to have sex with other men. He also met some very cool transgender women who gave him lots of praise for the special way he lined his hairline. Over the coming months, he became tight with this group and joined the local chapter of the House of Givenchy. Soon he would be competing in ball competitions of behalf of that legendary house, but for now he was very fulfilled to help his house mother with the construction of her ball gowns. He also met some older men who offered to help him out if he needed a summer job. Within the house—which wasn't a literal house, but was a social network, like a supportive family—he found acceptance and encouragement. Some of the "aunts" and "uncles" in the house, along with the other ball children like him, Darius, and Ginger, gave him advice on how to sensitively reveal his sexual identity to his dear mother—his birth mother.

They spoke to him often about how true love will love you no matter what, and without judgment.

Jaylen learned how to express himself sexually without losing control. While he was not always as careful as he should have been, he did practice safe sex "most of the time." He was annoyed that the voice of his social worker would appear in his mind at the worst times, reminding him to use a condom and that he "is worth it."

Jaylen's freshman year was eventful. He earned passing grades in all but one of his classes, lost his "ball virginity" by walking in the biggest ball on the circuit, told one of his sisters and one of his brothers about being gay (as a warm-up to telling his mother), learned terms like "empowerment," "boundaries," "self-defeating," and something called "re-authoring your narrative" from the social worker, and decided to get into a same-sex relationship. To his delight, Ginger dumped Darius, who was the cute one, and Darius and Jaylen have planned to share a dorm room next term.

Questions for Reflection

1. Based on his age and his dilemmas, which of Erikson's stages of development is Jayden working through?

2. At the start of this case story, what stage is Jaylen at in the Cass Model of sexual identity development? At what stage is he as the story concludes?

3. In this chapter, we learned that adolescents and young adults commonly exhibit the following developmental traits: invulnerability, low or unregulated self-esteem, identity formation, and the search for autonomy. Which of these traits do you identify in Jaylen's story? Describe how these traits present themselves.

4. How did drugs and alcohol impact Jayden's ability to protect himself from HIV or STD infection?

5. Imagine you were like Jaylen and awoke to the realization that you had been sexually victimized. What would you have done differently from Jaylen, if anything?

6. How did Jaylen's spirituality affect his identity development?

7. What sexual behaviors presented above do you identify as risk-taking in Jaylen's story?

8. Jaylen received mental health services from the social worker on campus. Which of the practice approaches that she used with Jaylen were most effective? If you were the social worker, what would you have done differently with Jaylen, if anything?

9. What role did the house/ball community serve in Jayden's identity development?

10. Do you think Jaylen ever told his mother that he is gay? If so, what do you think happened?

11. What do you think might cause Jaylen to be more cautious about protecting his HIV-negative status?

References

AIDS Education and Training Centers. (2007). *Psychosocial assessment: Getting a good HEADSS start.* Retrieved from http://www.hivcareforyouth.com/adol?page=md-module&mod=01-02-03-01

Bailey, M. (2009). Performance as intravention: Ballroom culture and the politics of HIV/AIDS in Detroit. *Souls: A Critical Journal of Black Politics, Culture, and Society, 11*(3), 253–274.

Barrett, B., & Logan, C. (2002). *Counseling gay men and lesbians: A practice primer.* Pacific Grove, CA: Brooks/Cole.

Bopp, P. J., Juday, T. R., & Charters, C. W. (2004). A school-based program to improve life skills and to prevent HIV infection in multicultural transgendered youth in Hawaii. *Journal of Gay and Lesbian Issues in Education, 1*(4), 3–21.

Cass, V. (1979). Homosexual identity formation: A theoretical model. *Journal of Homosexuality, 4*(3), 219–235.

Centers for Disease Control and Prevention (CDC). (2011). *HIV among youth.* National Center for HIV/AIDS, Viral Hepatitis, STD, and TB Prevention, Division of HIV/AIDS Prevention. Retrieved from http://www.cdc.gov/hiv/youth/pdf/youth.pdf

Chabon, B., Futterman, D., & Hoffman, N. D. (2001). HIV infection in parents of youths with behaviorally acquired HIV. *American Journal of Public Health, 91*(4), 649–650.

Futterman, D., Lewis, S., Stafford, S., & Johnson, R. (2007). *Fundamentals of adolescent care and cultural competence.* Retrieved from http://www.hiv careforyouth.com/adol?page=md-module&mod=01-02-03-01

HIV InSite. (2011). *HIV transmission and prevention in adolescents.* University of California, San Francisco. Retrieved from http://hivinsite.ucsf.edu/InSite? page=kb-07-04-03

Murrill, C., Liu, K., Guilin, V., Rivera Colon, E., Dean, L., Buckley, L., . . . , Torian, L. (2008). HIV prevalence and associated risk behaviors in New York City's house ball community. *American Journal of Public Health, 98*(6), 1074–1080.

Phillips, G., Peterson, J., Binson, D., Hidalgo, J., & Magnus, M. (2011). House/ball culture and adolescent African-American transgender persons and men who have sex with men: A synthesis of the literature. *AIDS Care, 23*(4), 515–520.

Rowan, D., Long, D. D., & Johnson, D. (In review). Identity and self-representation in the house/ball culture: A primer for social workers. Manuscript submitted for publication.

World Professional Association for Transgender Health (2011). *Standards of care for the health of transsexual, transgender, and gender nonconforming people: Seventh version.* WPATH Publication. Retrieved from http://www.wpath.org/ documents/Standards%20of%20Care%20V7%20-%202011%20WPATH.pdf

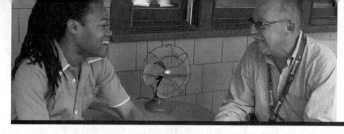

8

Over Fifty and Living with HIV

Susan Grettenberger and Mary Boudreau

If I would have known I'd live this long, I'd have taken better care of myself!

—Anonymous

Discourse about the first baby boomers reaching the magic age of sixty-five has permeated public venues in the United States and driven questions about their impact on health care, Social Security, volunteerism, religion, and even the stock market. As of 2010, the U.S. Census Bureau reported 5.7 million people over the age of eighty-five. Approximately 40 million people were sixty-five years or older (U.S. Census Bureau, 2011). Work with persons who are older touches every facet of social work practice, including that with persons living with or affected by HIV/AIDS (human immunodeficiency virus and acquired immune deficiency syndrome). A social worker in HIV/AIDS services must consider and be prepared to meet the needs of older persons. Social workers who primarily focus their efforts in gerontology must likewise understand and be prepared to work with clients who have HIV/AIDS–related needs.

Although not a new trend, substantial numbers of people living with HIV and AIDS (PLWHA) are older. To many, HIV associated with older people seems a contradiction, with HIV still thought of as a disease of younger people. Yet, this is clearly not the case. According to the Centers for Disease Control and Prevention (CDC, 2011), persons fifty-five and older accounted for 8.6 percent of new HIV diagnoses in 2008. If the age is dropped to include those fifty and older, the percentage nearly doubles to 16.4 percent. Most citizens would be surprised to learn that of all the people who tested positive in 2008 for the first time, 16.4 percent were at least fifty years old. The CDC further estimates that, of the entire population of persons living with HIV/AIDS in the United States, 24 percent are fifty and older. This is considerably higher than the percentage of persons over the age of fifty known early in the epidemic, in part because treatment is extending the lives of those with the disease and perhaps in part because more persons who are older are becoming infected.

So what exactly does this mean in terms of what social workers need to know about HIV and more mature populations? Let's start with a basic overview of who these individuals are.

Older Populations in the Epidemic

The statistics given above are for person fifty and older. Given that people today can live over one hundred years, this is a broad age range. Those working with older populations typically separate this wide span into several subgroups. The parameters of these vary, but three subgroups tend to be the norm. The youngest group, often called the young old, includes persons from fifty to about seventy. The oldest group includes persons more than eighty or eighty-five years of age, depending on the source. These distinctions are important as the functioning of persons in their early sixties, on average, will be quite different from functioning of persons in their early eighties. On a related note, some health-care professionals are beginning to suspect that HIV may accelerate some of the processes of aging.

At present, the majority of people with HIV classified as older adults are actually in their fifties. This means that there are many individuals over the age of sixty living with HIV, with growing numbers as those in one decade age into the next. Social workers must be prepared to differentially work across the older age spectrum, since, as a group, persons in their fifties have needs and lifestyles that are quite different from needs and lifestyles of persons, for example, in their seventies. However, a significant number of older adults are newly diagnosed each year. From 2006 to 2008, the largest percentage increase in the number of people living with HIV infection was among people sixty to sixty-four years old. From a slightly different perspective, from 2006 to 2009, the rate of new HIV diagnoses increased among people fifty-five to fifty-nine years old (CDC, 2011).

Diversity among Older People with HIV

Other characteristics are relevant in working with older populations as well. Increasingly, the epidemic includes persons who are heterosexual, female, poor, and persons of color. Just as is true with younger populations, social workers in

HIV must be prepared to work with a diverse group of people including, for example, straight African-American men, people who are poor, people who are executives, White women, or Latino gay men; virtually, every group is represented in the older population living with HIV or AIDS. As the saying goes, "HIV does not discriminate."

Among the characteristics on which people will vary are the circumstances that have led them into having HIV as an older person. These circumstances can have direct bearing on what the client's needs are because they include both how the client was probably infected and the age at which he or she was infected. The circumstances of an individual can include the following:

- Long-term survivor. With the development of effective treatments (e.g., highly active anti-retroviral therapies [HAART]), people with HIV are living into their older years. While there are older people being newly diagnosed with HIV, aging is the main reason for the increasing number of HIV-infected people over the age of fifty. People with HIV are living longer.

- Gay men or men who have sex with men (MSM). The tendency of the service community to identify people based on the risk behavior that likely led to infection comes from the CDC's methods of collecting data. However, these risk categories are not always helpful when it is used to generalize about someone's life situation. This is true for MSM. Some men clearly identify as homosexual and live quite openly as gay. Among the issues for this group is that a large number of gay identified men who were their peers and friends when they were younger died early in the epidemic. HIV has been a part of their lives since they were young adults. Although most have come to terms with their own survival when so many friends and former lovers died young, it seems likely that the transition into older years evokes and will continue to evoke feelings of grief and reflection about those who did not have the opportunity for a longer life.

A second general group of MSM is those who do not embrace an identity of homosexuality or being gay. It is probably more common for older MSM to still be married to or to have been married to a woman than it is for younger MSM. The sexual relationships of these MSM outside the marriage may or may not be known to their wives, suggesting concerns about the risk for HIV transmission to their female partners or wives. These MSM may seek sex in more casual relationships or have dual lives, one as a married man and the other as a gay man. MSM may be long-term survivors or recently infected. Issues for this group include the role of their family, including adult children, in their treatment and support. Disclosure of status, particularly if the man has recently been diagnosed, may be challenging if the family is unaware of his dual relationships or lifestyle.

• Straight men or women who had sex outside their primary relationship. While this includes the MSM discussed above, seeking sex outside the primary relationship may take many forms. It can involve commercial sex workers, people who have sex partners while traveling, or people who have multiple sex partners. In this age group, men are more likely than women to have been sexually active outside their primary relationship as they have aged, but one should never make assumptions about people's behavior.

• Older widows or widowers who had sex with dates. The threat of pregnancy was often the reason couples used birth control when they were younger. That threat removed, and having often been in a long-term and often monogamous relationship throughout their mature adult years, widows and widowers may be ill prepared to engage in or even know about safer sex when they begin to date again. They also may be ashamed of having sex or reticent to talk about sex. Their religious beliefs may mediate their willingness to talk or even acknowledge their behavior.

Prevention

These characteristics or behaviors are important to consider when providing treatment and services for persons with HIV. They are also important to consider with respect to prevention. Certainly, some individuals with whom social workers have contact will be engaged in risk behaviors without knowing it. Providing appropriate prevention interventions is a responsibility of the social worker as well. One of the challenges for many social workers is letting go of assumptions about people's behaviors given other things known about them. For example, simply because a person is a successful businessperson doesn't negate the possibility that the person was once an injection drug user. Similarly, simply because a person is aging does not mean they do not have an active sex life, possibly with multiple partners. In Karpiak, Shippy, and Cantor's (2006) study of older adults with HIV in New York

City, about half of participants had had sex in the prior three months, few of them with a live-in partner. It is the responsibility of the social worker to address prevention issues with all clients and to provide the resources they need. Assessment is most effective if completed with an open mind, laying aside worker assumptions about clients. Social workers should examine themselves for bias in this area.

Affected Others

One additional group of people who may seek services from HIV providers are affected others. Some of the people who are living with HIV are not those who are infected, but those who have a close relationship with a person or persons who are infected. Throughout the epidemic, parents and even grandparents have played a significant role as caregivers, and they may approach the social worker or agency for assistance. Some caregivers have been providing assistance for years and even decades, and may be fearful of their continuing ability to fill this role as they themselves age. For example, Betty and her husband are in their seventies, and she is a carrier of the gene that causes hemophilia. (In the early years of the epidemic, the blood supply was not thoroughly tested. As a result, many hemophiliacs, whose treatment requires blood products, became infected with HIV and other blood-borne pathogens. Some of these individuals have survived and have had HIV for decades.) Betty has already lost her second son, who was increasingly ill, and a brother to the HIV epidemic She rarely sleeps more than a few hours a night because of her care giving, and they drive hundreds of miles a week for his medical appointments. She needs emotional and tangible support as a caregiver, and reassurance that this role will be filled for her son if she is unable to physically continue. These needs require that the social worker understand a myriad of community resources.

Life Stage Factors

The client's life stage is always a consideration in providing social work services. Changes in physiology, life circumstances, and emotional needs occur across the entire life cycle. Significant life events tend to occur at certain ages and are relatively predictable. People fifty and older face several such life stages. Consider that many people will live into their eighties or nineties. While the aging process for persons with HIV is not well researched and understood, this suggests that people with HIV who are over fifty still have many years left.

Often, people in their fifties and even early sixties find themselves still having significant responsibility for their children while potentially having increasing responsibility for their own aging parents. Lengthening life spans in the United States can mean caring for one's parents well into one's own older years. For example, the authors know of several instances where persons eighty years of age and older are still caring for mothers who are one hundred years of age and older.

Among the other developmental tasks for older years is retirement. On the one hand, retirement brings changes in a person's life situation. On the other hand, many older people have planned to retire at a certain age only to find that they are either forced into a early retirement for which they are financially unprepared or unable to retire when they would like due to financial concerns. Retirement brings emotional adjustments that can be both positive and negative. These can include new living arrangements due to a need to reduce costs or a desire to simplify life, less-meaningful work, relationship changes with significant others, reduced income, and increased time for leisure or volunteering.

With passing years, there is more and more loss to face, as friends and family members die and the aging person is confronted by his or her own limitations. Needless to say, living these years with a chronic illness confounds these transitions. For example, the deaths of family and friends may significantly weaken support networks on which the HIV-positive person has relied.

Gender Differences

The average age for women to reach menopause in the United States is about fifty-one years. Since women who are postmenopausal can no longer get pregnant, they may not feel a need to use contraceptives, including condoms. Stereotypes about HIV and gay men abound and older heterosexual populations (female or male) have not been exposed to the same types of sex education, including education about risks of unprotected sex. Both the risks and hence prevention education about it have become the norm for younger adults but are new to older populations. People who are older are likely to approach relationships quite differently from how they did when they were younger.

Gay Men

Gay men over the age of fifty have seen a revolution in their lifetimes in that the gay culture is a part of the media, internet, and social and political discourse.

Despite the greater amount of information available to them, many gay men continue to feel isolated, whether they live in small towns, rural areas, or large urban enclaves. Some of the support networks that once existed for people with HIV are no longer viable options for social support. Factors contributing to this decrease in support systems are the deaths of peers, changes in the overall context of the epidemic, and changes in how HIV services are conceptualized by providers and policy makers. Many older gay men have lost peers to the HIV epidemic and older age. Furthermore, changes in who is affected by HIV and the policy responses to those changes, have reduced the focus on gay men and shifted the way services are provided. An additional factor in the lives of gay men is that much of gay media focuses on handsome young gay men, and older men may have a hard time identifying with these images. They may feel inadequate for not living up to perceived societal expectations.

Death and Dying

The prospect of death challenges most people. The younger a person, the less real the prospect is, with the death of a friend or family member coming as an occasional shock. Over the course of one's life, death becomes more and more a real and immediate presence in a person's life. For an older person, even someone fifty to sixty, the imminence of death becomes inescapable. Parents, perhaps even siblings, are becoming more frail and vulnerable. Many people's parents and siblings have already died. Each day, people of the person's age are listed in the obituaries. As the decades pass, more and more contemporaries and loved ones die.

Yet while the certainty of death becomes more real for everyone over time, people handle the prospect of losing others and facing death themselves in different ways. Some accept death while others fear or dread death. Religious beliefs often color the way people feel about death. For example, people who have a deep sense of judgment from God may fear death, particularly if their lifestyle has included behaviors judged unacceptable in their religious tradition.

Facing a potentially fatal illness often changes the way people approach both life and death from the moment of discovery on. It would be helpful to review Elisabeth Kübler-Ross' works on death and dying and AIDS for her interpretation of these life stages, which include denial, bargaining, depression, anger, and acceptance. (See chapter 14 for more about the stages of grief with respect to integration of spirituality in social work practice.) Though people do not always progress through these stages chronologically, the stages are a helpful framework for understanding many people's experiences. People who have been living with HIV or who have been affected by HIV for decades have progressed through these stages several times and continue to gain new insights.

> **Box 8.1. You and Death**
>
> 1. What personal experiences have you had with death?
>
> 2. Have you ever imagined your own death or that of someone close to you? What was that like?
>
> 3. What feelings generally come to you when you consider the idea of death?
>
> 4. What do you think happens when people die?
>
> 5. How do your own religious beliefs (or lack of beliefs) influence your thoughts and feelings about death?

Medical Issues

Older people with HIV encounter specific health concerns that social workers are not expected to treat but of which they should have a reasonable understanding. A major concern is the impact of both HIV and aging on the neurocognitive system. HIV not only has an impact on the immune system, but also is harbored in the cells of the central nervous system (the brain and spinal cord). Therefore, HIV over the long term can have a profound effect on a person's cognitive ability. When an older person with HIV develops memory issues, a health-care practitioner should thoroughly assess that person for dementia to determine if there is an organic cause, possibly related to HIV. In fact, some health-care practitioners advocate for cognitive evaluation of all people with HIV to assess for subtle changes.

Comorbidities such as hypertension, diabetes, cardiac issues, neuropathy, and peripheral vascular disease are exacerbated in people with HIV. These conditions are found in some people who are aging, and the impact of having HIV disease for many years may be a factor in their severity. In addition, a high percentage of people with HIV (50 to 70 percent) are cigarette smokers (Reynolds, 2009). This can lead to cancer and chronic obstructive pulmonary disease, as well as to an increase in the previously mentioned conditions.

Specifically, HIV increases the likelihood of the following:

- Hypertension and cardiac disease: HIV or the medication that treats it may cause an increase in blood pressure, cholesterol, and general heart disease. Since these are also problems of aging populations, people with HIV are at higher risk.

- Diabetes: Many of the early HIV medications caused increased glucose intolerance, and therefore a number of people developed diabetes. Diabetes can also lead to peripheral vascular disease (see below).

- Peripheral vascular disease: HIV, diabetes, neuropathy, and smoking can lead to damage of the arteries. This in turn causes pain and loss of blood supply. Unfortunately, this can lead to the need for amputations.

- Neuropathy: Both HIV and the early meds that treated it can cause damage that leads to pain in the peripheral nervous system (feet and hands). This is burning, searing, debilitating pain that is very difficult to relieve. It is severe enough to affect mobility and general functioning.

- Many older people with HIV are being treated for multiple conditions, and may be on dozens of medications. The conflicting side effects of the latter are not well researched or understood. It is known that polypharmacy (taking many medications) may lead to medication errors (taking the wrong medication or dose) and increasingly dangerous effects. Since older people metabolize medications more slowly than do young people, the risk of toxicity or liver damage is increased with more medications and is higher for older than for younger adults.

Men who are older often experience erectile dysfunction (ED). The extent to which this is a concern to many men seems reflected in or perhaps encouraged by the proliferation of ads for this problem. Viagra and Cialis, the two most popular name-brand prescription drugs for ED, ranked thirty-second and fifty-fifth, respectively, in total sales of pharmaceuticals in the United States in 2009. These meds and improved treatment allow older men to be sexually active in ways that probably would not have been possible in the past. This reality in turn increases their likelihood of becoming infected with sexually transmitted diseases (STDs), including HIV. Since men using these ED meds are able to have a more extensive sex life, there is increased need to include STI prevention messages in interventions with them.

Finally, HIV disease can cause changes in one's body image that increase with age, including lipodystrophy, a condition where one's body fat is redistributed from the extremities to the trunk. Many people who were on early HIV medication experienced changes such as "buffalo hump" (fat accumulation in the upper back), "Crix belly" (fat accumulation in the torso that was related to the med Crixivan), and "AIDS face" (fat depletion in the cheeks). Although these are somewhat treatable through medication, surgery, or injections, the impact on self-esteem can be significant, and an important social work role is to help the client cope with his or her feelings about these changes.

Unfortunately, the nature of the immune system means that healing and immune responses are significantly affected as one ages. This process, called immune senescence, means that the thymus gland and other immune organs no longer produce cells to fight infection. This aging mechanism may explain the fact that half of adults over the age of fifty who are diagnosed with HIV, are diagnosed with AIDS within one year of diagnosis (Hab/HRSA).

Box 8.2. Self-Reflection and Application

Make a list of five older adults you know who are not family members. Do that before you read the reflections below. Once you have the list, consider these ideas:

- Think about sex and being sexual, then picture each of those five people being sexual.

- What is your reaction to that idea?

- Can you imagine talking to any of them about sexual behaviors?

- What might you say? How do you imagine them responding?

Psychosocial Needs

Older persons living with HIV have a variety of needs that they share with younger populations. Some are likely more pressing due to the interface of HIV with aging. Depression is common among older people who often face isolation and significant loss within their personal lives and in their relationships with others. Depression is often missed or ignored by both families and service providers, including physicians and social workers. Data from a large study in New York suggest that depression is linked to other problems such as financial problems, limited emotional support, living alone, and stigma. Depression also is more likely to be linked to suicide ideation. Finally, depression, when there is greater stress in the person's life, is related to poorer health indicators such as lower CD4 counts (Karpiak et al., 2006).

The Research on Older Adults with HIV study (Karpiak et al., 2006) further suggests that loneliness, which many older adults experience, is even more likely among older people living with HIV and likely contributes to depression. Karpiak and colleagues suggest that the findings relate to the quality of support people have, not to how often they interact with others or how big their support network is. They also suggest that the stigma of HIV is a factor in the sense of loneliness. (Stigma is discussed in more detail in a later section of this chapter.) Developing interventions that reduce loneliness by improving the quality of support for and acceptance about the HIV status of the older person is likely to be quite important when developing programs and when working with individuals. The same study suggests that past substance abuse is quite prevalent among older persons with HIV, at least those in urban settings. Current use of unprescribed mood-altering drugs, including alcohol and illicit drugs, was not uncommon with more than half smoking, and nearly one-third actively drinking or using illicit substances, or both. Aside from the mood-altering effects of these drugs, the interactions between them and HIV medications can be problematic. Substance abuse is often ignored in older populations or simply not recognized as a potential issue. It is very important for workers to explore and consider possible substance misuse and abuse. Substance use and abuse, including accidental abuse due to prescription meds, can mimic dementia and physicians can easily miss it. Social workers can help identify these concerns.

Bias and Lack of Competency as Barriers

As always, bias lurks in many places in the lives of our clients. There is ageism and ignorance about the concerns and needs of aging persons within HIV support systems, while conversely there is stigma and ignorance about HIV in the supports associated with aging. The social worker is often the person who ensures the environment is appropriate, so that clients are treated fairly and receive competent services. The social worker also may be the person who works with the informal support systems people have to make sure they are actually helpful and supportive of their aging family member or friend.

Let's start with the HIV service delivery system. HIV is primarily transmitted through sexual behavior or drug use at present. Many social workers focus efforts of prevention and identification of infected people on those who are perceived as most likely to be sexually active. Workers may have limited training and experience working with older populations. If workers are younger, their experience with older populations may be limited to relationships with grandparents, people at church, and social work professors. Among younger workers whose clients are older persons affected by HIV, there may be limited understanding of aging needs.

Even those experienced with older populations may not recognize the possibility of HIV for their clients or residents. On a related note, although programs serving older populations may recognize that there are potential HIV-related needs amongst their clientele, overall they are ill prepared to work with those needs (Emlet, Gerkin, & Orel, 2009). For example, a social worker at a local nursing home met with a patient and his adult children when he was admitted, and was surprised to learn the patient was HIV positive. He had been sexually assaulted many years before and had never been tested until an astute emergency room doctor realized he had been admitted with pneumonia several times. He was in his seventies, and due to his state of confusion was unable to live on his own. The nursing home administration was reluctant to allow him to live in their facility for fear other families would be concerned. Fortunately, the social worker had spent considerable time learning about HIV and was able to advocate for the patient.

Stigma, Fear, and Denial

The prior section focused on potential bias in the service delivery system but bias in communities and families also plays a role in access to and effectiveness of prevention and intervention for older persons. One such form of bias is stigma. The stigma associated with AIDS has diminished somewhat since the early days of the disease. Stigma associating the disease with being gay has been mediated by increased acceptance of same-sex sexuality in many quarters of the United States. Fear, which once led even nurses to avoid contact with patients known to have HIV, has been mitigated to some extent by understanding about transmission of the virus and, optimistically, increased compassion for persons who are infected. Still, stigma and fear are not gone. Stigma seems to be especially strong in certain communities or for certain populations, including communities of color, rural areas, and older people. There is some reason to believe that there are also regional differences in stigma and fear. Urban areas may offer more safety from these twin challenges. When two or more of these intersect, the impact on the client can be significant. Stigma and fear also affect the delivery of services, both (1) prevention and (2) treatment or intervention. It is essential for the social worker to understand the community context in which he or she is providing services to this population and to assess the amount of stigma present, along with the factors contributing to it.

One effect of stigma can be unwillingness of older persons to disclose their status to others. Karpiak and colleagues (2006) found that two-fifths of participants in their study had not told someone they wanted to tell about their status. Who were they most like to have told? Their health-care providers (more than 90 percent). Who were they least likely to have told? People in their place of worship (about 35 percent).

Box 8.3. Popcorn Exercise

Take out two pieces of paper. On one write, "older people." On the other write, "people living with HIV."

Without taking a lot of time to think about your answers, under each heading jot down all the words that come to mind for you when you think about each of these. Don't be shy! Let's just get it out there so you can deal with it!

If you did this exercise in class, compare notes with one other person to see where your knowledge shows and where you might have some bias. You may also do this on your own.

Rural versus Urban Issues

Much of the research and many of the service models for working with general populations of people who have HIV were developed in urban settings. Particularly early in the epidemic, urban areas were epicenters of the epidemic, and policy makers and service providers paid little attention to how the needs of persons in rural areas were being met. Rural areas have their share of persons with HIV. Rural areas are also unique service delivery areas with characteristics that influence the ways in which clients believe they can access services and address their HIV generally.

Rural health systems are typically less sophisticated than those in urban areas, which are often affiliated with university-based medical schools. Probably because the population is more sparse, health-care facilities are more spread out, with clients sometimes having to travel hours to reach an infectious disease health-care team. Specialized health care in general is less readily available in rural areas due to the relatively lesser amount of demand. Other systems of formal services and supports are similarly limited. Compounding this barrier, older people often lose mobility and may be less confident about their ability to drive safely. Driving between communities or even within counties in rural areas is nearly always on local highways, county roads, or even, in some areas, unpaved roads. Public transportation may be limited within counties and nonexistent across counties, even as clients may need to travel through several counties to reach health-care providers. These factors combine to make transportation a very important component of the services needed in rural areas.

Poverty, substandard housing, few jobs that offer health insurance, and isolation add to the risks of being HIV positive in rural communities. Stigma about homosexuality, sex outside marriage, or drug use may be greater in rural communities, which may discourage people who are at risk from finding out their status. Additional concerns regarding confidentiality in small communities, where everyone knows everyone else, increase the isolation. People who know that they are HIV positive may avoid seeking treatment and social services due to realistic concerns about others finding out. In rural areas, people may recognize each other's cars, noticing the person is parked outside the infectious disease clinic or wonder why the social worker is visiting the person's home. There may be only one pharmacy and the pharmacy might have to order the HIV meds rather than having them in stock. Each point of accessing services is a potential point where an individual may be exposed.

For older persons, particularly those who learn their status later in life, the picture may be even more complicated. Little research exists for older persons with HIV in rural areas. However, many older people in rural areas have lived in the same area, even in the same house, all of their lives. If there are younger adults with HIV living in the area, the older adult may have known them as children. This may decrease the ability of older adults to gain support from other people with HIV who live locally.

Resource Issues

As aptly expressed by the character in *Fried Green Tomatoes,* "I'm older and I have better insurance," one of the benefits of aging is a higher rate of medical coverage. In the United States, the rate of insurance coverage increases with age, and nearly all older adults can access Medicare after age sixty-five. However, many people face gaps in coverage, especially in their medication or pharmaceutical coverage. While at the time of this writing there is a federally funded program to assist people with the cost of securing their HIV medication, the budget for such programs is increasingly under fire in Congress. Direct advocacy and supports for clients in advocating for their own programs are important roles for social workers to take.

As people age, they are less likely to find work that will meet their financial needs or that they are physically able to do. As a result, even those who were previously self-sufficient may become more financially strained than in previous years. Working with older people with HIV requires that the social worker understand local, state, and national benefits programs. Nationally, policy makers are coming to recognize the treatment and social support needs of older adults with HIV as a significant concern. There is now a National HIV/AIDS and Aging Awareness Day. However, stigma and bias at all levels, including at the policy-making level, continue to plague this age group.

Box 8.4. The AIDS Institute

One organization interested in issues of HIV/AIDS and aging is The AIDS Institute (http://www.theaidsinstitute.org/). In 2011, The AIDS Institute hosted the HIV/AIDS and Aging Awareness Day. Links to presentations made for the event can be found at http://www.theaidsinstitute.org/education/hivaids-and-aging-awareness.

Effective Implementation of Social Work Principles

Social work values include self-determination and respect for the dignity of the client. Yet, their professional training can sometimes lead social workers to trust their own judgment over that of the client. Older clients who have had HIV for a number of years typically know much more about their own disease and needs than the worker does. Treatments for HIV and related disorders can be complex and sometimes idiosyncratic. Additionally, the structure of services requires the involvement of the social worker in securing some benefits, even if the client is completely competent to access services on his or her own. Less-experienced workers, in particular, need to be very attuned to the client. Younger workers' primary relationships with older persons may be within their own families, with aging grandparents, and they may unwittingly use these relationships as a point of reference in their work. One approach in addressing this bias is to solicit the client's input on an ongoing basis. Trusting clients to know their own situation and respecting their decisions about themselves is a fundamental tenet of social work, yet workers are sometimes tempted to impose their own ideas or, particularly with older clients, interact in ways that the client interprets as patronizing.

Assessment

Assessment is always a key to effective work with clients. Concrete needs such as insurance status, future financial security, and adequacy or appropriateness of living arrangements are relevant. Health conditions that may emerge as people age include diabetes, cardiovascular disease, osteoporosis, cancer, and dementia. While medical concerns such as these are properly addressed by health-care professionals, the social worker must be attentive to the additional needs that emerge when these health conditions intersect with HIV in order to ensure that the client secures appropriate services. Furthermore, supports are often needed as people negotiate living with these health conditions.

The social worker should carefully assess the possibility of depression in an aging person, as was discussed earlier in this chapter. Since depression is linked to such problems as less support, lack of HIV-related information, suicide risk, and a suppressed immune system, it is essential for social workers to identify and promptly treat depression. Depression is not necessarily evidenced by sadness, but may be seen in other affective expressions and physical health symptoms. Unfortunately, depression is still stigmatized and therefore both clients and their service providers or caregivers may ignore or miss its presence. Tools are available to assess depression, such as the Beck Depression Inventory.

Older women are often an invisible population in HIV work. Furthermore, even though the proportion is not quite as high as in the general population of women with HIV, older women tend to be disproportionately of color. Emlet, Tangenberg, and Siverson (2002) proposed the use of a feminist approach to work with women, particularly older women, as the challenges they face due to sexism, racism, and ageism in combination with their HIV status are significant and unique to them. These authors' work enumerates those challenges and suggests services that promote connection (such as women-only support groups and facilitation of social opportunities) and that teach relational skills (empathy and mutuality) while affirming the bias that the women face. Settings in which women can discuss their unique needs, such as needs surrounding menopause, negotiating sexual relationships with male partners, and caregiving not related to young children, are needed. While an empowerment approach is a general principle of social work, it is especially important with this population to listen to the needs expressed by the women themselves.

Models for prevention, such as that proposed by Pamela Foster (2007), may be useful. While Foster proposed this model for African Americans in rural settings, many of the issues facing older persons with HIV, particularly in rural areas, are quite similar to those she describes. Stigma, fear, and denial are the barriers identified in this model as areas to target for improved prevention. Three core elements are identified to reduce or eliminate stigma, fear, and denial.

The first element is a community-based empowerment approach. For application to the aging population, this approach would likely involve reaching and educating clergy, leaders of women's groups at religious congregations, and groups that tend to be older, such as service clubs (e.g., Rotary and Kiwanis) and groups that are even less formal that reach women, such as the Red Hat Society (www.redhatsociety.org, and on Facebook).

The second element is cultural sensitivity, which seeks to reduce stigma, fear, and denial through increasing awareness among service providers about the presence of these three barriers for older people (stigma, fear, and denial).

The third and final element is to create social action to actually remove the conditions that promote stigma, fear, and denial. It is always a big challenge to change social conditions. However, the principles of social work consistently and readily identify facilitating social change, whether funded or not, as the duty of an ethical social worker.

Developing Effective and Helpful Support Systems

Social workers should always consider both formal and informal support systems in work with clients. Most clients need both. Informal systems are particularly helpful to older persons because they include people with whom the person has often had a long-standing relationship. Informal systems typically have little cost, making them feasible where formal systems of support, with their greater cost, may not be available. As noted elsewhere, informal support systems can be especially important in rural areas where formal systems are spread out geographically and where people have limited resources.

Often people who are older have relied on informal support systems heavily, and those support systems are beginning to unravel. Adult children, although often well connected to their aging parents, have other responsibilities and may live too far away to be of help with day-to-day needs. Friends who have been a natural helping network often are becoming less functional themselves or may need to focus their energy on a spouse who is experiencing illness or dementia. Many people in older people's social and support networks are simply gone, having moved away to be closer to children, or having died. Some fortunate older adults have continuing support from their religious congregations, but this support may be limited because many friends in their congregation are likely to be their age, with related limitations.

Increasingly, funders such as the federal government expect and require cooperation and coordination between different service domains. This expectation is institutionalized in agreements, coordinating agencies, and interagency structures. This mandated coordination is less visible between aging and HIV services. Social workers must be actively aware of the need for collaboration between service delivery systems. Their role is often that of facilitating coordination and then ensuring implementation of increased, ongoing collaboration both in the overall service delivery system and on behalf of individual clients.

Summary

Older populations have always been a part of the HIV epidemic yet are historically under-recognized and underserved. The medical and psychosocial needs of older people are unique, and must be carefully addressed by social workers, whether or not the setting in which they work is HIV specific. Furthermore, these needs are often a constellation of related and even interlocking factors that together are overwhelming to the older person. Isolation and loneliness lead to depression, which is exacerbated by the losses of aging. Stigma and fear may discourage the use of services, including those that might address the depression and loneliness.

Often the social worker will be the one person who recognizes the complexities of the older person's situation and who is equipped and willing to address that situation. This action includes addressing factors such as the extent of isolation and stigma as well as the discrimination facing the older person with HIV. Respect and genuine regard, careful listening and assessment, thoughtful planning and intervention, and assertive advocacy are among the competencies social workers need to bring to their work with older populations. Work with older adults is a growing area of social work practice, and the area of HIV with older adults can be a particularly rewarding social work practice setting.

Case Example

"Happy Holiday" is a seventy-year-old man who has lived with HIV for thirty years. As a younger man, he studied for the priesthood and before that was married briefly to a woman. He has two adult children from that marriage, which ended amicably. Happy Holiday came out as a gay man in the 1970s. Originally from a medium-sized city in the Midwest, he moved to San Francisco when he realized he was gay. He had many partners at that time and worked as a bartender and stripper. When he first tested positive, he was told he had two years to live. Despite many setbacks, he has beat the odds and survived three decades.

Recently, Happy lived in a senior housing project. He was uncomfortable there because he felt like an outsider, perceiving that his neighbors were uncomfortable with him. He moved into a small apartment complex where he now lives. Still, he is very isolated. He worries that if he becomes ill his guardian will move him into a nursing home where he will not be accepted as a gay man. He has some contact with his two children, who live in a nearby state. However, he is not confident he can count on them to be there for him on a regular basis.

Happy keeps somewhat busy with his collection of Christmas ornaments, which he plans to donate to a local museum. However, he is frustrated because he misses socializing with other people. He tried to write an autobiography recently, but it reminded him of his many losses and he became depressed. Sometimes he feels that his life is over, and questions why he survived the early years of the pandemic when so many others did not.

For about two years, Happy has struggled with health issues. The neuropathy in his feet became so painful he fell a number of times, which particularly dismayed him when he broke some of his Christmas ornament collection. He also became diabetic and had to start managing his diet and tracking his blood sugar. His health has improved significantly, but he now struggles with depression. Additionally, practical issues such as transportation to events and medical appointments continue to challenge him. He no longer drives due to the cost of maintaining a car as well as to the neuropathy in his feet. He relies on public transportation and two friends. None of these is a reliable means of getting to appointments, as the public van is often late and his friends both work during business hours when most of his appointments are. He is in significant pain, for which he takes a high dose of narcotics (morphine derivatives). Unfortunately, his pain meds sometimes cause him constipation and drowsiness. He is dependent on these medications and feels frustrated because his nurse constantly questions his use of high doses of meds.

He and his most recent partner broke up several years ago, and although he would like to date, Happy does not know anyone whom he could date. He has few friends his age in the gay community and few friends sharing his sexual orientation in the aging community. He sometimes reminisces with the social worker about all the men he knew at the bathhouses when he first came out. Of the twenty-five or so men he knew back then, including many with whom he was sexually involved, only three are still alive. He wonders why he survived when so many did not. He feels alone in part because so few of his contemporaries survived the early days of the HIV epidemic. Happy does keep in touch with some people via the internet, mostly Facebook, which has allowed him to reconnect with people he had not talked to or seen in years.

Questions for Reflection

- What are some of the challenges Happy faces because he is both aging and homosexual?

- What would be the appropriate roles of the social worker in Happy's life?

- What specific needs must the social worker address to assist Happy?

- What long-term plans should be in place?

- How comfortable would you be to work with Happy? Examine any biases you have. How might these impact your work with him?

Web Resources

National Institutes of Health (NIH): http://aidsinfo.nih.gov/ General information about HIV that is reliable and evidence based.

AARP (formerly American Association of Retired People): www.aarp.org. Numerous articles and resources, such as "HIV/AIDS Prevention Pushed for the 50+": http://www.aarp.org/relationships/love-sex/info-02-2008/aids_prevention_for_50plus_pushed.html.

HIV Wisdom for Older Women: http://www.hivwisdom.org/

AIDS Education Global Information System: www.aegis.com. This site is not exclusively about aging and HIV, but includes detailed information about HIV. There are research reports, news articles, and statistics and data about the epidemic in the United States and around the world.

References

Centers for Disease Control and Prevention (CDC). (2011). *Basic statistics.* Retrieved from http://www.cdc.gov/hiv/topics/surveillance/basic.htm#hivaidsage

Emlet, C. A., Gerkin, A., & Orel, N. (2009). The graying of HIV/AIDS: Preparedness and needs of the aging network in a changing epidemic. *Journal of Gerontological Social Work, 52,* 803–814.

Emlet, C. A., Tangenberg, K., & Siverson, C. (2002). A feminist approach to practice in working with midlife and older women with HIV/AIDS. *Affilia, 17,* 229–251.

Foster, P. H. (2007). Use of stigma, fear, and denial in development of a framework for prevention of HIV/AIDS in rural African American communities. *Community Health, 30,* 318–327.

Karpiak, S. E., Shippy, R. A., & Cantor, M. (2006). *Research on older adults with HIV (ROAH).* New York: AIDS Community Research Initiative of America.

Reynolds, N. R. (2009). Cigarette smoking and HIV—More evidence for action. *AIDS Education and Prevention, 23* (Suppl. A), 106–121.

U.S. Census Bureau. (May, 2011). *Age and sex composition: 2010 census briefs.* Retrieved from http://www.census.gov/prod/cen2010/briefs/c2010br-03.pdf

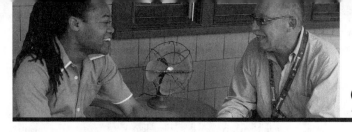

9

HIV-Affected Populations:
A Ripple Effect

Kimi Fey Powers and Diana Rowan

If you find it in your heart to have cared for someone else, you will have
succeeded.

—Maya Angelou

Introduction

Over the past three decades, the face of the HIV/AIDS (human immunodeficiency
virus and acquired immune deficiency syndrome) pandemic has changed. What
was once considered gay-related immune disease (GRID), or the gay plague, is now
more accurately understood as an illness that has deeply affected people from all
walks of life. The day-to-day impacts of HIV on society can be illustrated as having
a metaphorical ripple effect, starting with the HIV-positive individuals, and con-
centrically spreading to their families, friends, and communities. HIV-affected populations encompass everyone whose lives are impacted by the HIV/AIDS pandemic.

This chapter addresses the scope of the unique challenges of serving HIV-affected
(as opposed to HIV-infected) populations from a social work perspective. The
HIV-affected groups that social workers encounter in practice can be divided into
broad categories: spouses and partners, children, parents, friends, formal caregivers, and communities of HIV-positive persons. The needs of HIV-affected populations are as diverse as their members, though there are commonalities: stigma-
related issues, emotional strain, financial hardships, role conflicts, and health
issues. As such, social workers must employ an eclectic approach to meet the many
challenges that arise. This chapter explores several social work roles for interventions with HIV-affected individuals, including medical case management, individual and group psychotherapy, advocacy, and modeling of self-care.

Overarching social work values and ethics are invaluable in guiding practitioners to "meet the client where they are," and in developing effective therapeutic relationships. Of these, the profession of social work's respect for confidentiality and belief in the worth and dignity of all individuals are paramount. Stigma is a powerful divider of communities. Fear of contracting the virus still exists in HIV-negative communities, and this fear drives the perpetuation of stigma. In turn, stigma instills fear in those who are HIV positive—that they will be labeled, then discriminated against by strangers, employers, health-care providers, friends, and family members. Stigma has lessened over the past two decades, but it is still a powerful silencer (Gilbert, 2001; Mason, Berger, Estwing Ferrans, Sultzman, & Fendrich, 2010). For this reason, confidentiality is an essential ethical consideration for social workers in HIV/AIDS work. Before a meaningful therapeutic relationship can be formed, social workers must convince their clients that without exception they will handle clients' personal information with confidentiality.

A majority of HIV-positive and HIV-affected populations are likely to have encountered discrimination. Historically, groups experiencing discrimination include ethnic or racial minorities, low socioeconomic status, same-sex or bisexual orientation, single mothers, and substance abusers (Adamsen, 2002; Flores, 1997; Heckman et al., 2004; Sikkema et al., 2005). Social workers who interface with these clients must believe in the inherent worth and dignity of all people, regardless of ethnicity, socioeconomic status, sexual orientation, religion, cultural beliefs, lifestyle choices, and, equally, HIV status.

There are two important caveats for the readers of this chapter. The first is that the biopsychosocial issues of HIV-affected individuals identified will not be present in all HIV-affected populations. Indeed, every family member, friend, loved one, formal caregiver, and community affected by HIV must be treated as an individual; these populations embody all socioeconomic statuses, ethnicities, levels of functioning, and health statuses. The second caveat is that the focus of this chapter is social work practice with HIV-affected populations within the United States, and thus represents only a fraction of the global impact of HIV and AIDS.

Who Is HIV Affected?
Racial and Ethnic Minorities

HIV in the United States disproportionately affects racial and ethnic minorities (Heckman et al., 2004; Sikkema et al., 2005). Some African Americans and Latinos face life challenges of poverty, substance abuse and dependence, lack of access to health care, and inadequate educational and employment opportunities (Snell-Johns, Mendez, & Smith, 2004). And, the wide array of HIV-related issues further exacerbates the complexity of the socioeconomic obstacles faced by these under-served and economically disadvantaged populations (Rotheram-Borus, Stein, & Lester, 2006).

Social workers should value cultural competence when working with racial and ethnic minorities. It is helpful to acknowledge that within African-American com-munities there may be a stigma on receiving mental health services that is greater than the stigma present in White communities. A culturally sensitive social worker will be aware of this potential for stigma and resistance to services. In practice set-tings with socioeconomically disadvantaged populations, stigma was identified as a significant barrier to using a service. In these situations, social workers can reach the client through creative engagement of their natural support systems. Outreach programs, such as culturally relevant partner counseling and support groups, can be promoted through churches and other community-based institutions (CBOs) in communities of color (Poindexter, 2003).

Among all races and ethnic groups, women are more likely than men to be care-givers. African-American women, in particular, have been providing care for others for many generations, in both informal and formal helping roles. They are often seen as strong, supportive resources in their communities, and often "live lives of self-sacrifice and dedication to the needs of others" (Land, 2010, p. 317). With African-American women at high risk for HIV transmission, HIV caregivers may also be HIV positive themselves. Supportive services for caregivers should "be gen-der-sensitive and focus on the needs of the African American female experience" (Land, 2010, p. 319).

Partners of HIV-Positive Individuals

Partners of HIV-positive individuals may themselves be HIV negative; such cou-ples are termed sero-discordant, as opposed to sero-concordant, where both are HIV positive. Couples of mixed HIV status (sero-discordant) face unique and complex realities. HIV disease imposes drastic emotional and sexual difficulties for affected partners and demands a constant shift in relationship dynamics. Stigmas both from within and imposed on the relationship are inversely related to relation-ship satisfaction and stability. HIV-related stigma also influences the partners' perceptions of self-worth, sexual functioning, and power in making reproductive decisions (Talley & Bettencourt, 2008).

Many emotional conflicts may arise in an HIV-affected intimate relationship. In some situations the relationship existed prior to the HIV transmission and in some cases it did not. Upon disclosure of HIV-positive status, among the first emotions to surface are distrust and frustration about the means by which a partner has acquired HIV (Beckerman, 2002; Poindexter, 2003). The uncertainty of the progression of a partner's illness is a primary concern of the HIV affected. An HIV-negative individual is often acutely aware that a partner may get sick at any time, which often leads to emotional distancing as a protective mechanism (Beckerman, 2002). Psychosocial factors significantly impact the prognosis for the HIV-infected person. Historically, there are higher rates of morbidity and mortality for non-White and socioeconomically challenged individuals with HIV. In association, HIV-positive men who have sex with men (MSM) and their partners are more likely to perceive HIV/AIDS as a terminal condition, rather than one that is life-long, but manageable. If they are of lower education level and have a higher level of perceived race-based discrimination, they are also more likely to see AIDS as a death sentence, not a chronic, manageable condition. Studies have suggested that those who can find positive meaning in illness have higher levels of well-being and long-term survival (Hoy-Ellis & Fredriksen-Goldsen, 2007).

Sexually active sero-discordant couples face the risk of transmitting HIV to the uninfected partner. The fear and anticipatory guilt associated with potential transmission can significantly alter their sexual relationship (Beckerman, 2002). The HIV-negative partner may actively engage in unprotected intercourse because of feelings of invincibility, a desire to have children, or because the individual may consciously or unconsciously want to contract HIV from his or her partner, to feel closer and stop living in fear of transmission (Beckerman, 2002; Stevens & Galvao, 2007). Reasons for this wish can be a desire to feel closer to a partner, to put an end to the fear associated with HIV transmission, or a desire to share access to the special financial and health-care-related benefits for those living with AIDS. While none of these seems outwardly logical, they all may appear that way in the context of the situation.

There are some ways in which HIV can strengthen partner relationships. Hope regarding further medical advancements and improved care keeps couples active in supporting each other. HIV/AIDS, to varying degrees, has forced partners to embrace death as an inevitable part of life. The realization of the fragility of life can first lead to emotional drifting between partners, then ultimately lead to strengthened commitment to one another, as they place more value in the time spent as a couple (Beckerman, 2002; Poindexter, 2003). Gay men in sero-discordant relationships are reported to have longer relationships than those in concordant-negative and concordant-positive relationships (Hoff et al., 2009). Overall, shared identity as an HIV couple increases strength and intimacy of a relationship (Talley & Bettencourt, 2008).

Key components to social work care for HIV-affected couples include providing interventions focused on improving dyadic communication (Talley & Bettencourt, 2008). Therapy aimed at helping couples communicate openly will be most helpful. Encouraging couples to openly discuss with each other their HIV-related emotional burdens is effective in strengthening their relationship, which in turn strengthens the natural support system for the HIV-positive partner(s). Social workers can also assist in formulating strategies to decrease their sexual risks of transmission, and assist with family planning (Adamsen, 2002; Beckerman, 2002; Corey, 2000; Stevens & Galvao, 2007).

Couples and Children

Antiretroviral therapy (ART) has improved the prognosis of those living with HIV and reduced the risk of vertical transmission (from mother to child) to less than 2 percent in the United States. As such, many more couples where one or both members are HIV positive are inspired to conceive (Matthews & Mukherjee, 2009). However, HIV-affected couples often encounter multiple obstacles to their reproductive freedoms. Health concerns of couples with HIV include fear of transmission of HIV to the HIV-negative partner during intercourse, fear of transmission of HIV to the infant during delivery, and stigma within the health-care system, which does not always outwardly assist HIV-affected couples in having children (Beckerman, 2002; Matthews & Mukherjee, 2009). HIV-affected couples desiring to have biological children are increasingly looking to health-care providers for solutions (Tschudin, 2008).

For couples wanting to conceive, the multidisciplinary health-care team can discuss harm-reduction techniques that reduce horizontal HIV transmission (from partner to partner) such as treating genital infections prior to intercourse. Social workers and other health-care providers can suggest to HIV-affected couples wishing to conceive that they limit intercourse to fertile periods, times of optimal antiretroviral (ARV) medication adherence, and times when lab results show low or undetectable viral loads (amount of HIV in blood). Costly options like artificial intrauterine insemination after sperm washing can be explored for those with adequate resources. Intensive multidisciplinary counseling is the best conduit for managing complex perceptions, realities, and fertility options of HIV-affected couples (Matthews & Mukherjee, 2009; Tschudin, 2008).

Creation of partnerships between the client, his or her support system, the social worker, and other health-care providers maximizes the quality of care. Social workers can help their clients frame their perceptions of HIV through a family-centered approach. In HIV work, an unfortunate reality is that because of stigma, clients may not receive much support from their natural family. In these cases, clients form new familial support systems with others who are not judgmental about their HIV status, sexual orientation, drug use, or lifestyle choices. Using a family-centered approach, social workers can work with health-care providers to effectively educate both patients and their families about the complexities and advancements in treating their chronic but manageable illness (Hoy-Ellis & Fredriksen-Goldsen, 2007). The social worker should be aware that affected couples can be opposite-sex couples or same-sex couples, involve transgender partners, be married or not, and be living in the same home or not.

Children and Adolescents with HIV-Positive Parents

Compounded by the typical growing pains of childhood and the subsequent tumultuous transition from puberty to adulthood, children with HIV-positive parents face unique challenges. HIV-affected children and adolescents are defined as young persons with one or both parents diagnosed with HIV or AIDS, who may themselves be HIV positive. A glimpse into their situations shows that many HIV-affected children are at risk for marginalization either before or in addition to HIV entering their lives. Historically, HIV has disproportionately impacted inner-city, single-parent people of color who are more likely than non-HIV-affected populations to be living at or below poverty level and to have a history of substance abuse. In fact, 80 percent of children in the United States who have lost their parents to HIV/AIDS are members of ethnic minority groups living in low-income communities (Linsk & Mason, 2004; Rotheram-Borus, Lee, Gwadz, & Draimin, 2001).

Parents with AIDS have a disproportionately high incidence of substance abuse. A study by Rotheram-Borus and colleagues (2006) found that 84 percent of the parents of HIV-affected adolescents had been involved in heavy illegal drug use. The role of the family in American culture has a significant impact on the health, socialization, beliefs, and feelings of self-worth of individuals, especially during childhood and adolescence. Many children of substance abusers are at a high risk to continue in their parents' footsteps (Tinsley, Lees, & Sumartojo, 2004). A recent study has shown that if a parent is both HIV positive and has an active drug addiction, the adolescent children had increased maladjustment and substance use (Brook, Brook, Rubenstone, Zhang, & Finch, 2010).

Although stigma is dissipating and the typical life span of HIV-positive individuals is increasing, HIV-affected children still face considerable challenges imposed by their parent(s)' illness. Unlike children of diabetics or cancer patients, children of parents with HIV/AIDS often suffer in silence during an already vulnerable and impressionable phase of their lives. Many affected children are left on their own to face the stigma of HIV and the consequences of unpredictable and prolonged parental illness. Sometimes they have help, but it can be in the form of unreliable guidance from makeshift caregivers from their extended family (Gunther, Crandles, Williams, & Swain, 1998; Linsk & Mason, 2004; McKay et al., 2004). Having a supportive outlet for their varied emotions is critical. However, they may be reluctant to disclose the cause of their parent's illness for fear of isolation from their peers. As Gunther and colleagues (1998, p. 252) state, "These individuals experience a double abandonment, one from the parent leaving them and one from a society that shuns them for being associated with AIDS." Thus, stigma often has a silencing impact. Affected children and adolescents may lack a supportive outlet to confront their grief, which can lead to multiple unresolved stressors (McKay et al., 2004; Pivnick & Villegas, 2000).

These stressors manifest in the form of mental health issues such as anxiety and depression at a significantly higher rate than in unaffected peers (Havens & Mellins, 1996). These stressors can be directly observed through high-risk behaviors such as noncompliant or aggressive behavior in school, truancy, family violence, early sexual encounters, and suicidal ideation (Forehand, Steele, Simon, Morse, & Clark, 1998; Gilbert, 2001; Gunther et al., 1998; Linsk & Mason, 2004; Rosenblum et al., 2005; Rotheram-Borus et al., 2006). These externalizing behaviors are more common in HIV-affected male adolescents and older adolescents than they are in female adolescents, who are likely to suffer from internalizing behaviors such as social withdrawal and isolation more than noninfected peers and HIV-affected males (Rotheram-Borus et al., 2001; Rotheram-Borus et al., 2006).

HIV complicates typical adolescent issues; future growth and personal development may be diminished during this sensitive phase of life. In relation to their peers, HIV-affected adolescents have additional obstacles to overcome in order to develop their identities. According to Erickson, identity formation occurs through many factors such as parental support and encouragement to explore, peer interaction and attachment to friends, as well as to schools and communities (Berk, 2004, p. 385). In regards to identity formation, HIV-affected adolescents who suffer from depression and anxiety, and who isolate themselves from their peers, will not have the same benefit of exploring friends' beliefs and value systems.

Self-determination theory states that when parents promote their adolescents' volitional (autonomous) functioning, the adolescents have a higher level of well-being and academic functioning (Soenes et al., 2007). In many HIV-affected families, adolescents have fewer opportunities to develop autonomous skill sets due to HIV-related family crises. HIV-positive parents may not be able to adequately support their adolescent's exploration of the outside world, especially when home life becomes tumultuous due to illness. Instead of being encouraged to attend after-school activities or to participate in sports or youth groups, many HIV-affected adolescents prematurely are encouraged to take on caregiver roles and family responsibilities, especially if there are younger siblings to look after. In this respect, it is vital that other supplemental authority figures in the adolescents' lives step in to bolster parental support in the promotion of volitional functioning (Berk, 2004; Soenes et al., 2007).

Social workers who practice in schools, hospitals, mental health clinics, community support agencies, and substance abuse facilities are likely to encounter HIV-affected children and adolescents. An overarching theoretical approach is essential to meet the unique needs of these individuals. The strengths perspective, cognitive behavioral therapy, reality therapy, and solution-focused therapy are all valuable frameworks for use in these settings (Adamsen, 2002; Flores, 1997; Gilbert, 2001; Rotheram-Borus et al., 2006). Access to peer support groups, religious youth groups, and afterschool extracurricular activities should be explored (Berk, 2004).

For continuity of care, social workers must be knowledgeable about and connected to outside resources that may serve to bolster the normalcy of the child's life (Kulic, Horne, & Dagley, 2004; Snell-Johns et al., 2004).

The social work strengths perspective demands a shift in focus from problems and deficits to personal strengths and opportunities for success (Corey, 2000; Lietaer, 1984; Saleebey, 1996; Thyer, 2002). Clinicians can help HIV-affected children claim empowerment by helping them identify untapped resources within themselves that can lead to resilience and transformation (Saleebey, 1996). Adolescent clients are very sensitive to the opinions of others, especially authority figures. Once rapport with their social worker has been established, adolescent clients who are questioning their identities will benefit from becoming aware of their personal strengths. The social worker and peers can point these out to them in individual and group counseling.

Parents of HIV-Positive Children

Social workers encounter parents of HIV-positive children in a variety of contexts. HIV-affected parents can be divided into groups, dependent on the age of their HIV-positive children: young children and adolescents, adult children, or grandchildren. Parents of HIV-positive adult children face challenges such as revisiting the role of caretaker both to their adult children as they become ill and to surviving HIV-affected grandchildren. The HIV-affected parent suffers a loss of off time normally afforded to persons of advanced age. These parents face increased stress in caring for others, often when on a fixed income. This dynamic can lead to increased health risks as they put their family's medical needs above their own. With the layering of hardships, parents of adult HIV-positive children find it even more difficult to deal with the typical anticipatory losses of their life stage. The denial of the potential loss of their children to HIV can pose a significant barrier to permanency planning for their grandchildren (Capobianco Boyer & Poindexter, 2005).

Parents of HIV-positive young children and adolescents face daunting challenges; they must manage complex pediatric HIV adherence issues and confront real and perceived stigma directed at their family. These parents may be concurrently ill and may put their children's needs first, to the detriment of their own health. HIV disproportionately affects marginalized populations who may already be overwhelmed by poverty, domestic violence, substance abuse, or a combination of these factors (Davey, Duncan, Foster, & Milton, 2008). These family features make it difficult for parents to place life-saving ARV treatment regimens for their children at the top of their family hierarchy of survival (Childs & Cincotta, 2006).

All HIV-affected parents, regardless of their child's age, battle stigma. Many take on protective roles by defending their child's dignity and encounter associative stigma as a consequence. Even if they are not personally experiencing discrimination, parents still feel the hurt and anger associated with witnessing what occurs in their child's life. This may lead to, even on a subconscious level, managing outside relationships by grouping people according to various dichotomies: safe or betraying, accepting or discriminatory. Social workers can assist family members to handle their anxieties about perceived stigma by helping them anticipate situations where stigma may arise, such as disclosure to extended relatives and friends. The practitioner and family members may rehearse how they want to respond. Social workers can help empower HIV-affected family members who decide to be open about their loved one's diagnosis by encouraging them to speak out publicly against stigma, and to serve as peer advocates (Poindexter, 2005).

Being in a constant state of fight or flight leads to social isolation (Poindexter, 2005). Also, caregivers can repress emotions perceived as taboo. Often the parent develops anger and resentment about the constant demands of the child and the family, which leads to feelings of guilt. The caregiver can repress feelings of hopelessness, disappointment, and waves of overwhelming nonspecific emotions, and the affected parents can develop a skewed discrepancy between their real and ideal selves. Eventually, self-worth becomes synonymous with how well they provide care (Capobianco Boyer & Poindexter, 2005; Gurney, 1995).

Social workers can form a therapeutic alliance with HIV-affected parents by addressing both medical and nonmedical family concerns (Gurney, 1995). The family care-giving dynamics can become very complicated if both a parent and a child are HIV positive. If the positive parent's health declines, he or she may need to access help from the older generation, introducing grandparent caregivers to the system. Important social work roles are to mediate sessions between HIV-affected grandparents and HIV-positive parents, and to raise the question of who will provide care for the HIV-positive child should the parent become too ill. The HIV-affected grandparent(s) are assessed to determine both willingness and capability for providing the complex care for an HIV-positive child. The social worker can help the family make difficult formalized legal guardianship transitions and help navigate the legal system by brokering pro bono or low-fee legal services (Capobianco Boyer & Poindexter, 2005).

Several factors have been identified that lead to less medication adherence in adolescents with HIV. These include advanced HIV disease, being out of school, higher-than-usual alcohol use, depression, and social crises such as a death, a break-up with a boyfriend or girlfriend, a family fight, or a problem in school or on the job (Wiener & Taylor-Brown, 2010). During periods of stress, they are also less likely to practice safe sex. Social workers can assist parents and other caregivers by assisting them to understand that the adolescent will be at higher risk during periods of stress. They also can help assess the youth for these risk factors and provide additional psychosocial support during these times.

Friends and Communities

Social support is vital for ensuring positive psychological outcomes of HIV-positive populations (Talley & Bettencourt, 2008). Valuable support networks include friends, neighbors, church groups, family members, and partners' families. HIV-positive Latinos and African Americans are more likely to rely on social support and religious or spiritually based coping resources than are White Americans. In addition to positive psychological outcomes, stronger connections within communities of color yield higher levels of medical treatment adherence (Sunil & McGhee, 2007). How, in turn, are friends and communities of HIV-positive individuals affected? The positive individual does not want discrimination to carry over to his or her loved ones and may withdraw from valued relationships without disclosing their sero-status. Even still, HIV-affected friends are subjected to stigma by association, referred to as courtesy stigma (Goffman, 1963). When one's status is disclosed, the fear of rejection carries over to HIV-affected friends and leads to their social isolation. Friends pull away from social networks according to the real or perceived threats of discrimination to either themselves or their HIV-positive loved one(s) (Linsk & Gilbert, 2007; Poindexter, 2005).

HIV-positive communities serve as a valuable foundation for normalization of identity for HIV-positive individuals, their families, partners, and friends. Experiencing the comfort and encouragement offered by a supportive community often strengthens bonds inside of family systems affected by HIV. Advocacy against discriminatory stigma is put into action when individuals publicly embrace the HIV-positive community. Such activism has been shown to provide beneficial effects on psychological adjustment and interpersonal functioning of HIV-positive and HIV-affected persons. Identification with a larger group that shares in the common struggles and victories helps shield the HIV-affected individual from potentially debilitating stigma (Talley & Bettencourt, 2008). Social workers can serve as brokers of these supportive communities by facilitating linkages (Snell-Johns et al., 2004).

Formal Caregivers

Addressing the health and mental health needs of the HIV affected is a relatively new focus, since the HIV pandemic is only three decades old. As social workers, it is our ethical obligation to meet these challenges as educators, mediators, group facilitators, psychotherapists, advocates, and community support specialists. This population can be served by social workers in related overarching micro and macro settings, not necessarily just in AIDS service organizations (ASOs).

Clinical social workers comprise a majority of the mental health professionals in North America (Thyer, 2002). A serious consideration for social workers in mental health care, especially in practice with HIV-positive clients, their families, loved ones, and other professional colleagues, is burnout. In order to maintain their own health and mental health, social workers in this setting must believe in the self-efficacy of their client, and maintain hope for continuously improving quality of life of people living with HIV, as well as those affected by HIV. Working in this field can be an emotional, tedious struggle. To combat burnout and compassion fatigue, social workers must adhere to their own treatment plans of self-care and maintain quality supervision.

In the face of limited professional resources, cultivating collaborative relationships with colleagues is essential to creating a supportive workplace. Good teamwork benefits not just the workers, but also the client systems. Cohesive interdisciplinary teams allow all team members involved to glean a more comprehensive scope of issues that their clients have, and to gain valuable professional relationships with which to gain referral sources for their clients (Gilbert, 2001). Though physicians and nurses provide an abundance of technical knowledge, their practice will benefit from the skills of social workers that provide the psychosocial support necessary for comprehensive, quality health care for the patient and the patient's family (Gehlert & Browne, 2006; Oliver & Dykeman, 2003). In many nonprofit agencies, such as ASOs, social workers are usually the dominant professionals. Collaborating social workers in these settings should use one another to process difficult client cases, ventilate, and find common strength through a shared code of ethics and social work values.

Case Example

When the Disease Intervention Specialist (DIS) from the county health department visited her boyfriend to tell him he tested HIV-positive, Chelsea thought she had experienced a huge shock. When she learned the next day that not only was she HIV positive as well, but also that she was pregnant, she called that the shock of her life. The year was 2003. Chelsea was twenty-one years old, a senior in college, and had no idea how to proceed with her life. She lost the support of her boyfriend when he was sent to jail soon after his HIV diagnosis, and she was reticent to tell her family not only that she was going to be a mother, but also that she unknowingly had a life-altering medical situation thrust upon her. She sought support on her college campus. Her university counselor connected her with an advocate at a local ASO in the city. With support, determination, and a steadfast spirit, Chelsea gave birth to a beautiful baby boy, and stayed in school to earn her bachelor's degree. She had no inkling at that time that her introduction to AIDS services would lead to the start of her important career. She kept in touch with her HIV case manager; less than one year later her case manager offered Chelsea a position as a case manager at the ASO. Her responsibilities were to run educational sessions and support groups, broker medical services, and advocate for people living with HIV and AIDS. She discovered that she was able to develop very productive working relationships with the younger clients, and her supervisor began to refer many of the adolescents and young adults to Chelsea, since the other case managers found them to be high maintenance.

As a newcomer to the human services field, Chelsea was eager to make a difference; she was emotionally invested in the personal successes of her clients. One client in particular taught her a valuable lesson about the importance of professional boundaries for human service workers. It was the Christmas season. A new mother, who was recently diagnosed as HIV positive, called Chelsea in a panic. Through sobs she told Chelsea she was about to have her electricity shut off because she couldn't pay her bill. Chelsea tried to calm her client down and spent the whole afternoon trying to tap into Ryan White emergency financial funds. She pled with the power company, and even solicited private donations on behalf of this client. Well past the end of her workday, Chelsea was finally successful in helping the client pay off her balance at the power company. Chelsea felt good about her Christmas victory.

Two months later, she heard from this client again, who was desperate for more money to keep her power on. This time, Chelsea checked the client's chart carefully; she saw she was noncompliant for medical visits, never showed up for support groups, and never came in for her scheduled and rescheduled case management appointments. When Chelsea confronted her about her apparent lack of effort, the client shouted at her angrily then hung up on her, never to call again. From this encounter Chelsea gained perspective that every client, no matter how sad their story, has a role to play in changing his or her own situation; the clients must be held accountable for what they can reasonably control. She knew she had played a part in allowing the client to become dependent on her for finding solutions, rather than empowering her to problem solve for herself. She also learned that it is most beneficial for everyone that she empathize with, not sympathize, with her clients. Chelsea actively decided to be invested in the work she accomplished, to celebrate her clients' successes, and yet not feel responsible for personal outcomes. She has learned to protect the clients' self-determination. She admits that it is a difficult balance, but gets a bit easier with experience. She is also more conscious to let clients assist in finding their own solutions, so that they are more self-sufficient in the future.

> **Box 9.1. The Differences between Sympathy and Empathy**
>
> Sympathy. A feeling or expression of pity or sorrow for the distress of another; commiseration. (Social workers should avoid telling a client that he or she is sympathetic, because the word can be disempowering.)
>
> Empathy. The action of understanding, being aware of, being sensitive to, and vicariously experiencing the feelings, thoughts, and experiences of another. (Often there is a misperception that one must actually have shared the same experiences in order to express empathy.) (National Association of Social Workers [NASW], 2005)

Over time, Chelsea learned to set other boundaries. She was available to her clients through her personal cell phone, but let them know at the start of their working relationship that she would not take calls past 7:00 p.m. Chelsea was eager to educate her community about HIV/AIDS and had powerful messages to deliver, but she soon began feeling overwhelmed with requests for speaking engagements. She learned to decline offers to guest speak and teach at events that were either not scheduled far enough in advance, or were not aligned with her commitment to serving affected youth.

As she took more and more initiative in meeting the unique needs of her clients and their families, Chelsea's job title quickly evolved from case manager to adolescent services coordinator to director of adolescent programs. She conducted parent training sessions and child training sessions, and offered comprehensive medical case management by helping families apply for the AIDS Drug Assistance Program (ADAP), Ryan White emergency financial funds, vision services, and dental services. She helped her patients navigate their medical appointments, from scheduling appointments with trusted medical practitioners to providing bus passes to get there. Chelsea helped provide HIV-affected families access to basic necessities like diapers, clothing, and furniture. Whether it is the young person who is HIV positive or a parent or sibling, many of these affected families struggle to get by. Sometimes they were struggling before the diagnosis, and sometimes having HIV or AIDS is what brings on financial troubles. Chelsea spent time not just with individuals, families, and support groups, but also with community development activities. She participated in a stigma-reducing campaign, "See No AIDS, Only People," and conducted local and national trainings to empower HIV-affected or HIV-positive youth.

Chelsea was developing confidence as a case manager when she first met Alex and his mother, Yvonne. (Some names and details have been altered to maintain confidentiality, but Chelsea's story is a true account of determination and initiative.) They arrived at her office with an interest for Alex to participate in support groups for HIV-positive youth. Alex was a nineteen-year-old African-American college freshman. On his first visit in Chelsea's office, he sat quietly and politely, but not timidly. Chelsea liked him immediately. She liked most of her clients, but not all of them. She knew it was easier to serve clients fairly when she liked them, but realized that was not always possible. In the chair beside Alex, Yvonne sat wringing a tissue in her hands, choking back tears. She began rapid-firing questions about the support group program, and frequently interrupted herself to impress upon Chelsea the direness of their circumstances. When Alex's routine HIV test taken at the family practice physician's office came back positive, he decided to come out of the closet as a gay man. Yvonne had been shocked. Shortly after she learned of Alex's homosexual lifestyle and HIV diagnosis, Yvonne's oldest son died in a car accident. "Alex made it into college, he had so much going for him and now I feel like I've lost both sons." Chelsea immediately looked to Alex, saw him wince, and feared that he was losing his willingness to participate in work with Chelsea. She gently asked Yvonne to wait in the lobby, assuring her that it was customary to screen youth in a one-to-one interview for readiness for support group participation.

Chelsea spoke to Alex candidly, like a capable adult, to which he responded well. They discussed what they both wanted him to get from group, what to expect, logistical details, and the value of confidentiality.

In the group sessions to follow, Alex rarely discussed how his mother's disappointment in him had affected him, but he drew strength from his HIV-positive peers. During one group session, Chelsea hosted a guest who spoke about college grant opportunities for people who are HIV positive. Alex took advantage of that opportunity and received help paying his way through college.

Though she felt she gained ground with Alex, Chelsea sensed that Yvonne was taking Alex's diagnosis harder than he was and was in greater need of support. Chelsea noticed this was a common finding in the parents of her HIV-positive youth and decided that the parents needed a separate support group. She brainstormed with her supervisor and coworkers during a team meeting; her colleagues encouraged her to create a group for parents of HIV-positive youth. She also began meeting individually with Yvonne. At their first session, Yvonne confessed, "I already bought Alex's tombstone. I know it's gonna happen! He's going to die. I bought a double plot engraved tombstone so when it happens he can be next to his brother." Yvonne was suffering from compounded, complicated grief. Over several weeks, Chelsea helped Yvonne compartmentalize and process through her issues; she was still mourning the loss of her oldest son, but was prematurely mourning Alex's death and harboring anger and resentment at the means by which Alex had acquired HIV.

The support group for parents that Chelsea started is still meeting. It operates similarly to Nar-Anon and Al-Anon, where members make an effort to refocus on themselves. It serves as a conduit to help parents feel they are getting control of their lives back. They challenge each other to focus on their own work and hobbies, and to take the opportunity to sleep in on their days off of work instead of setting their alarm clocks to their child's ARV medication schedule. They are encouraged to make peace, reconcile with their children's sexuality, and focus on the well-being of their own relationships. Group members help each other realize that they must allow children to make the transition to adulthood by making decisions for themselves and facing consequences for their own actions. The central empowering, at times frustrating, and ultimately liberating message to the parents is that they cannot control or take responsibility for their children's lives or their HIV. In order to be supportive and helpful parents, they must reestablish the balance in their own lives, which is the only thing over which they should exert control. Throughout the group process, HIV-affected parents are encouraged to gain strength from each other and always maintain hope for the future.

Yvonne became heavily involved in the parent support group and gradually accepted encouragement from other affected parents to do what was best for her. She decided to move back to her hometown to live near her sisters. Though she made significant progress and learned much about living with an HIV-positive son, she is still preparing for his death, though he's not currently sick. As his confidence grew, Alex joined the NAPWA (National Association of People with AIDS) youth conference, and was appointed as a national planner. After he graduated from college, he moved to a major city where he conducts youth HIV work. Alex has refused to allow the virus to slow him down. He blogs as an openly positive, empowered young man.

Chelsea is now married and the mother of two HIV-negative children. She continues to provide services to HIV-positive and HIV-affected youth and their families. Recently, she started a Master of Social Work program and plans to graduate and pursue clinical licensure. Chelsea's goals include communicating openly with her own children about sexual health, seeing comprehensive sex education put into schools, and further breaking down HIV-related stigma.

Questions for Reflection

1. Hindsight is always 20/20. How could Chelsea have handled her encounter with the young HIV-positive mother differently?

2. Yvonne is still having trouble coping with the diagnosis and lifestyle choices of her son Alex. Her care has been transferred to you. She tells you that her sisters forced her to see a counselor because she has been fired from her job as a preschool teacher. Yvonne reports, "I just have no energy. I am so angry and can't sleep because I worry about Alex, especially since he's all on his own now. Whenever I think about what's happened to our family I start crying and I just can't stop."

   a. What are appropriate treatment goals to discuss with Yvonne?

   b. What resources might be helpful to Yvonne?

3. Think about a person who you often turn to for support. In what ways would your life change if (s)he told you today that (s)he was HIV positive? How would your relationship with this person be affected?

4. Working in an emotionally intense field with limited resources but high demands is extremely stressful. What are some ways you can personally manage the risk of burnout?

5. Do you think it is an advantage or disadvantage for a worker at an ASO to be HIV positive? List some reasons why being HIV positive or negative would help a practitioner.

Web Resources

National Association of People with AIDS (NAPWA): www.napwa.org

Project Inform: www.projectinform.org/

Positively Aware: positivelyaware.com/

National Minority AIDS Council: www.nmac.org

Buzztracker.net

AIDS.gov

AIDS United: www.aidsunited.org

References

Adamsen, L. (2002). "From victim to agent": The clinical and social significance of self-help group participation for people with life-threatening diseases. *Scandinavian Journal of Caring Sciences, 16*(3), 224–231.

Beckerman, N. L. (2002). Case report: Couples coping with discordant HIV status. *AIDS Patient Care and STDs, 16*(2), 55–59.

Berk, L. E. (2004). *Development through the lifespan* (3rd ed.). Boston: Pearson Education.

Brook, D. W., Brook, J. S., Rubenstone, E., Zhang, C., & Finch, S. (2010). A longitudinal study of sexual risk behavior among the adolescent children of HIV-positive and HIV-negative drug-abusing fathers. *Journal of Adolescent Health, 46*, 224–231.

Capobianco Boyer, N., & Poindexter, C. C. (2005). Barriers to permanency planning for older HIV-affected caregivers. *Journal of Gerontological Social Work, 44*(3/4), 59–74.

Childs, J., & Cincotta, N. (2006). Pediatric HIV adherence: An ever-evolving challenge. *Social Work in Health Care, 42*(3/4), 189–208.

Corey, G. (2000). *Theory and practice of group counseling* (5th ed.). Belmont, CA: Wadsworth/Thompson Learning.

Davey, M. P., Duncan, T. M., Foster, J., & Milton, K. (2008). Collaboration in action: Keeping the family in focus at an HIV/AIDS pediatric clinic. *Families, Systems, & Health, 26*(3), 350–355.

Flores, P. J. (1997). *Group psychotherapy with addicted populations: An integration of twelve-step and psychodynamic theory* (3rd ed.). Binghamton, NY: Haworth Press.

Forehand, R., Steele, R., Simon, P., Morse, E., & Clark, L. (1998). The Family Health Project: Psychosocial adjustment of children whose mothers are HIV infected. Retrieved from PsycINFO database. *Journal of Consulting and Clinical Psychology, 66*(3), 513–520.

Gehlert, S., & Browne, T. A. (2006). *Handbook of health social work.* Hoboken, NJ: John Wiley & Sons.

Gilbert, D. J. (2001). HIV-affected children and adolescents: What school social workers should know. *Children and Schools, 23*(3), 135–142.

Goffman, E. (1963). *Stigma: Notes on the management of spoiled identity.* Englewood Cliffs, NJ: Prentice Hall.

Gunther, M., Crandles, S., Williams, G., & Swain, M. (1998). A place called HOPE: Group psychotherapy for adolescents of parents with HIV/AIDS. *Child Welfare, 77*(2), 251–271.

Gurney, S. (1995). Counseling the HIV 'affected' individual: A case study. *Counseling Psychology Quarterly, 8*(1), 17–25.

Havens, J. F., & Mellins, C. A. (1996). Mental health issues in HIV-affected women and children. *International Review of Psychiatry, 8*(2/3), 217–226.

Heckman, T. G., Anderson, E. S., Sikkema, K. J., Kochman, A., Kalichman, S. C., & Anderson, T. (2004). Emotional distress in nonmetropolitan persons living with HIV disease enrolled in a telephone-delivered, coping improvement group intervention. *Health Psychology, 23*(1), 94–100.

Hoff, C. C., Chakravarty, D., Beougher, S. C., Darbes, L. A., Dadasovich, R., & Neilands, T. B. (2009). Serostatus differences and agreements about sex with outside partners among gay male couples. *AIDS Education and Prevention, 21*(1), 25–38.

Hoy-Ellis, C. P., & Fredriksen-Goldsen, K. I. (2007). Is AIDS chronic or terminal? The perceptions of persons living with AIDS and their informal support partners. *AIDS Care, 19*(7), 835–843.

Kulic, K. R., Horne, A. M., & Dagley, J. C. (2004). A comprehensive review of prevention groups for children and adolescents. *Group Dynamics: Theory, Research, and Practice, 8*(2), 139–151.

Land, H. (2010). HIV-affected caregivers. In C. C. Poindexter (Ed.), *Handbook of HIV and social work: Principles, practice, and populations* (pp. 311–326). Hoboken, NJ: Wiley and Sons.

Lietaer, G. (1984). Unconditional positive regard: A controversial basic attitude in client-centered therapy. In R. F. Levant & J. M. Shlien (Eds.), *Client-centered therapy and the person-centered approach: New directions in theory, research, and practice* (pp. 41–58). New York: Van Nostrand Reinhold.

Linsk, N., & Gilbert, D. (2007). Attitudes, knowledge, behavior in the context of HIV/AIDS stigma. *Journal of HIV/AIDS & Social Services, 6*(3), 1–4.

Linsk, N., & Mason, S. (2004). Stresses on grandparents and other relatives caring for children affected by HIV/AIDS. *Health & Social Work, 29*(2), 127–136.

Mason, S., Berger, B., Estwing Ferrans, C., Sultzman, V., & Fendrich, M. (2010). Developing a measure of stigma by association with African American adolescents whose mothers have HIV. *Research on Social Work Practice, 20*(1), 65–73.

Matthews, L. T., & Mukherjee, J. S. (2009). Strategies for harm reduction among HIV-affected couples who want to conceive. *AIDS and Behavior, 13*(S5–S11).

McKay, M., Chasse, K. T., Paikoff, R., McKinney, L., Baptiste, D., Coleman, D., ..., Bell, C. C. (2004). Family level impact of the CHAMP family program: A community collaborative effort to support urban families and reduce youth HIV risk exposure. *Family Process, 43*(1), 79–93.

National Association of Social Workers (NASW). (2005). *NASW practice snap-shots: Mincing words—empathy vs. sympathy.* Washington, DC: Author. Retrieved from http://www.socialworkers.org/practice/behavioral_health/0605snapshot.asp

Oliver, C., & Dykeman, M. (2003). Challenges to HIV service provision: The commonalities for nurses and social workers. *AIDS Care, 15*(5), 649–663.

Pivnick, A., & Villegas, N. (2000). Resilience and risk: Childhood and uncertainty in the AIDS epidemic. *Culture, Medicine and Psychiatry, 24*(1), 101–136.

Poindexter, C. C. (2003). Sex, drugs, and love among the middle aged: A case study of a sero-discordant heterosexual couple coping with HIV. *Journal of Social Work Practice in the Addictions, 3*(2), 57–83.

Poindexter, C. (2005). The lion at the gate: An HIV-affected caregiver resists stigma. *Health & Social Work, 30*(1), 64–74.

Rosenblum, A., Magura, S., Fong, C., Cleland, C., Norwood, C., Casella, D., . . . , Curry, P. (2005). Substance use among young adolescents in HIV-affected families: Resiliency, peer deviance, and family functioning. *Substance Use and Misuse, 40*, 581–603.

Rotheram-Borus, M. J., Lee, M., Gwadz, M., & Draimin, B. (2001). An interven-tion for parents with AIDS and their adolescent children. *American Journal of Public Health, 91*(8).

Rotheram-Borus, M. J., Stein, J., & Lester, P. (2006). Adolescent adjustment over six years in HIV-affected families. *Journal of Adolescent Health, 39*, 174–182.

Saleebey, D. (1996). The strengths perspective in social work practice: Extensions and cautions. *Social Work, 41*(3), 296–305.

Sikkema, K. J., Hansen, N. B., Meade, C. S., Kochman, A., Lee, & Rachael, S. (2005). Improvement in health-related quality of life following a group intervention for coping with AIDS-bereavement among HIV-infected men and women. *Quality of Life Research, 14*, 991–1005.

Snell-Johns, J., Mendez, J. L., & Smith, B. H. (2004). Evidence-based solutions for overcoming access barriers, decreasing attrition, and promoting change with underserved families. *Journal of Family Psychology, 18*(3), 19–35.

Soenes, B., Vansteenkiste, M., Lens, W., Luyckx, K., Goosseens, L., Beyers, W., & Ryan, R. M. (2007). Conceptualizing parental autonomy support: Adolescent perceptions of promotion of independence versus promotion of volitional functioning. *Developmental Psychology, 43*(3), 633–646.

Stevens, P., & Galvao, L. (2007). "He won't use condoms": HIV-infected women's struggle in primary relationships with sero-discordant partners. *American Journal of Public Health, 97*(6), 1015–1022.

Sunil, T., & McGehee, M. (2007). Social and religious support on treatment adherence among HIV/AIDS patients by race/ethnicity. *Journal of HIV/AIDS & Social Services, 6*(1–2), 83–99.

Talley, A. E., & Bettencourt, B. A. (2008). A relationship-oriented model of HIV-related stigma derived from a review of HIV-affected couples literature. *AIDS and Behavior, 14*(1), 72–86.

Thyer, B. A. (2002). Evidence-based practice and clinical social work. *Evidence Based Mental Health, 5,* 6–7.

Tinsley, B. J., Lees, N. B., & Sumartojo, E. (2004). Child and adolescent HIV risk: Familial and cultural perspectives. *Journal of Family Psychology, 18*(1), 208–224.

Tschudin, S. (2008). Round-table multidisciplinary counseling of couples with HIV prior to assisted reproduction. *Reproductive BioMedicine Online, 17*(2), 167–174.

Wiener, L., & Taylor-Brown, S. (2010). The impact of HIV on children and adolescents. In C. C. Poindexter (Ed.), *Handbook of HIV and social work: Principles, practice, and populations* (pp. 231–252). Hoboken, NJ: Wiley and Sons.

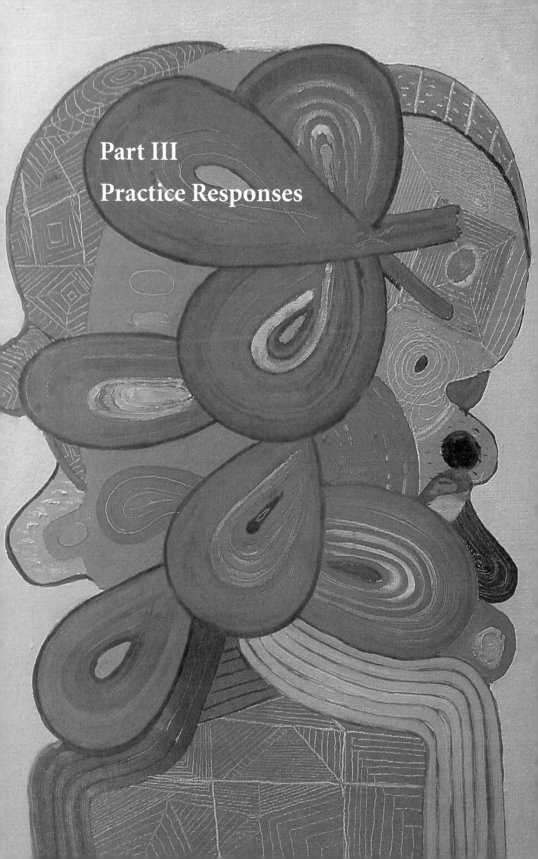

Part III

Practice Responses

10

HIV Case Management:
The Hub of Service Provision

Kevin Edwards and Diana Rowan

> The applause dies. Awards tarnish. Achievements are forgotten.
> Accolades and certificates are buried with their owners. . . . The people
> who make a difference in your life are not the ones with the most cre-
> dentials, but the ones who cared.
>
> **—Attributed to Charles M. Schulz (creator of *Peanuts* cartoon)**

Although social workers provide services to people living with HIV (human immunodeficiency virus) or AIDS (acquired immune deficiency syndrome) in varying types of agencies with varying missions, one of the most common and essential functions for a social worker is provision of HIV case management (Pugh, 2009). HIV case management is a systematic process of social work service delivery to persons living with HIV or AIDS. Case management for HIV focuses on the many medical and social services directly related to HIV and AIDS. The goal is to improve the quality of care for clients who are HIV positive or who have been diagnosed with AIDS through coordination of needed services. Evidence has shown that case management is associated with fewer unmet client needs and higher use of HIV medications by those who need them (Johnson, Polansky, Matosky, & Teti, 2010; Katz et al., 2001; Wohl et al., 2009).

Understanding Social Work Case Management

The case management process consists of eight components (steps) to ensure the consistency and quality of services to persons living with HIV or AIDS. These are listed below, and then expanded upon.

1. Client identification, outreach, and engagement

2. Biopsychosocial assessment and risk assessment

3. Development of the care plan

4. Incremental goal setting

5. Linkages with resources

6. Monitoring of service provision

7. Advocacy

8. Routine follow-up and evaluation.

Case management with clients with any type of physical or social need is important; given the numerous, complex, and interlocking social and medical needs of people living with HIV and AIDS, quality case management with this population is vital. Both newly diagnosed individuals and those who have lived with the virus for a while have needs that are not seen with any other population of clients. For example, they have needs related to stigma, disclosure of their status, and issues in negotiating multiple systems of services including medical, legal, and income maintenance. These multiple challenges can be confusing, and when serious medical needs are added, the combination can be overwhelming. It takes a savvy case manager to help people who are living with HIV, who are already marginalized, to navigate this bewildering maze of needs and resources (Brooks, 2010).

Client Identification, Outreach, and Engagement

Client identification, outreach, and engagement are the first core components of case management, and they set the trajectory for success through the next steps. Often community and government agencies, medical facilities, and AIDS service organizations (ASOs), have outreach staff that, through community testing sites, identify HIV-positive clients who need to be connected to case management services. Case managers may also receive referrals from private infectious disease practices, community clinics, hospitals, and public health departments. Potential clients may self-refer or be referred by family members or friends. A critical task of the case manager is engagement. To develop a trusting relationship centered in unconditional acceptance and a nonjudgmental attitude, it is important for the social worker to be mindful that the first encounter may be the first time the client has had an opportunity to talk about what it means to be HIV positive.

Biopsychosocial Assessment and Risk Assessment

Getting into medical care soon after diagnosis of HIV transmission is vital to longevity in living with HIV. Without a thorough biopsychosocial assessment, clients may be unsuccessful in staying in medical care, with negative impacts on their health and longevity. Adequately assessing psychosocial issues that may interfere with medical compliance is essential at this stage. Unaddressed issues such as housing needs, substance abuse, and mental health disorders can have devastating effects on treatment compliance and medication adherence.

For instance, clients who are living with friends or family members who are not aware of their diagnosis may have a difficult time taking HIV medications, for fear their friends or relatives will discover their HIV diagnosis. They may believe that they have to hide their pill bottles, which may cause them to skip doses. Failure to consistently take prescribed antiretroviral (ARV) medications reduces the effectiveness of the drugs and can lead to development of drug resistances. To take another example, a person who is homeless or using substances may be more concerned with housing problems or finding drugs than he or she is with taking ARV medications as prescribed and keeping medical appointments. Case managers, through the assessment process, must systematically gather information about all areas of the client's life, so a thorough plan can be created that has a high chance of leading the client to successful treatment compliance and better quality of life.

Risk assessment and education are also part of the assessment process. Case managers who incorporate prevention strategies into routine activities cannot only help prevent the spread of HIV, but also prevent their clients from becoming co-infected with hepatitis, or drug-resistant strains of HIV, or another sexually transmitted infection (STI), which can be difficult to treat in someone with HIV. Case managers should begin with a risk assessment during the initial assessment, using open-ended questions to ask about the client's sexual behaviors, perceived risks, and safer sex practices. This conversation also provides an opportunity to assess the client's knowledge of HIV transmission, universal precautions, and secondary HIV infection (i.e., reinfection with another strain of HIV). Information gathered from the risk assessment is vital to preparing an individualized prevention education curriculum for the client. While education of the client about prevention is ongoing, it begins with provision of basic information as early as the first session. While the social worker does not present the entire curriculum to the client during the assessment phase, he or she begins the process at that time.

The individualized prevention education curriculum begins with identifying the client's greatest risks for transmission and new infections. The case manager needs to educate the client on these risks and ways to protect himself or herself and others. For example, a heterosexual female client who enjoys performing and receiving oral sex should be educated on the proper use of condoms and dental dams and the ways in which HIV and other sexually transmitted diseases (STDs; such as genital warts) can be transmitted if these prophylactics are not used. The case manager must be comfortable in discussing sexual behaviors and safer sex practices with the client in a matter-of-fact manner, normalizing sexual behavior as a common human need and function. If the case manager is uncomfortable with this discussion, clients will perceive this discomfort and may wonder why the case manager brought up the subject, completely shut down the conversation, or tell the case manager what they think the case manager wants to hear. It is essential that case managers convey that they are comfortable with whatever the client shares.

Risk assessment entails assessing the client's awareness of the proper use of latex condoms, dental dams, polyurethane female condoms, and water-based lubricant. These are often misused, which can lead to prevention failures. Many case managers and HIV health educators have anatomical models that the client can use to demonstrate proper application of safer sex products. Exploring barriers to using condoms and safer sex products is crucial during the assessment. It may be advantageous to include partners, spouses, or significant others in this discussion.

The risk reduction curriculum may need to be modified if clients begin a new sexual relationship; the clients become co-infected with another STD or hepatitis; the composition of their HIV strain changes, indicating a possible infection with a drug-resistant strain of HIV; their alcohol or drug use increases; or there is a negative shift in their emotional state. Possible infection with a drug-resistant strain of HIV may be indicated by an unexplained decrease in the efficacy of the HIV medication regimen. Often at this point physicians will conduct a phenotype or genotype lab test of the virus to check for drug resistance. Resistance may also develop for other reasons, such as if the client is on a medication for a long period, or if he or she has poor adherence to the regimen.

Development of the Care Plan

Following a comprehensive assessment, the case manager and client are ready to complete a care plan to address the needs identified in the assessment. First and foremost, the case manager should look to the client for personal strengths and informal and formal resources to address needs and complete the goals the client develops. Operating from a strengths-based approach empowers the client and facilitates movement to self-sufficiency. The overall goal of HIV case management should be for the client to be his or her own case manager and not need the case manager's help any longer. An empowerment approach promotes self-awareness, self-responsibility, and commitment, and these in turn promote independence, personal power, self-trust, and reliance.

Incremental Goal Setting

Individual service plans should be developed on a case-by-case basis, to reduce obstacles to well-being. Case managers must bear in mind that while HIV might be the social worker's main focus, the client might see other problems as more important. To move from the need or problem to setting a goal, the case manager can simply ask a solution-focused question: "What will it look like when this problem is resolved or solved, or your need is met?" The client's answer then becomes the basic goal. The challenge often is making the plan SMART (specific, measurable, attainable, realistic, and timely) (Card, Solomon, & Berman, 2008). Considerate and careful confrontation is useful in helping clients become aware of unrealistic goals and prioritize goals. In order to achieve medication adherence, it is imperative for the social worker to explain to clients the importance of medical treatment. Goals should be written in positive achievement words—for example, "I will have access to HIV medical care" or "I will take my medications as prescribed 95 percent of the time." Interventions or tasks involved in reaching the goal should be both time and behavior specific.

The individual service plan (care plan) should be a workable contract indicating who will do what, using the client's strengths and supports first. After the case manager has assessed the client's resources, he or she should look at community resources available to provide specific services that aid in the accomplishment of the goal. A care plan is only as good as the periodic reviews of the plan. If both the case manager and the client do not periodically review the care plan, it becomes a useless piece of paper. These reviews afford evaluation and an opportunity to revise or discontinue the plan or change target dates because of unforeseen circumstances, changes in priorities, or the addition of new and better resources.

Case managers can include safer sex practices in risk reduction behaviors as a goal in the care plan. For example, a male client who has sex with other men (MSM) may enjoy both oral and anal sex. Perhaps prior to his HIV diagnosis he did not regularly use a condom. In order to reduce HIV transmission and further infection (which is the goal), the client should use condoms every time (100 percent) when engaging in anal sex. The client and case manager can brainstorm actions (strategies) that will make this goal happen (i.e., change the client's behavior). Strategies may include the client finding his preferred condom, deciding where to store condoms for easy access, identifying barriers to using condoms, and role-playing condom negotiation conversations.

Linkages with Resources

Case managers must be knowledgeable about community agencies and resources in order to link the client to services that will address their needs. Case managers also need to educate clients on how to access these resources, and provide information on eligibility requirements and service limitations. To link clients to resources, the case manager needs to build relationships with service providers and introduce the client to key personnel in agencies. Case managers must be up to date on resource availability and eligibility requirements in a wide range of systems. Making referrals and providing information is much more than giving a client a paper with a name and phone number of a resource on it. Sometimes social work case managers may need to make the contact along with the client, or write out a recommendation for the client to take when seeking the service.

Social work case managers should routinely double-check on resource availability before making referrals. Attempting to connect clients to a service for which they do not qualify or that does not exist will frustrate the clients, cause them to lose trust and confidence in the social worker, and waste the clients' limited time and energy. Offering a client what can be called a "dead lead" is a cardinal sin in all of social work case management; it can have even worse consequences in HIV-related work.

The case manager may often be the liaison between service providers and clients. For example, the case manager often deciphers medical information and puts it in an understandable format for the client. Likewise, the case manager often relays important information about the client's situation and psychosocial dynamics that may impact the client's medical treatment. The case manager's role as a liaison becomes less important as the client is empowered to communicate his or her own needs and as the client's knowledge of HIV/AIDS and community resources expands.

Monitoring of Service Provision

Monitoring the provision of services according to the care plan is another core component of case management. Asking clients if services are still relevant to their needs, if the services are being provided as planned, and if the services need to be altered or terminated puts clients in the role of expert and empowers them, boosting self-determination. Service monitoring also includes making contact with referral agencies to evaluate the clients' progress, and assessing whether the client requires more education.

As educator, the case manager provides information not only about resources but also about the nature of HIV disease. The case manager should provide information about medications, medical adherence, lab results, and HIV-related diseases as appropriate to the cognitive level of the client. Often pharmaceutical companies have brochures and handouts not only on medications, but also on adherence, lab tests, managing side effects, and ways to stay healthy. The more clients are informed, the more confident they will be in making decisions about their health care. The case manager's role also includes educating the client's family, friends, and partner. Since the case manager is often seen as the expert, her or she should educate persons associated with the client on transmission, risk reduction, and prevention practices. Also, by dispelling myths and misconceptions, the case manager can help the client forge relationships that move away from fear and rejection toward support and understanding. The social worker also should provide accurate information to service providers and the community at large.

Incorporating risk reduction strategies is an integral part of monitoring activities. When meeting with clients to review their care plan, the case manager should ask about relationships, and the client's use of safer sex practices, including condoms, female condoms, dental dams, and lubricants. Not all agencies keep on hand a wide variety of safer sex products, so the case manager should be aware of agencies or stores in the community where these can be obtained. The case manager should also review the proper methods for storage of latex products, including avoiding storage in warm places such as a car or wallet, and any newly identified barriers to safer sex practices.

Advocacy

Advocacy is one of the most important aspects of case management. It is an ongoing activity of service provision and programmatic evaluation. The case manager and client are best qualified to determine unmet needs and advocate for funding to provide the necessary services. Facilitating collaboration between several agencies may help create new services. Case managers can advocate for clients with housing officials, landlords, medical and mental health providers, substance abuse agencies, vocational training sites, and other agencies with resources. They can advocate for more and better services and for more equitable policies.

Advocacy in social work can focus on a case, a cause, or both. The social work profession has a dual focus: change in individuals and change in the system. Often the experiences of individual clients reveal the need to change the larger systems. Social workers, as opposed to some other professional helpers, engage these larger organizational, community-level, and political systems as targets for change. Therefore, social workers, depending on the needs of client systems, must intervene at multiple levels, including individuals, families, small groups, organizations, and communities.

In case advocacy a worker obtains resources for clients that would otherwise not have been provided. Cause advocacy involves attempts to effect changes in policies, practices, laws, and attitudes that affect all people in a specific class or group (Lens, 2004). Social workers often engage in both case advocacy and cause advocacy, especially in HIV and AIDS care, because of the marginalized status of their clients. For example, if social work case managers learn that there is a very long waiting list for new enrollees to the AIDS Drug Assistance Program (ADAP) in their state, they may start a petition campaign to put political pressure on legislators. If case managers observe a pattern of frustration in clients who use the public transportation system to reach the ASO, they may reach out to the city's transportation authority to ask for a bus stop to be placed near the agency. And if case managers learn that a housing manager appears to be discriminating against people living with AIDS, they may need to educate that manager on fair housing policies.

Clients are empowered when they are involved in evaluation and advocacy. Modeling effective advocacy for clients is important to teach them self-advocacy. In HIV, adding a consumer voice to dialogue about services is helpful to clients and to decision makers. Case managers can assist by recommending clients to serve on task forces, needs assessments, and program and policy evaluations (McIntosh, 2012).

Routine Follow-up and Evaluation

Depending on the policies of the agency that employs the HIV case manager, he or she makes routine follow-up contacts to ensure that clients are following their care plan. The case manager can conduct these follow-up sessions on the phone, in person at the agency, or during a home visit. The case manager will evaluate how well the care plan is working and make modifications if the client's needs have changed (new needs are identified, or previous needs are resolved); the array of resources and services available has changed (new resources or services that were not previously available now exist, or resources that were part of the care plan no longer exist); or further assessment reveals additional needs that were present but were not identified earlier. During follow-up and evaluation sessions, as with each step of the case management process, development of an effective partnership with the client will yield the best outcomes. Respectful partnerships are more easily developed when the case manager cares about the well-being of his or her clients.

Description of Supportive HIV Case Management Services

In 2010, Halkitis, Kupprat, and Pandley Mukherjee studied the frequency of use of various components of the services provided by HIV case managers. These are described in rank order below, from the most used services to the least accessed. The length of this list shows that HIV case managers must be knowledgeable about a wide array of resources in their community and in surrounding regions where clients may reside.

Transportation Services. In order to ensure that clients can get to necessary appointments, case managers can issue passes for the bus line or other public transportation; if medically necessary, case managers can arrange for ambulance transportation. Door-to-door shuttle service for people with disabilities may also be available in the region.

Primary Health-Care and Medical Specialty Services. Medically based agencies can offer care in-house, including specialty services such as eye care, dental care, family medicine, women's health, pediatrics, cardiology, podiatry, and dermatology. If not available in-house, the case manager can arrange for these services through referral or medical mobile units.

Support Groups. Support groups can be facilitated by social workers, other case managers, care technicians, and outreach workers. The groups can cover issues faced by men, women, and families living with HIV, such as disclosure of status, domestic violence, and peer advising; group attendance can be aligned with subgroups such as African Americans, Latinos, new arrivals, those over fifty years old, or adolescents. Some groups are co-ed and some are gender specific; some have open membership, and some start with a group of members and continue for a number of weeks without adding new members.

Prepared Meals, Food Vouchers, and Pantry. These services include preparation and delivery of hot meals, distribution of bag lunches, an emergency food pantry, referrals to free-standing food pantries, and provision of emergency food vouchers.

Recreational Activities. There are structured events and gatherings where families can bond and clients can network. Activities may include bowling, bingo and games, picnics, trips to parks, educational tours, or arts and crafts.

Personal Hygiene Assistance. Case managers may distribute hygiene kits that include soap, shaving cream, comb, razors, toothbrush and toothpaste, dental floss, an array of feminine hygiene products, and moist towelettes. Kits can be distributed upon request or through workshops that focus on self-esteem building, such as beauty tips, makeovers, manicures, pedicures, stress management, and positive body image.

Harm Reduction, Substance Abuse, Methadone Treatment. Treatment adherence programs can be offered in-house, through referral, or on the streets. Harm reduction initiatives include the distribution of bleach kits for cleaning injection tools, and distribution of condoms and lubricant. Case managers can make referrals to centers for safe detoxification of drugs or alcohol, and the control of cravings for drugs; and referrals to methadone clinics and treatment centers.

Workshops. Classes and psycho-education programs are offered to specific groups of clients, such as HIV-positive women, HIV-positive men, HIV-positive adolescents, caregivers and family of people with HIV, and people newly diagnosed with HIV. Classes and groups can address physical health, mental health, nutrition, stress management, domestic violence awareness, grief and loss, and supportive socialization groups.

Emergency Cash Assistance. This is provided on a case-by-case basis; the amount of benefit is determined by case managers who are aware of the details of a client's financial hardships. Emergency cash is given only to stave off eviction or utility shutoffs, or for rental assistance, moving costs, food, and basic furniture.

Financial and Entitlement Assistance. Services from case managers or outreach workers link clients with entitlement benefits; offer help with completing budget worksheets and the required forms for applying for benefits; and help with securing the required documentation necessary to qualify for benefits, including a birth certificate and driver's license.

Mental Health Services, Therapy, and Counseling. Psychiatric evaluations can be conducted in-house or by referral, and psychotherapy and counseling services can be offered on a one-on-one basis or in groups. Licensed social workers, counselors, psychologists, or other mental health professionals can provide mental health–related services. Case managers can refer clients to psychiatrists for psychotropic medications, and, for severe mental health concerns, can refer clients to inpatient psychiatric treatment centers.

Alternative Therapies. Case managers can link clients with complementary and alternative treatments such as acupressure, acupuncture, massage therapy, yoga, herbal treatments, and Eastern therapies.

Housing Services. Case managers can make referrals to housing opportunities, tenant-based rental vouchers, HIV/AIDS set-aside units, or transitional housing centers or shelters. These linkages can be for individuals, couples, or families with children.

Nutritional Counseling. Clinical nutritionists and registered dieticians can assist with issues related to health, weight control, and digestion, especially as they are impacted by medications and HIV disease.

Obstetrics/Gynecology. Routine OB/GYN services can be offered in-house, by referral, or through a mobile medical unit.

Budget Management. Case managers can provide help with handling finances, particularly if the client is having trouble paying bills. Cell phone bills are often a problem because charges can add up without notification. Discussing the importance of living within one's means and being financially responsible is important; ASOs can also offer emergency cash assistance.

Education Services. Training can be provided in-house or through referral, for life skills development, career development, GED preparation, money management, budgeting, vocational training, and positive health promotion.

Legal Services. Case managers can make referrals for legal advice on issues including health-care proxies, living wills, discrimination claims, housing issues, and immigration status.

HIV Prevention, Education, and Condoms. Case managers may offer prevention education through group activities, one-on-one counseling, or outreach events.

Case managers can make available male and female condoms, dental dams, and lubricants, as well as harm reduction kits and safer sex packets. Case managers emphasize HIV/AIDS prevention for HIV-positive clients.

Dental Care Services. Dental care can be provided either on-site or through referral.

Employment Services. Clients who are not eligible for benefits may receive help in finding work, including job interview training and résumé preparation.

Home Care. Case managers may arrange for help in the client's home with chores, cleaning, and shopping for those who have lost mobility.

Phone and Phone Cards. For those who do not have a telephone or cell phone, case managers may provide phones or phone cards so the clients can make calls about medical appointments or speak to a case manager.

Childcare Services. Childcare services can be provided on-site or through referral. Sometimes agency staff can watch clients' children to allow clients to attend case management services, groups, and workshops. Case managers may also accompany clients and their children to appointments for medical services or benefit consultations, to allow the client to speak privately while the children are in the waiting room.

Common Risks in People Living with HIV or AIDS

Social work case managers working with clients with HIV or AIDS have a challenging, complex, and multifaceted caseload consisting of all ages and races or ethnicities. They often work with highly vulnerable clients with high levels of physical and psychological risks, paired with limited resources for success. Social work case managers must be aware of the challenges in order to assess and serve clients effectively.

Physical Risks Associated with HIV/AIDS

People living with HIV and AIDS are at high risk for multiple physical threats and environmental stressors. Many are currently or have been inadequately housed, have lived in shelters, or have been evicted (Chernesky & Grube, 2000). Many are currently or have a history of being food insecure. Because they live marginally, their sense of control over their living situation may be low. Many are currently or have a history of being dependent on public assistance programs for medical and financial assistance. In addition, violence and HIV have been linked. Victims of violence, especially sexual violence, are at higher risk for HIV transmission, and those already HIV positive are at risk of violence upon disclosure of their HIV-positive status (Program on International Health and Human Rights, 2006). People living with HIV or AIDS may be injection (or intravenous) drug users. In 2008, injection drug users made up 19 percent of the people living with HIV (AIDS.gov, 2012). Furthermore, because there are disparities in HIV rates with respect to race and sexual orientation, people living with HIV and AIDS are more likely to be impacted by intersecting "isms," including racism, heterosexism, and classism.

Psychological Risks Associated with HIV

HIV case managers must be skilled in managing the multiple psychological impacts of the disease. The ways in which clients deal with their psychological stress and adjustment to an HIV diagnosis are most affected by their social support system. Since in society HIV is often associated with "antisocial behaviors," clients may isolate themselves from others and develop a negative self-image. The case manager should address psychological symptoms and link clients with mental health services as needed. Sometimes psychological distress can be so overwhelming that the only coping mechanism the client can use is denial. However, denial is dangerous because the client may then not seek medical care. Substance abuse and use may be an attempt to cope with an HIV diagnosis. The case manager should closely monitor persons with a history of substance abuse, and should invite clients to share feelings and consider support groups for added support.

Other psychological needs center around self-esteem, social isolation, intimacy, guilt, fear of the unknown, decision making, family relationships, and stress management. Because of the stigma associated with HIV/AIDS, a person may experience low self-esteem. This may translate into self-defeating behaviors such as not accessing services and medical care. It is important for the case manager to evaluate clients' moods and self-esteem and refer them for appropriate mental health treatment as necessary. Social isolation is not uncommon, but the case manager should monitor the situation if this continues for a longer period. Clients who are newly diagnosed frequently experience difficulty in making decisions because of the shock of the diagnosis, lack of knowledge about HIV, and feelings of being overwhelmed. Clients may experience a sense of urgency about decisions or may continually delay them. The case manager can assist clients in feeling more empowered about making decisions regarding treatment, disclosure, and lifestyle changes.

Family relationships can be either a source of support or a source of distress. Clients usually struggle with telling their family members about their diagnosis for fear of being rejected and ostracized. Case managers should facilitate discussions about disclosure with family members and should assess for additional supports in lieu of family supports. They should offer education for family members as a service to assist the client in his or her disclosure. Family members may view the case manager as an expert and may be more likely to listen to and accept what the case manager says, and follow the social worker's lead in feeling confident that the client can enjoy a high quality of life and not pose a risk to others.

Coexisting Psychiatric Disorders

Case managers must be aware that clients might have coexisting psychiatric disorders. Mental health practitioners can diagnose psychiatric disorders using the *Diagnostic and Statistical Manual of Mental Disorders (DSM)*. Licensed clinical social workers are among the mental health professionals who can diagnose and treat mental disorders. Case managers can serve clients by linking them with a mental health practitioner, preferably one with experience in working with people living with HIV or AIDS. Some mental disorders are treated with psychotropic medications prescribed by a physician, often a psychiatrist. Case managers can link the client with this component of their medical and mental health care.

Depression, mania, impulsivity, substance abuse, intoxication, cognitive impairment, and personality vulnerabilities are all associated with risk of HIV infection. However, not only does the presence of mental disorders increase the risk of HIV infection, but HIV also increases the lifetime presence of psychiatric conditions (Hammond & Treisman, 2007). It is important to note that psychiatric disorders may have preexisted or may have an onset after HIV diagnosis. Some of the most common co-occurring mental disorders are briefly described below.

Major Depression. Major depression is a common disorder in people living with HIV. During their lifetime, 22 to 45 percent of people with HIV or AIDS will experience depression, as compared to 5 to 17 percent of the general population (Kessler, Berglund, & Demler, 2005; Krishnan et al., 2002). Recognizing the symptoms of major depression can be difficult because "symptoms of fatigue, decreased appetite and libido, and poor memory are also symptoms of HIV infection" (Hammond & Treisman, 2007, p. 1). Case managers should involve mental health professionals in screening for depression.

New-Onset Psychosis. New-onset psychosis (i.e., psychosis that has not occurred prior to HIV infection) is a serious complication of HIV disease, and is more common in those with very low CD4 counts. The incidence of first psychotic episodes in HIV-positive clients is estimated to range from 1 to 15 percent (Hammond & Treisman, 2007). Psychosis in people with HIV is associated with drug abuse, affective disorders, cognitive impairment, dementia, and high mortality rates. Furthermore, people with schizophrenia are particularly likely to exhibit high-risk behaviors, perhaps because of their poor understanding of risks (Hammond & Treisman, 2007).

Anxiety Disorders. In an older study, the prevalence of anxiety disorders in people living with HIV and AIDS (PLWHA) was estimated to be about 38 percent (Elliott, 1998). In a more recent study, the rates appeared to be 16 percent for generalized anxiety disorder and 11 percent for panic disorder (Bing et al., 2001). Anxiety disorders have a significant negative impact on health-related quality of life for people with HIV (Hammond & Treisman, 2007).

Posttraumatic Stress Disorder. Posttraumatic stress disorder (PTSD) is more prevalent in people with HIV than in the general population. It is associated with lower medication adherence, magnification of symptoms, and catastrophic thinking (Delahanty, Bogart, & Figler, 2004).

Because people living with HIV have an increased prevalence of psychiatric disorders, it is important for case managers to frequently assess their mental state and quickly refer them to mental health professionals if symptoms are observed or reported by the client or family and friends.

What Are the Top Five Skills of an HIV Case Manager?

Case management with people living with HIV and AIDS is complex and demanding. What are the necessary skills for being successful? In a recent qualitative study, Brooks (2010) conducted interviews with five HIV case managers in order to gain their perspectives on the day-to-day activities of an HIV case manager and his or her interaction with clients. Brooks found that the top five skills were these: working from a person-centered perspective; negotiation and navigation of systems; task management, caseload management, and paperwork; effective communication; and modeling.

What Are the Top Five Attitudes of an HIV Case Manager?

Social workers new to HIV work or new to case management may find the role of HIV case manager both exciting and challenging. While working on development of skills described above, it may be helpful for these social workers to reflect on what veteran HIV case managers say are the necessary attitudes to be successful in their work. It is particularly important to preserve one's professional values and work to demonstrate to clients the qualities reported by Brooks (2010): an affirming attitude; patience; integrity and honesty; nonjudgmental attitudes; and authenticity.

Case Example

The following case example is written in the format of a client assessment.

Referral Information. Case manager, Brittany, from New Beginnings (Women's Homeless Shelter) called requesting HIV case management services for Teresa, a thirty-nine-year-old African-American female recently released from Camden Recovery Center, a residential twenty-eight-day substance abuse treatment center. Brittany reports that Teresa has no medical care, no insurance, and no income.

Intake and Assessment. Intake and assessment completed at New Beginnings with client. Case manager provided client with a description of HIV case management services, explained informed consent, rights and responsibilities, confidentiality, and case manager's role.

Client admits to a ten-year substance abuse history including crack cocaine, powder cocaine, and alcohol. She expresses a desire to remain drug free as evidenced by her communications with this case manager, her daily attendance in Narcotics Anonymous groups, and her current search for a sponsor. She states that she takes the bus to various meetings around the city at various times of the day. Her reasoning for this is to find a "home group" and a sponsor that she is comfortable with. Client reports that she has been clean for thirty-five days.

Client has been at the homeless shelter since her release from the recovery center. She states that she has a sister and two brothers, and her parents, all living in Charlotte. Client has a close relationship with one sister and her mother. She reports that she cannot live with anyone in her family due to her history of substance abuse, stealing, and conflict. Client would like to get her own apartment.

Client wants to receive medical care and have her HIV disease status assessed. Client is unaware of her CD4 count and viral load. She denies any other medical problems at this time. The only HIV-related symptom that the client reports at this time is night sweats. She denies ever being on HIV medication in the past. Client denies any allergies to medication and is currently not taking any medication except for over-the-counter ibuprofen occasionally for body aches and headaches.

Client reports being depressed over the past three months. She admits to a history of periodic depression but denies ever being clinically diagnosed or being on medication. She denies any suicidal or homicidal ideations, hallucination, or delusions. Client is willing to accept a mental health referral for evaluation.

Client denies any current legal issues but confides that she has worked as a prostitute over the past ten years and has been arrested and served jail time. She states that her prostitution was to support her drug addiction.

Client has no income, but is looking for a job. She reports she does not feel that her HIV status impedes her ability to work. She has worked for an uncle's catering business in the past. Client completed the ninth grade before leaving school. She reports not doing well in school. She would like to get her GED at some point.

Case manager provided risk reduction counseling. Client's greatest risk appears to be heterosexual intercourse without a condom. Client verbally agreed to use a condom when engaging in sexual activities. Case manager reviewed state public health laws with client.

Client was pleasant and cooperative throughout the interview process. Affect was congruent with her mood and demeanor. Client appeared to be focused and attentive. Client's thinking was logical and clear. Client did not appear to demonstrate any signs of distrust or paranoia and maintained good eye contact throughout the interview. She didn't demonstrate any signs of agitation or anxiety. She appeared calm and relaxed by her body posture and her tone and cadence. Her judgment and her short-term and long-term memory was intact. Client did not appear to be emaciated or malnourished. She was appropriately dressed for season and situation. She was neatly groomed and her clothes were clean and neat. She was agreeable to improving her situation and addressing her health care.

—Caseworker's signature and the date the report was written

Exercise 1: Identify as many client strengths as you can. Discuss in class with other students.

Exercise 2: Using the needs identified and prioritized, develop a SMART care plan with the client. Identify and address any barriers that would impede the client from achieving her goals.

Sample List of Client's Strengths

1. Client is willing to accept referrals for medical care, start medication if prescribed.

2. Client is capable, knowledgeable, and willing to use public transportation to get to her appointments.

3. Client has a good relationship with her counselor at the shelter.

4. Client has followed the rules at the shelter.

5. Client has remained drug free for thirty-five days.

6. Client is seeking a sponsor.

7. Client is going to Narcotics Anonymous meetings daily.

8. Client is open to mental health evaluation and treatment.

9. Client is interested in getting her GED.

10. Client is looking for a job.

11. Client made verbal agreement to engage in safer-sex behavior by using a condom every time she has sexual intercourse.

12. Client feels healthy enough to work.

References

AIDS.gov. (2012). *How are drug use and HIV related?* Retrieved from http://aids .gov/hiv-aids-basics/prevention/reduce-your-risk/substance-abuse-use/

Bing, L., Burnam, A., Longshore, D., Fleishman, J., Sherbourne, C., London, A., . . . , Shapiro, M. (2001). Psychiatric disorders and drug use among human immunodeficiency virus-infected adults in the United States. *Archives of General Psychiatry, 58,* 721–728.

Brooks, D. (2010). HIV-related case management. In C. C. Poindexter (Ed.), *Handbook of HIV and social work: Principles, practice, and populations.* Hoboken, NJ: Wiley & Sons.

Card, J., Solomon, J., & Berman, J. (2008). *Tools for building culturally competent HIV prevention programs.* New York: Springer Publishing.

Chernesky, R., & Grube, B. (2000). Examining the HIV/AIDS case management process. *Health & Social Work, 25*(4), 243–253.

Delahanty, D., Bogart, L., & Figler, J. L. (2004). Posttraumatic stress symptoms, salivary cortisol, medication adherence, and CD4 levels in HIV-positive individuals. *AIDS Care, 16,* 247–260.

Elliott, A. (1998). Anxiety and HIV infection, *STEP Perspective, 98,* 11–14.

Halkitis, P., Kupprat, S., & Pandley Mukherjee, P. P. (2010). Longitudinal associations between case management and supportive services use among Black and Latina HIV-positive women in New York City. *Journal of Women's Health, 19*(1), 99–108.

Hammond, E., & Treisman, G. (2007). HIV and psychiatric illness. *Psychiatric Times, 24*(14), 1–2.

Johnson, D., Polansky, M., Matosky, M., & Teti, M. (2010). Psychosocial factors associated with successful transition into HIV case management for those without primary care in an urban area. *AIDS and Behavior, 14,* 459–468.

Katz, M., Cunningham, W., Fleishman, J., Anderson, R., Kellogg, T., Bozzette, S., & Shapiro, M. (2001). Effect of case management on unmet needs and utilization of medical care and medications among HIV-infected persons. *Annals of Internal Medicine, 135*(8), 557–565.

Kessler, R. C., Berglund, P., & Demler, O. (2005). Lifetime prevalence and age of onset distributions of DSM-IV disorders in the national comorbidity survey replication. *Archives of General Psychiatry, 62,* 593-602.

Krishnan, K. R., Delong, M., Kraemer, H., Carney, R., Spiegel, D., Gordon, C., . . . , Otey, O. (2002). Comorbidity of depression with other medical diseases in the elderly. *Biological Psychiatry, 52*(6), 559–588.

Lens, V. (2004). Principled negotiation: A new tool for case advocacy. *Social Work, 49*(3), 506–513.

McIntosh, D. (2012). The difference between case and cause advocacy is U (you). *The New Social Worker Online, 17,* 44. Retrieved from http://www.social worker.com/home/index2.php?option=com_content&do_pdf=1&id=343

Program on International Health and Human Rights. (2006). *HIV/AIDS and gender-based violence (GBV) literature review.* Harvard School of Public Health. Boston: Author.

Pugh, G. (2009). Exploring HIV/AIDS case management and client quality of life. *Journal of HIV/AIDS & Social Services, 8,* 202–218.

Wohl, A. R., Garland, W., Witt, M., Valencia, R., Boger, A., Squires, K., & Kovacs, A. (2009). An adherence-focused case management intervention for HIV-positive patients in a public care setting. *Journal of HIV/AIDS & Social Services, 8,* 80–94.

11

Understanding HIV and AIDS Medical Care: A Primer for Social Workers

Diana Rowan and Lamont Holley

Once you choose hope, anything's possible.
—Christopher Reeve, Actor

A major role for social workers in HIV (human immunodeficiency virus) work is to help clients understand their disease and its treatment. Yet clients who have been HIV-positive for some time are likely to be more expert on HIV disease than are the social workers who work with them. Social workers often accompany clients to their medical appointments. With a better understanding of what to discuss during the visit, the social worker can more effectively prepare the client and review the information with the client.

The acronyms, medications, lab tests, and diseases that are routinely discussed in HIV and AIDS (acquired immune deficiency syndrome) care can be confusing, and most social workers do not have a background in medical terminology. This chapter provides a primer for social workers on information that is likely to be significant in the course of a client's medical care. It is, of course, not meant to replace expert medical care; rather, it is designed to help social workers navigate the complexities of HIV and AIDS diagnoses and care provided by medical professionals.

HIV/AIDS 101
What Are HIV and AIDS?

HIV is the acronym for human immunodeficiency virus, the virus that causes AIDS (acquired immune deficiency syndrome). There are two common errors in the use of these two abbreviations. First, because the "V" in HIV stands for virus, it is redundant to say "HIV virus." Also, note that HIV contains the word "immunodeficiency" and AIDS contains two words—"immune deficiency." Be sure to understand that no one becomes sick from either HIV or AIDS; instead people experience opportunistic infections that take hold because of a lowered immune response in the body brought about by the presence of HIV.

Prevalence of HIV in the United States

The most recent statistics on HIV prevalence from the Centers for Disease Control and Prevention (CDC) are from 2009. At that time, the CDC estimated that 1.2 million people in the United States were living with HIV and one in five were unaware that they had HIV. Each year, about 50,000 people in the United States learn that they are HIV-positive. Since the epidemic began in 1981, an estimated 1,108,611 people in the United States have been diagnosed with AIDS, and nearly 594,500 people with AIDS have died. About 16,000 people living with AIDS die each year (CDC, 2012).

Gay, bisexual, and other men who have sex with men (MSM) of all races and ethnicities are the population most affected by HIV (see figure 11.1). According to the

Figure 11.1. Estimates of New HIV Infections in the United States, 2009, for the Most-Affected Subpopulations

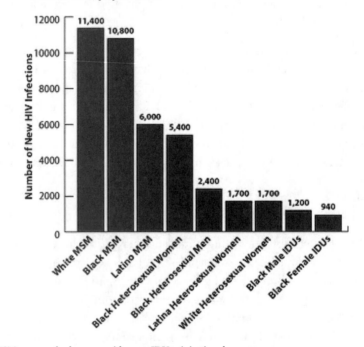

Notes: MSM = men who have sex with men; IDU = injection drug user.

CDC (2012), MSM account for 61 percent of all new cases of HIV and 49 percent of people living with HIV; young Black MSM were the only risk group in the United States to experience statistically significant increases in new cases of HIV. Heterosexuals and injection drug users also continue to be affected (see figure 11.2). Blacks represent approximately 14 percent of the U.S. population, but accounted for an estimated 44 percent of new cases of HIV in 2009. Latinos represent 16 percent of the U.S. population but accounted for 20 percent of new infections in that year (CDC, 2012).

Figure 11.2. Estimated New HIV Infections, 2009, by Transmission Category

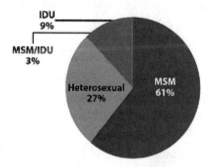

Notes: MSM = men who have sex with men; IDU = injection drug user.

Modes of Transmission of HIV

HIV is infectious, not contagious. It can be transmitted in three ways: (1) through blood transmission, (2) sexual transmission (through semen or vaginal fluid), or (3) from a mother to child, either at birth, which is called perinatal transmission, or through breast milk. HIV is not transmitted through casual contact, sneezing, coughing, sharing of utensils, swimming pools, public toilets, or mosquitoes. HIV is inactivated outside of a human host and therefore cannot survive in open air or water (AVERT, 2011a).

The CDC data presented above indicate that the most common route of infection is through sexual transmission. Yet the most efficient route of transmission is through infected blood or blood products (AVERT, 2011a). Prior to 1992, there was no reliable screening tool to detect HIV in the supply of donated blood. An estimated 10,000 people with hemophilia contracted HIV through tainted blood transfusions before screenings became mandatory for 100 percent of the supply of blood and blood products in the United States. Hundreds more people became HIV-positive through blood transfusions during surgeries (Cichocki, 2010). While the U.S. blood supply is now considered extremely safe, it is worth noting that not all countries, especially developing countries with weak enforcement of public health policies, can guarantee that their blood supplies are free from HIV.

Transmission of HIV through contaminated blood can occur when dirty needles, syringes, or other paraphernalia are used to inject drugs. Needle-exchange programs, which provide "no questions asked" exchange of dirty needles and syringes for new ones, were once highly controversial. Opponents believed that provision of injection drug paraphernalia would encourage and even endorse illegal drug use. In 1989, Congress banned the use of federal funds for use in syringe exchange programs. In 2005, however, the CDC reported that the National Institutes of Health (NIH) had concluded that these exchange programs contributed to an 80 percent reduction in risk behaviors in injecting drug users and a 30 percent reduction in HIV transmissions. They also concluded that there was a "preponderance of evidence to show that syringe exchange programs [did] not encourage increased substance abuse" (AIDS Action, 2007, p. 1). In 2009, Congress, at the urging of the Obama administration, reversed the ban so that federal funding could be used for syringe exchange programs. Then, in December 2011, federal funds for these programs were eliminated again as part of the 2012 budget cuts (Broverman, 2011).

Levels of Risk for Transmission Methods

HIV infection is acquired primarily through sexual intercourse. Anal, vaginal, and less frequently, oral sexual intercourse can result in transfer of the virus. The highest rates of transmission occur in unprotected receptive anal intercourse, especially with mucosal tearing. Unprotected receptive vaginal intercourse, especially during menses, and unprotected rectal or vaginal intercourse in the presence of genital ulcers, such as are found in primary syphilis or genital herpes, are also high risk for HIV transmission. Lower-risk sex practices include insertive anal or vaginal intercourse and oral genital contact (Saag, Chambers, Eliopoulos, Gilbert, & Moellering, 2011).

Transmission risk increases with the number of encounters and with a higher viral load in the person infected (Gray et al., 2001). The mode of transmission does not affect the natural progression of HIV disease, though those who acquire it through needle sharing may have a more complicated progression due to complications from substance use (May et al., 2007).

The virus can also be transmitted through contaminated blood in occupational exposures, for example in medical settings. There have been fifty-six confirmed cases of HIV transmission to health-care workers; more than 90 percent of these involved percutaneous exposure (such as accidental needle sticks); the rest involved mucous membrane or nonintact skin exposure (Sax, Cohen, & Kuritzkes, 2011). Anyone who suspects occupational exposure should consult with a physician as soon as possible to discuss postexposure prophylaxis, which usually involves placing the worker on certain antiretroviral (ARV) medications and administering HIV tests periodically over six months.

Sero-discordancy is the term given to sexual relationships in which one partner is HIV-positive and the other partner is HIV-negative. In 2011, exciting news was released by the HIV Prevention Trials Network (HPTN) with regard to a clinical trial called HPTN Clinical Trial 052. Across nine countries, 1,763 sero-discordant couples were enrolled in a study to measure the impact of placing the HIV-positive partner on ARV medications earlier than is called for in current protocols (Cohen et al., 2011). The randomized clinical trial found that provision of the early medication therapy to the HIV-positive partner reduced the risk of transmission of HIV to the HIV-negative partner by 96 percent. The study provides scientific proof that "treatment as prevention" is effective; *Science* magazine named the study the Breakthrough of the Year for 2011 (HPTN, 2011). The impacts of this study are not yet fully realized, however. Currently, the World Health Organization is using the study results to generate policies related to the global medical management of sero-discordant couples (HPTN, 2011).

Conditions that Facilitate HIV Sexual Transmission

Certain conditions facilitate the sexual transmission of HIV. These conditions vary based on the gender of the person with HIV, as noted below (Saag et al., 2011).

- Male-to-female transmission is facilitated by

  - Use of oral contraceptives

  - Use of a sub-dermal contraceptive implant

  - Candida vaginitis

  - Vitamin A deficiency

  - Low CD4 count in the male with HIV

- Female-to-male transmission is facilitated by

  - Lack of circumcision

  - Genital ulcers

  - Vaginal intercourse during menstruation

  - Genital herpes

  - Vitamin A deficiency

  - Low CD4 count in the female with HIV

Not all types of birth control are effective in preventing HIV and other sexually transmitted infections (STIs). Only latex and vinyl condoms are effective in preventing HIV and STIs. Natural condoms, which are made of animal intestine, are effective in preventing pregnancy, but not in preventing HIV transmission, because the membrane is permeable to viruses but not to sperm cells. Birth control devices called IUDs (intrauterine devices) are not effective in preventing STIs.

Stages of HIV Infection

HIV disease has a well-documented progression. If it is not treated, the virus will eventually overwhelm the immune system, and the person will be diagnosed with AIDS. The stages of HIV disease are briefly summarized below. (The people who experience exceptions to this progression, called chronic nonprogressors or elite controllers, are discussed in the next section.) The typical stages of HIV disease, and what happens at each stage, are described below (AIDS.gov, 2010; Sax et al., 2011):

1. Viral transmission. HIV is transmitted from a person with HIV to another person, through one of the routes of transmission listed above. The mode of transmission does not affect the progression of HIV disease.

2. Acute (primary) HIV infection. Acute HIV occurs one to four weeks after transmission. It is accompanied by a burst of viral replication and a decline in CD4 count (also known as T-cell count). Most people experience flu-like symptoms that they frequently overlook.

3. Sero-conversion. Sero-conversion, which is when an HIV antibody test shows a positive result, occurs between four weeks and six months after transmission of HIV.

4. Asymptomatic HIV infection. Asymptomatic HIV lasts a variable amount of time (usually eight to ten years) and is accompanied by a gradual decline in CD4 count and a relatively stable HIV RNA level (also known as one's "viral load"). The patient does not experience any symptoms during this period.

5. Early symptomatic HIV infection. This stage was previously referred to as "AIDS-related complex," or ARC. This stage is when symptoms begin to appear. Common symptoms at this stage are oral thrush, vaginal candidiasis, recurring herpes zoster, oral hairy leukoplakia, peripheral neuropathy, diarrhea, and constitutional symptoms (low-grade fevers, weight loss).

6. Acquired immune deficiency syndrome. AIDS is defined by a CD4 count of less than 200 cells per milliliter, and the occurrence of one of several AIDS-related opportunistic infections (OIs), including HIV wasting syndrome (see below for list of common OIs).

7. Advanced HIV disease. When the CD4 count is less than 50 cells per milliliter, the patient may die. Most AIDS-related deaths occur around this CD4 level.

Nonprogressors

Chronic or long-term nonprogressors are individuals who have been living with HIV for seven to twelve years, have stable CD4 counts of 600 or more cells per milliliter of blood, have had no previous ARV therapy, and have no AIDS-related diseases (Cichocki, 2007). It is estimated that about 1 percent of people living with HIV (PLWH) are nonprogressors, and a smaller number are elite controllers, who are capable of further suppression of their viral loads for extended periods. Chronic nonprogressors and elite controllers are of significant interest to medical researchers, since understanding why the disease does not progress in these individuals may hold the key to a new treatment or cure for AIDS. Although nonprogressors experience slowed or no progression of the disease, their health-care providers should routinely monitor their CD4 counts, to ensure that they are still in nonprogressor status (Health Central Network, Inc., 2011; Pogash, 2005; Smith, 2011).

Opportunistic Infections

When a person who is HIV positive has a CD4 count of 200 or fewer cells per cubic milliliter of blood and also has one of the twenty-four AIDS-defining illnesses (or opportunistic infections), the person is said to have AIDS. An opportunistic infection (OI) is an illness that affects a person who has a vulnerable immune system.

Early symptoms of worsening HIV infection include constitutional symptoms such as night sweats, fatigue, weight loss, and hugely swollen lymph nodes. Some of the most common life-threatening, AIDS-defining opportunistic infections are (PBS, 2006):

- Pneumocystis carinii pneumonia (PCP): PCP is a rare form of pneumonia seen in people with suppressed immune systems. The main symptom is extreme shortness of breath; treatment requires heavy doses of antibiotics combined with oxygen therapy. PCP is currently a common, but feared infection in people with AIDS, and many suffer several bouts of it before it causes their death.

- Candidiasis, or thrush: An explosive fungal growth that occurs in the mouth, throat, anus, or trachea, or on the skin. It appears most frequently in men as a white coating of the mouth and causes a burning sensation, a bad taste, and lack of appetite. Women can also get it in the mouth, but often one of the first warning signs of HIV for women is a problem with chronic vaginal candida that does not respond to treatment. The fungus naturally lives in the body in small quantities, but without a healthy immune system to keep it in check, it can run rampant. In rare cases, candidiasis can spread throughout the body and become a life-threatening condition.

- Toxoplasmosis (often called "toxo"): Toxo is a disease caused by a parasite that infects the brain and can cause both brain damage and blindness. In the United States, up to 60 million people are thought to be infected with the parasite, but for most, the body's immune system normally keeps it under control. Before AIDS, toxoplasmosis was considered a minor danger for pregnant women and was not seen as a serious public health threat.

- Cytomegalovirus (CMV): This virus is a member of the herpes family of viruses and one of the leading causes of blindness and death in people with AIDS. CMV is common in adults, but it is normally held in check by a healthy immune system. Almost everyone with HIV tests positive for CMV. However, it is very rare for CMV disease to develop unless the CD4 count drops below 50, a sign of serious damage to the immune system. CMV can infect any part of the body, but in people with AIDS, it generally attacks one or both eyes.

- Kaposi's sarcoma: Kaposi's sarcoma is a skin cancer characterized by purple lesions. Before AIDS, Kaposi's sarcoma (KS) was usually seen in older men of

Eastern European descent. This once highly visible sign of AIDS is less common in the United States now than it was during the 1980s and early 1990s because the medical profession has learned to prevent or control it. Internationally, KS is still frequently seen.

Physicians can treat these and other opportunistic infections, but when HIV has late stages of AIDS, HIV begins attacking other cells in addition to those in the immune system. Scientists do not entirely understand HIV's impact on the nervous system, but frequently individuals with AIDS begin to experience dementia, problems with balance, and an inability to move their legs and arms. HIV can also attack a person's internal organs.

AIDS-Defining Illnesses

The CDC in Atlanta are responsible for determining which opportunistic infections are included in the list of twenty-four AIDS-defining illnesses. These AIDS-defining illnesses are grouped in five categories (AVERT, 2011b):

1. Bacterial diseases such as tuberculosis, mycobacterium avium complex, bacterial pneumonia, and septicemia (blood poisoning)

2. Protozoal diseases such as toxoplasmosis, microsporidiosis, cryptosporidiosis, iso-psoriasis, and leishmaniasis

3. Fungal diseases such as PCP, candidiasis, cryptococcosis, and penicilliosis

4. Viral diseases such as those caused by CMV, herpes simplex, and herpes zoster virus

5. HIV-associated malignancies such as Kaposi's sarcoma, lymphoma, and squamous cell carcinoma

The Physician's Medical Assessment of Patients with HIV Disease

The outline below provides an overview of the content of the medical exam and assessment that a patient with HIV will encounter when meeting with a new physician. The exam protocol is similar whether the patient is newly diagnosed or is meeting with a new provider. This section is not meant to suggest that anyone other than a qualified physician (and ideally an infectious disease physician who specializes in HIV disease) should conduct the assessment. The assessment is well beyond the scope of the social worker's focus. The information provided here is meant to help social workers understand the assessment given to their patients. The social worker can use this information to help explain to the patient the purpose of the questions and tests.

Medical History and Physical

The information presented here is taken from the 2009 Primary Care Guidelines for the Management of Persons Infected with Human Immunodeficiency Virus, which are supported by the Infectious Diseases Society of America (Aberg et al., 2009; Saag et al., 2011). Short explanations are added to contextualize the significance of the information.

1. Documentation of a positive HIV antibody test, confirmed by a second HIV antibody test, a Western blot, or positive plasma viral HIV RNA PCR quantification.

2. History, review of systems, and past medical history

    a. General health status

        i. General well-being, symptoms

        ii. Infectious diseases (tuberculosis, leishmaniasis, cocci, histoplasmosis, etc.), childhood infections, infections in adult life, previous physician visits, hospitalizations (where, when)

        iii. Immunization history, e.g., hepatitis A, hepatitis B, BCG (Bacillus Calmette Guerin), pneumococcal

    b. Drug history

        i. Current medications and dosages

            (1). Prescription and nonprescription

            (2). Alternative therapies

        ii. Recreational drug use

            (1). Intravenous (or injection), smoking, oral, inhalant

            (2). Alcohol use—current and past

            (3). Cigarette use

   c. Sexual history

       i. Past and current sex practices

      ii. Past and current sexually transmitted diseases

    iii. Obstetric/gynecological history (for patients born as women)

    iv. Contraceptive use

     v. Risk factors for HIV and STDs

   d. Past or present HIV-related illnesses

   e. Risks for opportunistic infections (because some OIs are caused by bacteria that are more common in certain parts of the world and in certain environments, knowledge of the travel and activity habits of the patient can help create a clearer picture of risks)

       i. Travel history

      ii. Geographic location

    iii. Occupational history

    iv. Hobbies and recreation

     v. Tuberculosis status, history of BCG (Bacillus Calmette Guerin) vaccination, family members with or being treated for TB, contacts with people with known TB, results of chest x-rays

    vi. Pets, specifically cats: Bartonella henselae (cat scratch fever); and fish: M. marinum. Note that cat ownership has not been found to be associated with toxoplasma antibody sero-conversion.

   f. History of viral hepatitis and past history of herpes zoster

3. Comprehensive Physical Examination

   a. Height and weight, history of significant weight losses or gains

   b. Careful funduscopic and oral examination

   c. Dermotologic examination, including back, buttocks, and extremities

d. Examination of all lymph node areas, postoccipital, preauricular, cervical, submental, supraclavicular, axillary, epitrochlear, and inguinal

e. Rectal and genital examination, to include pelvic exam with Pap smear in women, and inspection for perianal or genital herpes simplex

f. Assessment of mental status for evidence of dementia

4. Laboratory evaluation

a. Baseline

i. Complete blood cell count (CBC) with differential (anemia may affect use of zidovudine)

ii. Electrolytes, blood sugar (diabetes may complicate use of protease inhibitor [PI] ARVs, which cause insulin resistance), renal function tests, BUN (blood urea nitrogen test), creatine (abnormal renal function may complicate use of tenovir or require adjustment in NRTI [nucleoside reverse transcriptase inhibitor] and NNRTI [nonnucleoside reverse transcriptase inhibitor] dosages)

iii. Liver enzyme tests, serum bilirubin, aspartate aminotransferase, alanine aminotransferase, alkaline phosphatase (indinavir and atazanavir can elevate indirect bilirubin levels)

iv. Creatine kinase (high level may indicate either HIV- or drug-induced myopathy)

v. Fasting lipid profile (elevated levels may indicate need for dietary or drug therapy or avoidance of certain protease inhibitors [PIs])

b. HIV staging (important for all future care decisions, including when to initiate ARV and prophylaxis)

i. CD4 and CD8 T-lymphocyte count

ii. Quantitative measurement of plasma HIV RNA: viral load or plasma viral burden

iii. Repeated measurement every three to four months

   c. Additional studies

      i. Purified protein derivative, a skin test for TB

      ii. Chest x-ray (baseline important for future comparisons)

      iii. VDRL (venereal disease research laboratory) or RPR (rapid plasma reagin) (test for syphilis) repeated annually (evidence of past or recent exposure requires treatment unless there is documentation of adequate course of treatment)

      iv. IgG (immunoglobulin G test) antibody test for toxoplasmosis

      v. Hepatitis B surface antigen (HBsAg), antibody to hepatitis B surface Ag (anti-HBsAg), antibody to hepatitis C (important in consideration of treatment decisions for chronic active infection and ARV), IgG antibody to hepatitis A

      vi. CMV antibody, IgG

      vii. G6PD Assay in African-American patients (glucose-6 phosphate dehydrogenase is a hereditary condition most common in African Americans, in whom red blood cells break down when exposed to certain drugs or infections)

      viii. Urine nucleic acid amplification test for C. trachomatis and N. gonorrhea

      ix. Type-specific herpes simplex antibody

      x. Serum testosterone level

5. Initial health care

   a. HIV risk reduction education

   b. Drug rehabilitation, safer needle use, needle exchange

   c. Smoking cessation (cigarette smoking increases the incidence of oral thrush, hairy leukoplakia, bacterial pneumonia, and coronary artery disease)

   d. Partner notification through the county health department

    e. Reproductive counseling

    f. Psychosocial support

    g. Immunizations (immunizations can temporarily increase HIV viral load)

        i. Pneumococcal vaccine

        ii. Influenza vaccine (annually)

        iii. Hepatitis B vaccine, hepatitis A vaccine

    h. Preventive dentistry

    i. Ophthalmologic evaluation if CD4 count is less than 100 cells per milliliter

    j. Cervical pap smear for females, anal pap smear for males and females

6. Primary care of patients infected with HIV

    a. Multiple studies demonstrate that physicians and other health-care providers who make care for large numbers of people with HIV a major focus of their practice, training, and continuing education have better outcomes. A team approach, with coordination of services around patients' needs and integration of acute and long-term care, is emerging as the most effective approach to HIV care (figure 11.3).

Common Laboratory Tests

A social worker may wonder why it is necessary to be knowledgeable about laboratory tests, when the field of medical technology falls outside the scope of social work practice. There are, in fact, several reasons. First, it is common for new, and even some veteran, HIV patients to be confused by the various types of tests that are administered during a medical office visit. It is also common for the social worker to be the person with whom the client feels most comfortable in asking clarifying questions. Some clients do not show much interest in understanding their lab tests and results, trusting that medical professionals are handling their care according to proper protocols. Yet others are very involved in their own care, learning about various aspects such as drug combinations, symptoms, possible side effects, and test results. Some clients are very sophisticated and educated about

Figure 11.3. Approach to HIV Testing

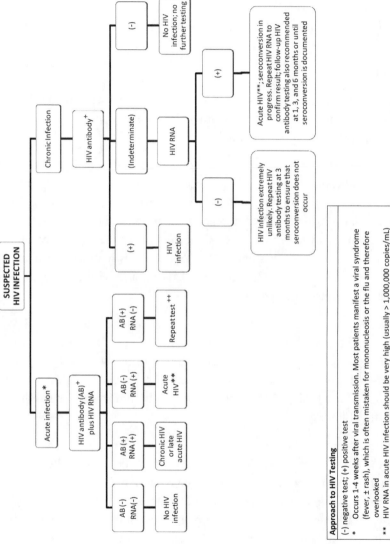

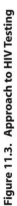

their conditions. When asked, social workers should be confident in any answers they share; it is better for them to ask others repeated times for clarification than to risk providing wrong information to a client even once. Furthermore, knowledge about HIV testing in particular is helpful for operation of AIDS service organization (ASO) HIV prevention programs, such as those that conduct counseling and testing on site.

HIV Testing

There are two main types of tests that determine whether a person has HIV: HIV antibody tests and plasma HIV RNA assays. Both are described below, followed by an explanation of when they are used.

HIV Antibody Testing. Most patients produce antibodies to HIV within six to eight weeks of exposure, and about 50 percent of people with HIV will have a positive antibody test within three to four weeks of exposure. Nearly all people with HIV will test positive for HIV antibodies by six months after infection (Sax et al., 2011). HIV antibody tests do not test for the presence of the HIV; instead, they test for the presence of antibodies to the virus that the body has made. Antibodies are made of proteins and are therefore much larger than a virus, and are therefore much easier to detect through testing.

There are two ways that HIV infection is determined: one is testing for HIV antibodies, and the second is testing for the virus itself. For the first way, there are two main types of HIV antibody tests: enzyme linked immunosorbant assay (ELISA) and Western blot (sometimes called protein immunoblot). ELISA is the usual screening test but positive ELISA results are usually confirmed through the use of the Western blot test.

ELISA detects antibodies, but not only HIV antibodies. It can be used to detect antibodies to other viruses, such as West Nile Virus, and to detect food allergies, such as allergies to milk, nuts, and eggs. Similarly, the Western blot is the term used for the approach to identification of proteins in a sample through the use of gel electrophoresis. This process separates the proteins present in the sample into separate bands. In HIV antibody testing, if bands are detected that match those standardized bands of known HIV antibodies, that is a conclusive determination that the sample from the person definitely contains HIV antibodies. HIV antibodies are only developed in response to HIV and therefore their presence indicates the presence of HIV. The Western blot test is also useful in testing for the presence of other proteins, such as antibodies to the viruses causing Lyme disease, hepatitis B, bovine spongiform encephalopathy (known as mad cow disease), and FIV (feline immunodeficiency virus) in cats.

HIV antibody testing can be done in settings other than medical clinics. A home test kit, called Home Access HIV-1 Test System, can be purchased without a prescription at a pharmacy or can be ordered by phone or website for less than $50. Users receive a kit that contains a stylet for obtaining a drop of blood from the fingertip, which they place on filter paper and mail to the company for testing. Using a code on the kit, the user calls the company to obtain the results of the test. This is considered anonymous testing, since no record of the name of the user is ever made. In contrast, health departments and clinics use confidential testing, where the name of the person being tested is recorded, but it is kept confidential. Once the user of the home test is given the result, the person can participate in optional phone counseling. If the test is positive for HIV antibodies, the person is told to seek care through a medical provider. It is important to note that the use of home test kits is controversial. Advocates support their use because those people who are too concerned about privacy to take a test through a provider can still find out their sero-status. Those not in support of home testing kits have concerns that people who learn they have a positive result may not seek care and will therefore not be tracked by the public health system. Furthermore, they may become emotionally despondent after learning their positive sero-status and without counseling may attempt to hurt themselves or others.

The OraSure test, which tests for HIV antibodies through a swab from the inside of the cheek, has been used since 1996. The sample is sent to a lab for ELISA testing, with positive results confirmed by Western blot. This test is still commonly used due to its accuracy, but since there is a delay in getting the results, the person being tested must return for the results.

Rapid HIV tests, such as OraQuick ADVANCE Rapid HIV Test and Uni-Gold Recombigen HIV, return results in ten to twenty minutes, thus not requiring that the person return for results. The OraQuick test was approved in 2004 and can test blood or cheek swabs. The Uni-Gold test only tests blood. The accuracy of these tests is about the same as with ELISA, so positive results must also be confirmed with a Western blot. A major advantage of these tests is that negative results can be given quickly, with no follow-up testing necessary.

An HIV diagnostic test called p24 Antigen is also approved for diagnosis of HIV but is rarely used because of its low sensitivity.

In the United States, donated blood is screened for HIV using nucleic acid based tests. The time between infection with HIV and detection of HIV with this test is twelve days. In 2010, a new test was approved that detects both HIV antibodies and the p24 antigen. It is ARCHITECT HIV Antigen/Antibody Combination Assay. This test provides accurate positive results sooner than standard ELISA testing.

Plasma HIV RNA Testing. Quantitative plasma HIV RNA testing, often called an HIV viral load assay, is used to measure the amount of HIV RNA in plasma. The high sensitivity of this assay allows for detection of the amount of actual HIV (the virus itself) present, not just the presence of antibodies to the virus. The assay can detect HIV in most people with HIV who are not on ARV medications at the time. The HIV RNA test, or "viral load," is used for two reasons. The first is to diagnose acute HIV infection. Determination of one's viral load at the time when the person is first determined to be HIV-positive is a helpful baseline for monitoring his or her response to ARV medications. The other reason the test is used is to monitor how well the medications are working at keeping the person's viral load low, with the goal being to have the virus be "undetectable." It is common practice to measure viral load two to eight weeks after initiation of ARV therapy, and then every three to six months after that.

There are several types of HIV RNA assays, with different levels of sensitivity. Any of these can be used to initially diagnose a person as HIV positive, but in order to monitor viral load over time, the same test should be used longitudinally, for the sake of comparison. The PCR (polymerase chain reaction) tests are the most common. The test takes a single piece or a few strands of DNA (or in the case of HIV, a few strands of RNA) and amplifies these into many copies. The RT-PCR Amplicor test can detect as few as 400 copies of the virus per milliliter, and the RT-PCR Ultrasensitive can detect as few as 50 copies of HIV per milliliter. The bDNA Versant test has a sensitivity of 75 copies per milliliter. The Nucleic Acid Sequence-Based Amplification test has a sensitivity of 176 copies per milliliter. The Real

Time HIV-1 assay is also a PCR-based assay; it has a sensitivity of 40 copies per milliliter.

Testing for viral load should be avoided while a patient is experiencing an opportunistic infection, such as bacterial pneumonia. As noted earlier, there can also be a slight increase in viral load after receiving immunizations, so tests may not be accurate then. Also, HIV RNA tests should not be used to diagnose HIV during the first three to six weeks after viral transmission because they have an unacceptably high false positive rate in the early weeks. Finally, if the patient is too sick for even deep salvage ARV regimens or when there are no medication options available, the common protocol is to not test viral load, since nothing can be done.

Correlation between HIV RNA (Viral Load) and CD4 Cell Count. In general, viral loads and CD4 counts are inversely related: if one is high, the other is expected to be low. However, in some situations, patients with high CD4 counts have relatively high HIV RNA levels, and vice versa. In response to ARV therapy, drops in viral load usually precede changes in CD4 cell counts. Figure 11.4 shows the levels of HIV RNA and CD4 cells through the typical progression of HIV disease.

Figure 11.4. CD4 Count and Viral Load across HIV Disease Progression

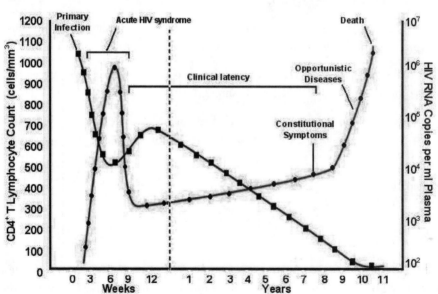

Typical Laboratory Tests for HIV Patients

Routine tests that the physician supervising the medical care of someone living with HIV orders are listed below. All of these tests are commonly conducted at the beginning of care, to record baseline values, and are repeated according to protocols.

- ELISA and confirmatory Western blot, to document HIV infection.

- HIV RNA assay (viral load).

- Complete blood count (CBC).

- Chemistry panel (SMA 20).

- Fasting lipid profile (the patient must be told not to eat anything after bedtime the night before blood sample is collected).

- CD4 cell count (table 11.1 gives details on the conditions associated with ranges of results).

- HIV resistance genotype (about 15 percent of newly diagnosed patients in the United States have some drug resistance).

- Tuberculin skin test (TB test).

- PAP smear. (The risk of cervical cancer is nearly twice as high in HIV-positive women; some advocate for anal pap smears to be given to HIV-positive men.)

- Toxoplasmosis serology (IgG). (This immunoglobulin test identifies patients at risk for cerebral or systemic toxoplasmosis.)

- Syphilis serology (VDRL or RPR). (This test identifies coinfection with syphilis, which is epidemiologically linked to HIV; syphilis progression can be accelerated in HIV patients.)

- Hepatitis A, B, and C serologies.

- Chest x-ray.

CD4 Cell Count

The CD4 cell count, also known as the lymphocyte subset analysis, is a routine test performed over the course of HIV care. It provides a quantitative measure of the degree of the patient's immunosuppression. Table 11.1 describes the conditions commonly associated with various ranges of CD4 cell counts.

Table 11.1. Conditions Commonly Associated with CD4

CD4 (cells/ml)	Associated Conditions
>500	Most illnesses are similar to those of people without HIV infection. There is increased risk of some bacterial infections, including pneumococcal pneumonia, herpes zoster, tuberculosis, and skin conditions.
200–500	All of the above, and Kaposi's sarcoma, vaginal candidiasis, and ITP (idiopathic thrombocytopenic purpura).
50–200	All of the above, and thrush, oral hairy leukoplakia, and HIV-related opportunistic infections, including PCP, cryptococcal meningitis, and toxoplasmosis.
<50	All of the above, and the final pathway opportunistic infections, including disseminated M. avium complex, CMV retinitis, HIV-associated wasting, and neurologic diseases, such as neuropathy and encephalopathy.

HIV Testing Brain Teasers

The questions below can be answered based on the information about HIV tests provided in the previous pages. These are difficult questions, even for veterans of HIV social work. Try your best to answer them. The correct answers appear at the end of the chapter.

1. Estelle is HIV positive and is new in town. Not long before moving, she gave birth to a baby boy she named Chance. Chance's new pediatrician, Dr. Baldwin, is not well versed in HIV testing, but upon learning that Chance's mother was living with HIV, she ordered that the ELISA test be performed on the baby's blood. The test results showed a positive result. Dr. Baldwin was aware that the Western blot test must be performed to confirm a positive ELISA test, so she ordered that the Western blot test be performed as well. Again, the results were positive. Dr. Baldwin called in Estelle for an emergency meeting in her office, and told Estelle that she has bad news: her baby had HIV, just like her. Dr. Baldwin began to explain that Estelle should have been taking prophylactic ARVs so that she would not transmit HIV to her baby during the delivery. Estelle quickly interrupted and said she did take nevirapine during the pregnancy and she was certain that Chance does not have HIV. Dr. Baldwin explained that she had already performed a confirmatory test called a Western blot, which is very accurate, and both the ELISA and Western blot tests showed positive results. Estelle began to laugh. She said to the pediatrician, "You need to learn more about HIV, Doctor. Of course he tested positive to the ELISA and Western blot! But, I am

sure my baby is not HIV positive and if you knew more about HIV testing, you would, too."

What fact about HIV tests is Estelle aware of that Dr. Baldwin isn't? (Check the answer at the end of the chapter.)

2. Booker notices a sign for "free and confidential HIV testing" outside the student union on his college campus. He thinks back to an exciting night of fun he had the previous semester. He had hooked up with at least two girls he didn't know, and it may have been more. He was concerned he might have caught a nasty sexually transmitted disease (STD), or even HIV. He considers participation in the testing, but decides to ask a few questions first. He would like to know how long the process will take and for how many days he will be kept in agony, waiting for his results. The counselor sitting behind the privacy screen in the student union tells him that they are using the OraQuick test, and he will be given his results in ten to twenty minutes. Booker is satisfied with that answer. He thinks of another reason why he might abandon the plan to be tested—needle phobia. Booker asks the counselor how long the needle is that will draw the blood sample. He is relieved when the counselor tells him that an oral sample is all that is necessary—just a swab on the inside of his cheek. Booker receives his results and is glad to hear he is HIV free. That weekend he attends a party and finds himself kissing a girl he just met. He wonders about HIV, then dismisses the thought, because he remembers from high school health class that you can't get HIV from kissing. Yet he thinks HIV must be present in the mouth, otherwise why else would saliva be used for an HIV test? He becomes mortified, thinking of the possibility of HIV all over this girl's kisses. On Monday morning, he calls the campus health center to ask if he can get HIV from kissing. The nurse chuckles, saying she hasn't heard that myth in years. But, he asks, if HIV is not present in saliva, then why does the OraQuick test use an oral sample?

How would you respond to Booker's question? (Check the answer at the end of the chapter.)

STIs and HIV
Sexually Transmitted Infections and Related Conditions

Having an STI (or STD) can make an individual more likely to get HIV (CDC, 2011). Indeed, individuals who are infected with an STI are two to five times more likely than uninfected individuals to acquire HIV if they are exposed to the virus through sexual contact. Furthermore, if a person with HIV is also infected with another STI (especially herpes), that person is more likely to transmit the virus than other HIV persons. Thus, STIs are factors in increased susceptibility and increased infectiousness.

The following is a list of sexually transmitted conditions, in alphabetical order:

- Bacterial vaginosis
- Chancroid
- Chlamydia
- Gonorrhea
- Hepatitis, viral
- Herpes, genital
- Human papillomavirus
- Lymphogranuloma venereum
- Pubic lice infestation
- Scabies
- Syphilis
- Trichomoniasis

Strong STD prevention, testing, and treatment play a vital role in comprehensive programs to prevent sexual transmission of HIV. Furthermore, STD trends can offer important insights into where the HIV epidemic may grow, making STD surveillance data helpful in forecasting where HIV rates are likely to increase. Better linkages are needed between HIV and STD prevention efforts nationwide in order to control both epidemics (CDC, 2011).

Treatment for HIV and AIDS
Antiretroviral Drugs for Treatment of HIV infection

Prior to 1987, there was no treatment for HIV disease, only palliative care. In 1987, the Food and Drug Administration (FDA) approved azidothymidine (AZT), the first ARV drug to address HIV. Since then, the protocols for treatment have advanced, first to a dual-drug therapy and now to highly active antiretroviral therapy (HAART). HAART is defined as treatment with at least three active ARV medications, typically two nucleoside or nucleotide reverse transcriptase inhibitors (NRTIs) plus a nonnucleoside reverse transcriptase inhibitor (NNRTI) or a protease inhibitor, or another NRTI called abacavir (Ziagen). HAART, consisting of the three classes of drugs named above, is often called the drug cocktail, or triple therapy. There are other classes of HAART, including fusion inhibitors (which are also called entry inhibitors), CCR5 (human chemokine receptor 5) antagonists, and integrase inhibitors. Table 11.2 lists the five main groups of ARV medications and how each group attacks HIV.

A list of all ARV medications, organized by class, is presented in table 11.3. Figure 11.5 shows where the various classes of ARV medications intervene in the life cycle of HIV. Since almost all ARV medications are now delivered in a triple cocktail, the abbreviation HAART is often replaced with ARV (ARV medications).

Table 11.2. Five Main Groups of ARV Medications

Antiretroviral drug class	Classifications and abbreviations	First approved to treat HIV	How they attack
Nucleoside/Nucleotide Reverse Transcriptase Inhibitors	NRTIs, nucleoside analogues, nukes	1987	NRTIs interfere with the action of an HIV protein called reverse transcriptase, which the virus needs to replicate itself
Nonnucleoside Reverse Transcriptase Inhibitors	NNRTIs, nonnucleosides, nonnukes	1997	NNRTIs also stop HIV from replicating within cells by inhibiting the reverse transcriptase protein
Protease Inhibitors	PIs	1995	PIs inhibit protease, which is another protein involved in the HIV replication process
Fusion or Entry Inhibitors	FIs	2003	Fusion or entry inhibitors prevent HIV from binding to or entering human immune cells
Integrase Inhibitors		2007	Integrase inhibitors interfere with the integrase enzyme, which HIV needs to insert its genetic material into human cells.

Source: AVERT, Introduction to HIV treatment (2011c). Retrieved from http://www.avert.org/treatment.htm.

Figure 11.5. Site of Disruption of HIV Life Cycle for Different Classes of Antiretroviral Medications

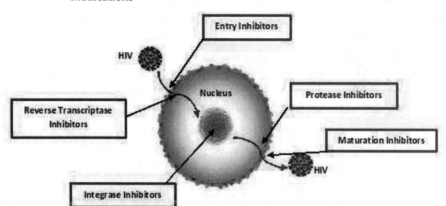

HAART affords physicians a potent way of suppressing viral replication in the blood while preventing the virus from rapidly developing resistance to individual ARV medications. Suppressing viral replication with HAART allows the body time to rebuild its immune system and replenish the destroyed CD4 cells (or T-cells). HAART has been clearly shown to delay progression to AIDS and to prolong life. Currently, there is no cure for HIV disease or AIDS. If the patient stops HAART, HIV becomes detectable in the blood once again. Once HAART is started in a patient, it must be continued throughout the patient's life. An exception to this is pregnant women with HIV disease who have high enough CD4 counts to avoid being on HAART but who take the drugs during their pregnancy to protect their child from HIV infection during birth. These women take HAART and then can stop the regimen after delivery, under supervision of their physician.

Numerous medications are now approved by the FDA for suppression of HIV. The treatment protocol developed by the physician for each patient depends on a number of factors. One of the most important is whether the patient is treatment naïve (has never been on HAART) or treatment experienced (has been on ARV medications in the past and may have failed on them). Other factors taken into consideration are the patient's CD4 count, viral load (HIV RNA), other health problems, life circumstances, and likelihood of adherence to a complicated drug regimen. Some regimens are simple: they require only one pill a day. Others are more complicated and require multiple pills to be taken at numerous times during each day, some with food. The patient must adhere to ARV regimens consistently in order for the medications to be effective and to avoid development of drug resistance. Social workers can assist the health-care team by working with patients to help them understand and respect the importance of medication adherence to their health and long-term prognosis. Social workers can also provide information to the physician about the context of the patient's life situations and his or her ability to comply with the directions of the physician. In addition to ARV medications, other medications are routinely prescribed, depending on the patient's CD4 cell count. For example, people who have CD4 counts below 200 are susceptible to pneumocystis carinii pneumonia (PCP), but people who take trimethoprim-sulfamethoxazole (Bactrim) prophylactically significantly reduce the chances of developing this opportunistic infection.

Failure of HAART

Failure of therapy, defined as a sustained and high rise in viral load, can occur regardless of the patient's actions, though non-adherence to the regimen is frequently the cause of such failure. Patients fail in their adherence to HAART regimens for various reasons, including the severity of side effects, interruptions in their supply of medications, and life circumstances that make sticking to a set schedule difficult, such as an unstable housing situation. When this happens, the physician will need to change the regimen. The physician will frequently order a genotype or phenotype test to identify any drugs to which the patient has developed resistance. The outcome of the tests is helpful in devising the next best regimen, which is called a salvage regimen. The social worker should mitigate the words "failure" and "salvage," and can counter the negative tone of the terms by explaining them and pointing out that they are not statements about the patient as a person (HIVInfoSource, 2009).

The Evolution of ARV Protocols

The U.S. Department of Health and Human Services (DHHS) guidelines for the use of ARV agents have come nearly full circle. In 1995, world-renowned AIDS researcher Dr. David Ho recommended a "hit early and hit hard" approach (Ho, 1995). This initial approach to the use of ARV was thought to eventually "cure" HIV (Jefferys, 1999).

The approach began to develop critics, however. People were becoming concerned about drug side effects and development of multidrug resistances (AIDSmeds, 2009) associated with taking ARV medications. There was special concern about the use of protease inhibitors, considered the "backbone" of HAART, being associated with abnormally high levels of fats (triglycerides and cholesterol) in the blood and changes in body fat distribution called lipodystrophy. This was the era when people taking ARVs worried about developing the "buffalo hump" syndrome, an enlargement of the dorsocervical fat pad at the back of the neck, which was shown to be associated with protease inhibitor treatment (Lo, Mulligan, Tai, Algren, & Schambelan, 1998).

Structured treatment interruptions, or "drug holidays," became common. While viral loads were shown to rebound during breaks, they disappeared again once treatment was restarted (Jefferys, 1999). The "hit hard" philosophy was debated by those advising "stop and go" therapy or "FOTO," which stood for five days on medications followed by two days off (Miron & Smith, 2010). Another regimen was "wowo," for week on, week off.

Since then, researchers have recognized the survival benefits of starting HAART earlier (AIDSmeds, 2009) in asymptomatic patients. Furthermore, the current consensus is that once ARVs are started, they should never be stopped. (An exception is in prophylactic treatment of HIV-positive pregnant women.) The new protocol released by DHHS recommends ARV treatment to begin when the CD4 count drops below 350, instead of 200 as in earlier protocols. The adage of "hit hard, hit early" is back. Details of the current guidelines for treatment naïve patients are presented below (DHHS, 2011).

- ARVs should definitely be started in all patients with history of AIDS-defining illness or CD4 count < 350 cells per milliliter.

- ARVs are recommended in patients with CD4 of 350 to 500 per milliliter.

- ARVs for patients with CD4 > 500 per milliliter are optional, depending on clinical and psychosocial factors.

It is significant to note that the DHHS panel was divided on the recommendation for patients with CD4 counts over 500: 55 percent voted for ARV use at CD4 counts between 350 and 500 to be a strong recommendation and 45 percent voted for a moderate recommendation (DHHS, 2011). This is a significant departure from DHHS guidelines from a few years ago that only recommended ARVs to be used in patients with CD4 counts of 200 or below. The recent release of the data from HIV Prevention Trials Network (HPTN) Clinical Trial 052, which scientifically proved that early treatment has a significant impact on reduction of transmission rates (HPTN, 2011), only confirms that early and constant use of ARVs will remain the protocol of choice. Table 11.3 presents a list of all medications currently approved by the FDA for use as ARV medication.

Table 11.3. Antiretroviral Medications Currently Approved for Use by the FDA

Brand Name	Generic Name	Manufacturer Name	Approval Date
Multiclass Combination Products			
Atripla	efavirenz, emtricitabine tenofovir disoproxil fumerate	Bristol-Myers Squibb and Gilead Sciences	12-July-06
Complera	emtricitabine rilpivirine tenofovir disoproxil fumerate	Gilead Sciences	10-Aug-11
Nucleoside Reverse Transcriptase Inhibitors (NRTIs) ("nukes")			
Combivir	lamivudine and zidovudine	GlaxoSmithKline	27-Sep-97
Emtriva	emtricitabine, FTC	Gilead Sciences	02-Jul-03
Epivir	lamivudine, 3TC	GlaxoSmithKline	17-Nov-95
Epzicom	abacavir and lamivudine	GlaxoSmithKline	02-Aug-04
Hivid	zalcitabine, dideoxycytidine, ddC (no longer marketed)	Hoffmann-La Roche	19-Jun-92
Retrovir	zidovudine, azidothymidine, AZT, ZDV	GlaxoSmithKline	19-Mar-87
Trizivir	abacavir, zidovudine, and lamivudine	GlaxoSmithKline	14-Nov-00
Truvada	tenofovir disoproxil fumarate and emtricitabine	Gilead Sciences, Inc.	02-Aug-04
Videx EC	enteric coated didanosine, ddl EC	Bristol Myers-Squibb	31-Oct-00
Videx	didanosine, dideoxyinosine, ddl	Bristol Myers-Squibb	9-Oct-91
Viread	tenofovir disoproxil fumarate, TDF	Gilead	26-Oct-01
Zerit	stavudine, d4T	Bristol Myers-Squibb	24-Jun-94
Ziagen	abacavir sulfate, ABC	GlaxoSmithKline	17-Dec-98
Nonnucleoside Reverse Transcriptase Inhibitors (NNRTIs)			
Edurant	rilpivirine	Tibotec Therapeutics	20-May-11
Intelence	etravirine	Tibotec Therapeutics	18-Jan-08

Brand Name	Generic Name	Manufacturer Name	Approval Date
Rescriptor	delavirdine, DLV	Pfizer	4-Apr-97
Sustiva	efavirenz, EFV	Bristol Myers-Squibb	17-Sep-98
Viramune (Immediate Release)	nevirapine, NVP	Boehringer Ingelheim	21-Jun-96
Viramune XR (Extended Release)	nevirapine, NVP	Boehringer Ingelheim	25-Mar-11
Protease Inhibitors			
Agenerase	amprenavir, APV	GlaxoSmithKline	15-Apr-99
Aptivus	tipranavir, TPV	Boehringer Ingelheim	22-Jun-05
Crixivan	indinavir, IDV	Merck	13-Mar-96
Fortovase	saquinavir (no longer marketed)	Hoffmann-La Roche	7-Nov-97
Invirase	saquinavir mesylate, SQV	Hoffmann-La Roche	6-Dec-95
Kaletra	lopinavir and ritonavir, LPV/RTV	Abbott Laboratories	15-Sep-00
Lexiva	Fosamprenavir Calcium, FOS-APV	GlaxoSmithKline	20-Oct-03
Norvir	ritonavir, RTV	Abbott Laboratories	1-Mar-96
Prezista	darunavir	Tibotec, Inc.	23-Jun-06
Reyataz	atazanavir sulfate, ATV	Bristol-Myers Squibb	20-Jun-03
Viracept	nelfinavir mesylate, NFV	Agouron Pharmaceuticals	14-Mar-97
Fusion Inhibitors			
Fuzeon	enfuvirtide, T-20	Hoffmann-La Roche & Trimeris	13-Mar-03
Entry Inhibitors: CCR5 co-receptor antagonist			
Selzentry	maraviroc	Pfizer	06-August-07
HIV integrase strand transfer inhibitors			
Isentress	raltegravir	Merck & Co., Inc.	12-Oct-07

Source: Adapted from FDA (2011).

Basic Medical Terminology

Social workers have an ethical responsibility to practice within their area of competence. Social workers are not trained as medical professionals and should therefore be careful to never attempt to give medical advice to a client. However, social workers are able to educate clients on how to comply with the medical care delivered by medical professionals. Case managers and medical social workers can be helpful to clients and their families by helping to clarify the instructions and explanations given by medical staff. Social workers in HIV and AIDS care will be more effective in assisting clients if they become more knowledgeable about care for HIV and AIDS. One requirement for understanding medical explanations is understanding basic medical terminology. An understanding of terms can help the social worker follow conversations and clarify details with nurses, physicians, or other medical providers.

Some medical terms are easily understood if one has a background in the study of Latin. For others, a list of terms with explanations can quickly provide much clarification. For learning basic medical terminology, Elgin (1994, pp. 205–209) and Gant (1998, pp. 23–25) pose four questions:

1. Which body part is being referred to in the term or phrase?

If the problem is located . . .	Look for this prefix:
stomach	gastro
liver	hepato
kidney	nephro
gall bladder	cholcyst
intestine	enter, ili, ile
uterus	hyster
ovary	oophor
vagina	colpo
testes	orchilo
bladder	cysto, vestic
rectum/anus	procto
colon	colo

2. Where is it located?

If the problem is located . . .	Look for this prefix:
inside	endo, eso, intra
outside	ecto, exo
on, above, or over	epi, supra
under, below	infra, sub
between	inter
beside, around	para

behind	retro
away from	ab
near	ad
through, across	dia
beyond	meta
with, together	syn, sym, syl, sys
against	anti, contra

3. What is wrong with it?

If the complaint is . . .	Look for this prefix:
It hurts.	algia, dynia
It's inflamed and/or infected.	itis
It's diseased.	osis
It's got a tumor or swelling.	oma
It's hardening.	sclera
It's bleeding or pouring out.	rhage, rhagia, rhea
It's growing, maybe too much.	plasia
It's developing wrong.	trophy
It's too (X).	hyper
It's not (X) enough.	hypo
It's without (X).	a, an, in
It's big.	macro, mega
It's small.	micro
It's bad or wrong.	mal
It's fake.	pseudo
It's fast.	tachy
It's slow.	brady
It's double.	ambi, amphi
It's changing.	meta
It's red.	eryth
It's white.	alb, leuko, leuco
It's blue.	cya

It's abnormal.	dys
There's only half, or half is relevant.	hemi
There's more than one, or a lot of it.	poly, multi

4. What are they proposing to do to it?

If the solution is to . . .	Look for this prefix:
Remove it.	ectomy
Look inside it.	oscopy
Make an opening in it.	ostomy
Free it up.	lysis
Fuse it.	desis
Fix it, or sew it up.	pexy
Make it, or reconstruct it.	plasty

Case Example

Rosalind's phone rang and Tierra, her coworker from the health department clinic, was on the other end: "Hey, Roz. You have a minute?" Tierra's voice was purposefully sweet and gentle. Rosalind felt a wrenching in her stomach because that greeting meant that Tierra had a client who just tested HIV positive who needed to talk with a case manager. Rosalind had noticed that the only time that Tierra ever called her Roz was when she had a new positive. Rosalind had a great rapport with clients and was known for being very professional and thorough as a case manager.

"Of course I have a minute, for you. Do you have someone for me to meet?" Rosalind took a deep breath and grabbed a pad she kept by her phone. "You are a life-saver Rosalind!," Tierra said with a sigh of relief. "Well, I have a young man for you to meet. I delivered the news and started talking to him about resources. He started crying really hard because he is new to Anytown. He lives with his mother, but he doesn't want to tell her his status. He is just really going through it over here."

"Okay, what room are you in?" Rosalind started grabbing her clipboard to go to the other side of the health department to speak with the young man. "Thanks so much, Rosalind. We are in room 2B. I'll meet you there. I left him alone in there to come call you. I need to get right back." Tierra was emotionally gathering herself to introduce the young man to Rosalind.

Rosalind was the intake manager for the HIV division of the Anytown Health Department. She also was a case manager for a few clients. Her caseload was composed primarily of people who had just found out that they were HIV positive. As she walked across the clinic to where the young man awaited her, she took some deep breaths and focused her mind. She liked her job, but these moments were particularly difficult.

Tierra was waiting outside of the room with a forced smile on her face. Rosalind returned the smile and asked what the young man's name was just before Tierra opened the door. "PJ," she said in a hushed voice. As she opened the door, Rosalind looked down at a very young-looking man whose puffy red eyes showed the pain he was feeling. He held balls of wadded up tissues in his hands. Rosalind looked down and smiled at PJ and said, "Hello, I'm Rosalind." She reached behind the desk and grabbed the small wastebasket and passed it over to PJ. PJ halfway smiled and sort of giggled as he threw the wet tissues into the trashcan. Tierra took a seat on the other side of the desk and Rosalind sat beside her, directly in front of PJ. She reached over and lightly put the tissue box down in front of PJ. In a very calm voice, she asked PJ, "How are you?" with a very kind smile.

PJ looked up at her with tears in his eyes and opened his mouth to reply, but only an inaudible cry came out, and PJ began to cry again. For the next hour, Rosalind took her time talking with PJ and assuring him that his life was not over. She was not able to complete the intake paperwork that she needed, but she did set up another appointment with him for the following Tuesday.

The following Tuesday PJ came in to meet Rosalind to complete his intake interview and start a maintenance plan for his HIV care. He waited in the front clinic reception area after checking in with the receptionist. Rosalind came out to the front after she was paged; the receptionist told her that PJ was waiting. PJ was looking around the lobby nervously when Rosalind rounded the corner. PJ immediately hopped to his feet and began walking toward Rosalind. They greeted each other and Rosalind took him back for his intake session. Rosalind introduced herself again and explained her role to PJ. He listened attentively with a smile on his face. Rosalind informed him why she would be asking him the questions that she had to ask during the intake session. She informed him what the next steps would be after the session. When she asked if he had any questions, PJ looked at Rosalind with tears in his eyes, and asked, "Can you go with me to the doctor when I go?"

Rosalind smiled and said, "It would be my honor to go with you once we get it all set up." Rosalind shuffled some papers around while PJ wiped his eyes. After a moment, she quietly asked, "Why do you like me to go to the doctor with you? I'm just curious! I will go regardless of your answer."

PJ giggled at Rosalind's question and said, "Because you said you would the other day when we first met." The both laughed a little and Rosalind began her intake paperwork. When the intake interview was complete, PJ and Rosalind called the doctor's office together to set up his first appointment with an infectious disease physician.

A month later, Rosalind called PJ to remind him about the appointment and to inquire if he had any questions. PJ was nervous and asked Rosalind questions about the following day. "So what exactly is going to happen tomorrow?"

"You are going to go to the doctor!" Rosalind said with a slight chuckle. "They are going to take blood for labs and then we'll come back in two weeks to learn the results of those labs." "Labs? How will they do labs?" PJ's voice began to get a little more intense on the phone.

"They will draw blood to determine your viral load and T-cell counts. Do you remember when we spoke during intake about how...." Rosalind was interrupted by PJ. "Yeah the T-cells fight infection and viral load is how much virus is in my blood that can infect the T-cells," PJ proudly replied.

Rosalind smiled as she replied, "Yep! That's it. So tomorrow you will have labs done for those tests, to check your complete blood count, your genotype, and to have other labs drawn in preparation for your next doctor's visit in two weeks." There was silence on the phone. Rosalind replied, "Are you there, PJ?"

"Yeah, yeah I'm here." PJ stammered. "I just don't get all the labs." "Ohhh, I'm sorry, PJ," Rosalind replied. "The complete blood count checks your overall health by looking at your white and red blood counts and your hemoglobin counts. The genotype test is the test that determines which medicines will work best to stop the duplication of the HIV strand that you have. Does that make sense?"

"Yeah ... yeah it makes sense," he replied after a moment of thinking. "We did talk about that during the intake, but we talked about a lot and I don't remember all of that!" He chuckled.

"You are right about that PJ!" Rosalind laughed with PJ. "If you ever have any questions, please do call me. I will see you tomorrow at your appointment, unless you have more questions. And you don't need a ride there, correct?"

"No … But … I mean, what will really happen tomorrow?" PJ asked, with intensity in his voice. Rosalind calmly replied, "Tomorrow I will meet you at the clinic. You will check in and they will call you back to get your blood pressure checked, your temperature, weight, and all those things. Then the nurse will see you. The nurse will ask you a few questions. I think you are seeing Dr. Emmil. He will come in just to introduce himself, but primarily this first visit is to get your initial lab work done."

PJ was a bit relieved. "So when do they do the labs?" "After you speak with the nurse, they will send you to get labs done. Then we will come back in two weeks to meet with the doctor and talk about the results. Now, one thing to note, this is how things work in Dr. Emmil's office. In some offices, you may go in to give blood samples and never talk with a nurse or a doctor until the results come back weeks later. Some doctors order the lab work and only call you afterwards if something needs to be addressed. It just depends on the doctor."

"Okay. Well, I'll see you tomorrow," PJ replied. "Okay. Are you sure you don't have any more questions?" Rosalind asked. "Not as of right now, but maybe tomorrow," PJ replied with a chuckle. "Don't forget the paper that we filled out during our intake session. Do you have it? If you have lost it, I have a copy." Rosalind waited for a reply from PJ.

"I have it Ms. Rosalind" PJ replied. "See you tomorrow."

"Okay, I'm just making sure! See you tomorrow." They both hung up the phone and Rosalind laughed.

A few months before, she had started handing out to her clients a list of questions to take with them to the infectious disease clinic. The list included questions that the physician would probably ask the client. Rosalind gave the client the questions ahead of time so that they would not be shocked by them and would answer them more honestly. It also provided an opportunity for Rosalind to have a conversation with her clients about the importance of being honest about their behaviors with their medical doctor. The paper had questions such as, "Do you smoke? What do you smoke? How often do you smoke?" She discussed the questions with clients either during the intake session or before their first medical appointment. Then she asked them to take the list home with them, in order to think about the answers before their first appointment. She started this practice to help her clients be prepared for the questions to be asked of them in their first appointments. She had seen too many of them appear shocked and embarrassed.

Rosalind's phone rang again. "Hello, Anytown Health Department. This is Rosalind." "Hello. It is PJ again. I have one more question." Rosalind could sense the hesitation in PJ's voice. "Sure, PJ. Ask away. I'll either know the answer or know how to find it for you. What's up?"

PJ's voice began to shake, "Will I have to tell anyone that I'm positive?" He began to cry. Rosalind took a deep breath. "Yes, you will. You will need to put it on the paperwork that you fill out and the nurse will probably verify the documents with you and ask you about it." Rosalind could hear PJ sob a little harder. "But I will be right there with you and can help you through it. Remember, these are health-care professionals. They are there to help you, not judge you. They also will respect your right to privacy."

There was a period of silence on the phone. PJ finally replied with a broken voice, "Okay, thank you. Sorry to bother you. I'm sorry." He began to sob again. Rosalind cut him off. "You are not a bother to me, PJ. That is what I am here for—to help answer your questions. Please call me back if you have any questions." "Okay. Thank you. See you tomorrow." PJ hung up the phone.

The next day at the clinic PJ seemed a bit nervous, but chatted with Rosalind about the weather and how cold the office was. The small talk seemed to make time go by a bit faster for PJ until it was time to meet Dr. Emmil. He had already been through registration, filled out his medical history paper, had his vitals taken, and spoke to the nurse about his medical history. The physician was there to speak with him about the next steps in his care.

Dr. Emmil asked if he had any questions. "Will I have to go on meds?" PJ asked him, while looking at Rosalind for validation. Rosalind smiled and nodded. PJ looked back to Dr. Emmil for a reply.

"It depends on the results of your lab tests. We will analyze your lab results to determine your T-cell count—which is the amount of immune fighting agents you have in your blood—and correlate it with your viral load—or amount of HIV virus you have in your body." PJ looked at Dr. Emmil and smiled, looking back at Rosalind. The doctor continued, "At your next visit I will do a complete physical examination of your body, as well as look at the results of the lab tests that we started today."

"What about this?" PJ pulled out the paperwork that Rosalind had given him, with the questions about his behaviors. Dr. Emmil looked at the paper and then over to Rosalind. Rosalind chuckled and explained, "Oh, he doesn't need the paperwork, PJ. That is just for you to have thought about before the appointment." Dr. Emmil interrupted and said, "I'd like to make a copy of this for your records. You have done a lot of work here, making notes about your answers to all of these questions. Good work being so engaged in your medical care, PJ!" he praised.

When Dr. Emmil left to make a copy of the information for his chart, Rosalind added her praise. "That is so great, PJ—the more that the doctor knows about you, the better he will be able to deliver services to you. That is why it is good for him to understand all about your current and past history with smoking, sex, exercise, and all the other details on that list."

Dr. Emmil returned, verified PJ's appointment in two weeks, and asked if PJ had any questions. PJ and Rosalind left the clinic together. Rosalind once again gave PJ her business card, let him know that she was proud of him, and said that she would be happy to accompany him to his next appointment.

"Okay, one more appointment, Mrs. Rosalind. Then I have a feeling I'll be just fine."

Questions for Reflection

1. Rosalind had worked at the health department for several years. Do you think it is realistic that she would have a physical reaction to meeting a new client who just tested HIV positive? Why or why not?

2. Why was Tierra uncomfortable about leaving PJ alone for too long?

3. How effective is the practice of letting the client know ahead of time the questions the physician may ask?

4. Imagine that Rosalind had not explained the concepts of T-cell counts and viral loads to PJ before the first medical appointment. What might have been different about that appointment?

5. Rosalind demonstrated great patience in responding to PJ's questions. Would you be that patient with him? If she had not been so patient, how might he have responded?

6. If you were Rosalind and PJ was your client, would you have done anything differently?

7. Imagine that PJ had been rude and demanding with his care providers. How might his attitude have affected the quality of his care from Tierra, Rosalind, and Dr. Emmil? Should a client's demeanor have any effect on services? If not, why? If so, when?

8. Anytown Health Department has just undergone a large budget cut, due to the reduction in the tax base of the county. Rosalind and the other case managers have been affected by having their caseloads increased by 30 percent. How might Rosalind's delivery of services to clients like PJ change?

References

Aberg, J. A., Kaplan, J. E., Libman, H., Emmanuel, P., Anderson, J., Stone, V. E., Oleske, J., . . . , Gallant, J. E. (2009). Primary care guidelines for the management of persons infected with Human Immunodeficiency Virus: 2009 update by the HIV Medicine Association of the Infectious Diseases Society of America. *Clinical Infectious Diseases, 49*(5), 651–681.

AIDS Action. (2007). Syringe exchange and HIV/AIDS: Policy brief. Retrieved from http://www.aidsaction.org/attachments/518_Syringe%20Exchange.pdf

AIDS.gov. (2010). Stages of HIV. Retrieved from http://aids.gov/hiv-aids-basics/diagnosed-with-hiv-aids/hiv-in-your-body/stages-of-hiv/

AIDSmeds. (2009). DHHS Guidelines: Return of "Hit hard, hit early." Retrieved from http://www.aidsmeds.com/articles/hiv_dhhs_guidelines_1667_17645.shtml

AVERT. (2011a). How can HIV transmission be prevented? Retrieved from http://www.avert.org/prevent-hiv.htm

AVERT. (2011b). What are opportunistic infections? Retrieved from http://www.avert.org/hiv-opportunistic-infections.htm

AVERT. (2011c). Introduction to HIV treatment. Retrieved from http://www .avert.org/treatment.htm

Broverman, N. (2011). Gay Men's Health Crisis on needle exchange funding ban. TheAdvocate.com. Retrieved from http://www.advocate.com/News/ Daily_News/2011/12/25/Gay_Mens_Heatlh_Crisis_on_Needle_Exchange_ Funding_Ban/

Centers for Disease Control and Prevention (CDC). (2011). The role of STD detection and treatment in HIV prevention. *CDC fact sheet.* Retrieved from http://www.cdc.gov/STD/hiv/STDFact-STD-HIV.htm

Centers for Disease Control and Prevention (CDC). (2012). HIV in the United States. Retrieved from http://www.cdc.gov/hiv/resources/factsheets/us.htm

Cichocki, M. (2007). Long-term non-progressor. Retrieved from http://aids.about .com/od/hivaidsletterl/g/nonprogdef.htm

Cichocki, M. (2010). Hemophilia and HIV. Retrieved from http://aids.about.com/ od/hemophilia/a/hemohiv.htm

Cohen, M., Chen, Y., McCauley, M., Gamble, T., Hosseinipour, M., Kumarasamy, N., . . . , Fleming, T. for the HTPN 052 Study team. (2011). Prevention of HIV-1 infection with early-antiretroviral therapy. *The New England Journal of Medicine, 365,* 493–505.

Elgin, S. H. (1994). *Staying well with the gentle art of self-defense.* Englewood Cliffs, NJ: Prentice Hall.

Gant, L. (1998). Essential facts every social worker needs to know. In D. Aronstein & B. Thompson (Eds.), *HIV and social work: A practitioner's guide* (pp. 3–25). Binghamton, NY: The Harrington Park Press.

Gray, R. H., Wawer, M. J., Brookmeyer, R., Sewankambo, N. K., Serwadda, D., Wabwire-Mangen, F., Lutalo, T., . . . , Rakai Project Team. (2001). Probability of HIV-1 transmission per coital act in monogamous, heterosexual, HIV-1 discordant couples in Rakai, Uganda. *Lancet, 357*(9263), 1149–1153.

Health Central Network, Inc., The. (2011). HIV long-term nonprogressors and elite controllers: Personal stories. *The Body: The complete HIV/AIDS resource.* Retrieved from http://www.thebody.com/index/treat/nonprog.html/

HIVInfoSource. (2009). HIV treatment options. NYU Medical Center. Retrieved from http://www.hivinfosource.org/hivis/hivbasics/treatment/index.html

HIV Prevention Trial Network (HPTN). (2011). HPTN named top scientific breakthrough of 2011. Retrieved from http://www.hptn.org/web%20 documents/IndexDocs/052NamedScientificBreakthrough2011.pdf

Ho, D. D. (1995). Time to hit HIV, early and hard. *New England Journal of Medicine, 333*(7), 450–451.

Jefferys, R. (1999). Partial eclipse of the HAART: New treatment strategies to overcome roadblocks. *HIV plus, 5,* 11–13.

Lo, J. C., Mulligan, K., Tai, V. W., Algren, H., & Schambelan, M. (1998). "Buffalo hump" in men with HIV-1 infection. *The Lancet, 351*(9106), 867–870.

May, M., Sterne, M. M., Sabin, C., Costagliola, D., Justice, A. C., Thiebaut, R., Gill, J., . . . , Antiretroviral Therapy (ART) Cohort Collaboration (2007). Prognosis of HIV-1-infected patients up to 5 years after initiation of HAART: Collaborative analysis of prospective studies. *AIDS, 21*(9), 1185–1197.

Miron, R. E., & Smith, R. J. (2010). Modelling imperfect adherence to HIV induction therapy. *BMC Infectious Diseases, 10*(6), 1–16.

PBS. (2006). Frontline: The age of AIDS. Retrieved from http://www.pbs.org/ wgbh/pages/frontline/aids/virus/virus.html

Pogash, C. (2005, May 5). AIDS and the secret of long-term survivors. The *New York Times.* Retrieved from http://www.nytimes.com/2005/05/04/health/ 04iht-snlive.html

Saag, M., Chambers, H. F., Eliopoulos, G. M., Gilbert, D., & Moellering, R. C. (2011). *The Sanford guide to HIV/AIDS therapy.* Sperryville, VA: Antimicrobial Therapy.

Sax, P. E., Cohen, C. J., & Kuritzkes, D. R. (2011). *HIV essentials,* 4th ed. Sudbury, MA: Jones & Bartlett Learning, LLC.

Smith, S. E. (2011). What is a non-progressor? Retrieved from http://www .wisegeek.com/what-is-a-non-progressor.htm

U.S. Food and Drug Administration (FDA). (2011). Anti-retroviral drugs used in the treatment of HIV infection. Retrieved from http://www.fda.gov/ForConsumers/byAudience/ForPatientAdvocates/HIVandAIDSActivities/ucm118915.htm

U.S. Department of Health and Human Services (DHHS). (2011). Guidelines for the use of antiretroviral agents in HIV-1-infected adults and adolescents. Retrieved from http://www.aidsinfo.nih.gov/contentfiles/AA_Recommendations.pdf

Answers to Brain Teasers

1. Estelle knew that both the ELISA and Western blot tests checked for the presence of HIV antibodies, and not the presence of the virus itself. Babies, until they are about two years old, will test positive for the HIV antibodies that their bodies developed before birth in response to their mother's HIV. However, because the blood of the mother and fetus never mix, the virus is never passed to the fetus before birth. The only way to test a baby for HIV is to test for the virus itself, using an HIV RNA test. The PCR test is commonly used on newborns to determine if they were infected with HIV during the birthing process.

2. Booker is correct. HIV is not present in saliva. The OraQuick test does test oral fluid, but not for the presence of HIV. Instead, it tests for the presence of HIV antibodies. These are present in oral fluids. The actual virus, however, is only present in blood, semen, vaginal fluids, and breast milk. That is why viral load assays are performed on blood samples. Note that even though Booker tested negative for HIV, he still needs to be tested for other STDs.

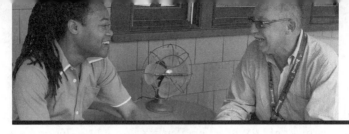

Sex, Drugs, and HIV
Diana Rowan and Lamont Holley

"People do stupid things. That's what spreads HIV." ... This is a headline in a UK newspaper, *The Guardian*, not that long ago. ... I am now going to argue that this is only half true. People do get HIV because they do stupid things, but most of them are doing stupid things for perfectly rational reasons. ... And although I'm sure you all know that HIV is about poverty and gender inequality, ... actually, HIV's about sex and drugs, and if there are two things that make human beings a little bit irrational, they are erections and addiction.

—Elizabeth Pisani, epidemiologist, journalist, and author of *The Wisdom of Whores*, speaking at TED Talks, 2010

Social workers working with HIV (human immunodeficiency virus) prevention and care must be comfortable discussing, thinking about, and providing interventions focused on sex and drugs. There is no way around the fact that this type of work requires a high level of comfort with the topics of human sexuality and drug use. The profession of social work requires one to be desensitized to many topics, but with HIV and AIDS (acquired immune deficiency syndrome) work, the need to exude comfort discussing sex and drugs is not just helpful, but essential. The purpose of this chapter is to assist social workers with increasing their comfort with and knowledge of these areas, which are sometimes avoided in social work education. This chapter will introduce some key elements of the process of conducting a sexual history interview and a sexual risk assessment. Next, the chapter will present a description of the continuum of sexual risk behaviors. This discussion will contain graphic descriptions of sexual behaviors so that social workers are informed, in case these are familiar activities of their clients. Injection drug use and use of club drugs will be discussed as well. Social workers in HIV- and AIDS-related positions often discuss condom education and condom negotiation skills with clients; therefore, information helpful to this process will be presented.

Sex and HIV

The most common form of transmission of HIV is by sexual intercourse. Thus, prevention of transmission of the virus is firmly linked with the topic of sex. A social worker or other health or mental health practitioner who is unwilling to become comfortable talking to clients about sex would do best to select a different area of specialization. A new social worker who is either unknowledgeable about or uncomfortable with discussion of sex behaviors should know that it is possible to learn how to be comfortable, and reading this chapter is a step in the correct direction.

The Sexual History Interview

Taking a candid and nonjudgmental sexual history is the cornerstone in HIV preventive education (Maurice & Bowman, 1999), yet many health or mental health practitioners and social service providers tend to move quickly through the sexual history section of a psychosocial assessment interview. Why is this? Research shows that there are a variety of reasons why social workers avoid discussions of sexual topics during assessments (Maurice & Bowman, 1999). These reasons, plus others, are presented below. The interviewer might

- Be afraid of receiving a graphic answer

- Be uncertain about how to phrase questions and what words to use

- Be concerned about opening Pandora's box, and eliciting too much information

- Be worried that a question might offend a client or patient

- Want to avoid being seen as intrusive or nosy

- Be uncomfortable with an age difference between the interviewer and interviewee and the perception of generational obstacles

- Be concerned that the questioning might be characterized as sexual misconduct, resulting in licensure problems

- Be unfamiliar with the sexual behaviors mentioned by the client

- Have a lack of personal experience with sex

- Make assumptions about cultural and religious diversity variables

- Have a different gender, gender expression, or sexual orientation from the client or patient, and so believe that he or she can't understand the client's answers

- Have his or her own sexual hang-ups, or be a sex abuse survivor with unresolved issues

- Misperceive sexual history and current behaviors as irrelevant

- Assume that if there is something to report, the client/patient will bring it up

The volume of these reasons for avoidance of the topic of sex with clients is not an excuse for a social worker to move quickly through the sexual history section of a biopsychosocial assessment. The long list of reasons why the social worker may avoid the topic of sex is offset by the list of reasons why it is important that the social worker address the client's sexual history completely and skillfully. Social workers should pose sex-related questions to clients for the following reasons:

- Such questions provide an opportunity to introduce HIV transmission prevention information.

- Disrupted sexual function can be a symptom of a medical condition requiring assessment, or may be a side effect of treatment of that condition.

- Past sexual history can help explain present behaviors.

- Sexual activity usually changes across the life cycle.

- The interviewer expressing comfort with discussing sex makes it easier for the client to open up.

- Discussing sex within the context of a professional conversation normalizes sex.

- Not asking these questions could be considered professional incompetence.

Beyond gathering information for a sexual history assessment, social workers in the field of HIV and AIDS are focused on reduction of risk behaviors with respect to sex. The Centers for Disease Control and Prevention (CDC) established three goals for individualized HIV prevention counseling. Counselors should (1) establish or improve the client's self-perception of risk, (2) identify and support behavior changes that a client has already attempted, and (3) negotiate with the client a realistic and incremental plan for reducing his or her risk of HIV infection or HIV transmission (Kinnell, 2002). To pursue these goals effectively, the social worker, or other type of counselor, must have both a comfort with discussing and a thorough understanding of sexual risk behaviors. This chapter provides detailed information that will be helpful toward building knowledge about the variety of sex practices in which clients may engage.

Comfort During the Sexual History Interview. Physical and emotional comfort when talking about sex are helpful for both the client and the worker. To assist with physical comfort, the worker should do what is possible to provide a suitable physical location for these conversations. Sexual risk assessment and counseling sessions should not be conducted in a public space or an open cubicle, if at all possible. Out of respect for the client's confidentiality, a location with a closed door is best. A physically comfortable seating area is helpful for putting the client at ease. Padded chairs are better than hard surfaces if the session is likely to last awhile. Social workers should know that clients who have been living with AIDS for a length of time may experience lipodystrophy, which is a redistribution of fat throughout the body. They may also experience wasting, a phenomenon where the person struggles to keep weight on. These physical symptoms can make sitting on a hard chair for a length of time very uncomfortable (Furman, Rowan, & Bender, 2009). Providing the client a chair with arms or a table to lean on is best for longer sessions. Social workers should pay attention to the temperature of the room, to make sure it is comfortable in all seasons. The temperature of the session location becomes even more important if the client is symptomatic for HIV and not feeling well. Furthermore, reduction of unnecessary noise can help the client focus on the content of the session. Having a restroom easily accessible is important because antiretroviral (ARV) medications often have side effects related to gastrointestinal problems, as does untreated AIDS.

A social worker can assess whether or not a client is nervous about the topic of sexual activity by observing his or her nonverbal behaviors when the topic is broached. Useful observations of the client's body language include frequent movement of hands and arms such as twiddling, fidgeting, or defensively crossing the arms. Some clients may exhibit the pectoral flush where redness creeps over the upper chest and neck, which can signify unease despite outward appearance of calm (Tomlinson, 1998). Clients may demonstrate a change in body position, such as a slump in posture or sitting upright when a sensitive topic is raised.

An effective way to put a nervous client at ease is for the social worker to model being comfortable. There is a saying in Alcoholics Anonymous that you should "fake it till you make it," or act as if something is already true. When talking with a client about sexually explicit topics, the saying applies as well. Even if the conversation drifts to discussions of sexual behaviors that are not in the social worker's current comfort zone, he or she should act as if they are, to encourage the client to continue sharing and learning about sexual risk reduction. However, the best defense can be a good offense when it comes to comfort with discussion of clients' sexual activities. It is best to be prepared rather than to be taken off guard. In preparation for this, the social worker can do some self-inventory work, to identify any unacknowledged biases that have to do with sexual behaviors, including same-sex activities and differences in gender expression. The following are some useful questions for the social worker to privately ponder prior to working with HIV prevention and care or with sexual minorities. And, since HIV prevention should take place in many social work settings, and sexual minorities are present across many populations, virtually all social workers can benefit from responding to the questions on the following list, some of which are adapted from Substance Abuse and Mental Health Services Administration (SAMHSA; 2000).

- Have you ever been to a gay or lesbian club, party, bar, or social event? If not, why not?

- Can you think of three positive aspects of a gay or lesbian life style?

- Do you believe that sex outside of marriage is a sin? If so, do you judge those who do this?

- How would you respond if a local minister told you that he is having multiple sexual relationships with men in the next county?

- A client reports to you that the cuts on her wrists are from being bound up by her boyfriend during sex. How do you respond? Would this be an uncomfortable conversation?

- Imagine talking to someone one or two generations older than you about his or her sex life. Is this uncomfortable?

- Imagine you ask a client if he or she has ever experienced sexual abuse and the client tells you a story about being a survivor of life-long incest. How will you respond?

- Are there any jobs you think transgender people should be barred from?

- Would you allow your young daughter to use a public restroom that a male-to-female transgender person is also using?

- A client asks you if you can get HIV from licking someone's anus. What do you say next? Is this topic too uncomfortable or odd?

- Do you think someone can influence a person's sexual orientation?

- Would you see a physician or a therapist that you believed to be gay or lesbian? Straight? Transgender?

- How would you respond if you were straight and someone thought you were gay or lesbian, or transgender? If you were gay or lesbian and someone thought you were straight?

Group Activity

Here is a group activity for a classroom setting or training session that is helpful for increasing comfort with discussing sex and using terms associated with sex.

Begin with asking the group to take turns shouting out words that can be used for a jail. Have a volunteer write these down on a whiteboard for the group to see. They will likely come up with terms such as prison, lock-up, pokey, slammer, the hole, and clink. Allow the group to become comfortable with the process. Next, ask them to shout out terms used to represent feces. Next, go through the same process for terms referring to sexual intercourse. Follow this with words to describe oral sex, and words used by people for penis, vagina, and semen. The process will start out more difficult and get easier as the group becomes normalized to these terms. It is important to do this in a group setting so that the more-vocal participants can model for shyer ones that it is okay to say these graphic terms. Writing them down publicly is important so that the participants can see the words written, as they may have to record these words as part of direct quotes in clients' progress notes. It is essential for social workers to develop comfort with a wide range of words, beyond clinical or medical terms, since many clients will not use formal terms or even know what they mean. For the best rapport and understanding, social workers should use the terms used by the client to describe genitalia and sex acts.

Case Example I

Consider the following example. Mason is an HIV-prevention counselor who works for the county health department. He is assigned to visit the county jail once per week to talk about HIV-risk reduction with inmates that have tested positive for HIV. Make notes on what mistakes you think Mason makes when he meets his client.

Hello, Mr. Santiago. My name is Mr. Kendall and I am here to discuss risk reduction in your intimate relations with women. You should always use a condom before you go to bed with a woman. Do you have any questions? I can't talk long because it is so noisy in here.

Now examine this example and see how Mason's approach has improved.

Hi, Mr. Santiago. I am Mason, from the health department. It's nice and quiet in here, compared to out in the pod, isn't it?

He waits to see if Mr. Santiago responds, indicating that he understands English.

I understand you speak Spanish and English—that's great, but I only speak English. Can you understand me okay, or shall I get a Spanish interpreter?

Mr. Santiago says he understands just fine.

Okay, great, then I just want to spend a little time talking about your HIV. I see from these notes that you have known you are HIV positive for about two years. Is that right?

Mr. Santiago says yes, but Mason notices that his body posture is closed, he is providing short answers, and he seems uncomfortable.

Just in case you are wondering why I'm here, it has nothing to do with immigration or anything legal. I am just here to talk about your health, and what we discuss is just for conversations at the health department. I come in and talk to guys all the time in your situation.

Mr. Santiago appears to relax.

So, let's talk some about your sex behaviors, just to be sure you have good information on how to keep yourself and your partners safe. Before you got arrested, were you sexually active?

Mr. Santiago says yes, that he is married.

Okay, so are you married to a woman?

He says that yes, of course she is a woman.

And do you have other partners for sex? Other ladies, or men?

Mr. Santiago says, "Yeah, some of each … but no one is ever at risk of HIV."

Why not? Do you always use protection?

Mr. Santiago looks confused.

Sorry—do you have sex with a condom? Do you use rubbers?

Mr. Santiago nods but says, "No, I am Catholic—we don't use rubbers."

Then how are you sure your partners aren't at risk?

Mr. Santiago says, "Because the ladies always have blood—I make sure that my wife is having her time with blood. And with the men, they ask me if I have HIV in my dick and they say they have it in their dick, too, so there is no worry."

Mason then proceeds to explain to Mr. Santiago that when women are menstruating (using the term "blood") they are not protected from HIV infection. He also discusses the risks of coinfections with different strains of HIV and the transmission of drug resistances that can occur when two people with HIV have unprotected sex. He is sure to use the same terms Mr. Santiago used, such as rubbers and dick. Mason makes some notes that on the next visit he will talk more with Mr. Santiago about his Catholic faith and discuss how he could respect it but also use condoms. He will also discuss arranging for an HIV test for his wife, if she hasn't been tested recently.

1. What was wrong with the first example?

2. In the second example, what did Mason do well with Mr. Santiago?

3. How could Mason have improved his interaction with Mr. Santiago?

4. What else should Mason discuss with Mr. Santiago in subsequent visits?

Assessing the 5 Ps

In assessing risk for sexually transmitted diseases (STDs), including HIV, the practitioner needs to gather information on Partners, sexual Practices, Past History of STDs, Pregnancy history and plans, and Protection from STDs.

The following is a basic template that can be adapted to a particular client, based on the client's age, cultural variables, and knowledge of the subject matter. The social worker should pay close attention to word choice in an effort to use words familiar to the client. This is not the time to use medical jargon or attempt to disguise or sanitize sexual terms with words that may be unfamiliar to the client. The following information has been adapted from the Chlamydia Care Quality Improvement Toolbox (California STD/HIV Prevention Training Center, 2006).

I am going to ask you some sensitive questions that are important for us to be able to keep you healthy. What we discuss is confidential.

1. Partners

For sexual risk, it is important to determine the number and gender of a patient's sexual partners. One should not make any assumptions about the gender of the person being interviewed or the gender of their sex partners. If there are multiple sex partners, explore for risk factors that are more specific, such as pattern of condom use and the partner's risk factors, such as injection drug use, and history of STDs and other partners. Ask about length of relationships. If the person reports having sex with both men and women, repeat the questions for each gender.

Do you have sex with men, women, or both?

In the past two months how many people have you had sex with?

In the past twelve months, how many sexual partners have you had?

2. Sexual Practices

In addition to asking about gender and number of partners, it is also important to ask about sex practices. The answers to these questions will guide risk-reduction strategies.

Do you have penis–vagina sex?

Do you use condoms never, sometimes, most of the time, or always for this kind of sex?

Do you have anal sex, meaning sex with the penis in the rectum or anus? If so, how often do you use condoms?

If anal sex: Do you prefer to put your penis in the other person's anus, or have a penis put in your anus? Do you do both?

Do you have oral sex, meaning sex with someone's mouth on a penis or vagina?

In what situations, or with whom, do you not use condoms?

3. Past History of STDs

A history of prior gonorrhea or chlamydia infections increases a person's risk of a repeat infection. Recent past STDs indicates higher-risk behavior.

What STDs have you had in the past, if any?

Have you been tested for STDs or HIV? When? What was the result?

Have any of your partners had STDs?

4. Pregnancy History and Plans

Based on information already obtained, you can determine if the patient is at risk of becoming pregnant or of causing a pregnancy.

What are your current desires regarding pregnancy and having a baby?

Are you concerned about getting pregnant or getting your partner pregnant? (This is dependent on if client is female or male, and if male, if they have sex with women.)

Are you trying to get pregnant?

Are you trying to get your partner pregnant?

What are you doing to prevent a pregnancy?

5. Protection from STDs

What do you do to protect yourself from STDs and HIV?

This is an open-ended question and allows for different avenues of direction for the rest of the conversation. Topics to be discussed can include condom use, monogamy, perception of risk, modification of risky sexual behaviors, and STD and HIV testing.

Additional Questions for Assessing HIV and Hepatitis Risks

The social worker can gather immunization history for hepatitis A and B at this point. Hepatitis A immunization is recommended for men who have sex with men (MSM) and injection drug users.

Have you or any partners injected drugs?

Have you ever had sex with sex workers?

Have you ever had sex in exchange for money or other goods?

Have you ever been forced to have sex with someone?

Have you ever forced someone to have sex with you?

Are you in an abusive relationship?

End the interview by asking if there is anything else about the client's sex practices that they think is helpful to discuss for good health care. Ask if there are any questions.

Social workers do their best work when they come from a neutral stance with a nonjudgmental attitude. While it is unrealistic to assume that a practitioner has no judgments, it is a more reasonable goal for the worker to set aside any judgments during work with a client, to prevent them from intervening with development of the therapeutic relationship.

HIV Infection Routes

HIV risk assessment is an essential component of primary care for all patients. Once the social worker has assessed the 5 Ps, he or she can provide education for risk reduction. As mentioned previously, when talking with patients, however, it is important to avoid use of medical or professional jargon. Terms such as "intercourse" should be replaced with "having sex," or better yet, with the slang term used by the client. Social workers should allow their clients to describe sexual behaviors in terms such as "fucking," or "butt-fucking." Rather than saying "unprotected" sex, the worker can ask about any use of "condoms" or "rubbers." The worker may need to explicitly define oral and anal sex by describing the act to clients, such as "sucking on his dick," to make sure they understand what is being discussed. The ideal with respect to sexual risk reduction is to listen to clients and learn what words they choose. When working with patients from a certain ethnicity or country of origin, it is wise to learn the terms used in that community. The setting may help inform the worker about what terminology will be most familiar. For example, a risk assessment session in a men's shelter may involve different terms than in an assessment in an up-scale retirement village clinic—though there are dangers in stereotyping and the social worker should assess each client independently. The worker should also make an effort to avoid judgmental terms, such as "promiscuous," or group designations such as "homosexual." Instead, he or she should assess for the presence and frequency of risk behaviors.

Most sexually active individuals are aware that sexual intercourse with a person who is known to be HIV positive is risky. Yet many people are unaware of the factors that make a partner of particularly high risk and the specific behaviors that are most risky for HIV transmission. Social workers can provide valuable information to clients by educating them on the risks involved in different sexual practices and in injection drug use behaviors.

The highest risk sexual partners are those who are HIV positive and have high viral loads. It is important to point out to clients that their sex partners may not volunteer to tell them that they are HIV positive, may not be honest if asked about their status, or may be unaware that they are HIV positive. Men and women who have a history of multiple partners are more likely to be HIV positive, as are MSM. If the partner has another STD, the risk for HIV infection is higher.

The Risky-Safer Sex Continuum

The next section presents the safe–safer sex continuum, which ranks sexual behaviors in order of most risky to least risky (Minnesota AIDS Project, 2012; National Native American AIDS Prevention Center [NNAAPC], n.d.). It is purposefully graphic to assist social workers to develop their knowledge of a wide array of sex behaviors, ranging from risky, to safer, to safe.

Highest-Risk Sex Practices

Unprotected Anal Receptive Intercourse. The practice of having anal intercourse without a condom is frequently called raw sex. People who engage in raw sex are often motivated by the experience of having intercourse without the encumbrance of a condom. Sometimes raw anal sex occurs not out of choice, but is forced or is done because neither partner has access to condoms.

Barebacking is a high-risk practice that has had a resurgence in recent years in MSM (Grov & Parsons, 2006; Halkitis & Parsons, 2003). In barebacking, partners do not use condoms for anal sex. The difference between raw sex and barebacking is that barebacking is purposefully engaging in high-risk sexual behaviors in an effort to become HIV infected. For example, an interview with a man active in the barebacking scene quoted the man as saying many barebackers consciously contract the disease or see it as simply a matter of time before they will belong to the HIV community and therefore be able to have even wilder unprotected sex with other infected men (Dabrowska & Lauer, 2011). Social workers therefore need to be aware that the mention of high HIV risk may not be enough to sway a person from engaging in high-risk behaviors.

Some barebackers may participate in a practice known as bug chasing, in which the intent is to become infected with as many STIs as possible (Grov & Parsons, 2006). Often bug chasers will seek out HIV-positive individuals to have a sexual encounter in an effort to become HIV positive themselves.

Fisting. A very high-risk form of anal intercourse is called fisting, or handballing. It involves fully inserting the hand (or hands) into the anus during sexual intercourse (McCarthy, Wagner, & Jacques 2010). (When this occurs during vaginal intercourse, it is called vaginal fisting.) The behavior is becoming more popular both in practice and in pornography because of its dangerous and alternative nature. Because of the danger of tearing of the mucosal lining of the anus or vagina, it is a high-risk behavior for HIV transmission, since the tearing provides direct access to the bloodstream. Beyond HIV risk, the practice is dangerous to the health of the recipient, who is at risk for infection, hospitalization, and need for reparative surgery. Fisting can be performed on oneself, or with a partner or multiple partners. Though still highly risky, the damage to the recipient can be reduced through the use of latex gloves, which protect the anal or vaginal lining from scratches from fingernails and rings (McCarthy et al., 2010).

When working with a client who reports barebacking, fisting, bug chasing, or other high-risk sex practices, the social worker must strive to avoid any judgmental attitudes. Judgmentalism will not be helpful in the development of a trusting helping relationship. The key is to present factual information, including persuasion that HIV infection is not inevitable for all MSM or heterosexual people who have HIV-positive partners, thus providing hope that the client can avoid HIV.

Unprotected Vaginal Receptive Intercourse. Female clients may be unaware that they are HIV positive. If they are menstruating with blood present, they are more likely to transmit HIV to a partner who is unprotected. As noted above, vaginal fisting is a very high-risk practice because it has a high likelihood of tearing the vaginal mucosa. It is particularly high risk if the recipient is HIV positive, since it will introduce the blood-borne virus into the activity. It is also high risk for an HIV-negative woman to engage in fisting, followed by unprotected vaginal intercourse with an HIV-positive man.

Medium-Risk Sex Practices

Unprotected Anal Insertive Intercourse. A male partner who inserts his penis into the anus of a person with HIV is at medium risk for becoming infected. Because he is not being anally penetrated, however, he is at lower risk for transmission of the blood-borne virus. The penis, unless it has open sores or ulcers, does not provide the best route for viral infection. The most vulnerable place on the penis for infection by an STD is at the end of the urethra, the opening at the tip of the penis. Because of differences in risk levels between receptive and insertive anal sex, it is very important to ask clients whether they prefer to engage in topping, bottoming, or using both positions during intercourse. Their answer will help the social worker to assess risk and negotiation of a risk reduction plan.

In a transgender man, the surgically created penis may have been constructed out of moist membranes, which is where vagina secretions were produced when he was a female. The man should be aware of where the moist membranes are and keep these protected with the use of a condom, dental dam, or plastic wrap during intercourse (McCarthy et al., 2010). The moist membranes are at risk of transmitting HIV and being infected by HIV.

Unprotected Vaginal Insertive Intercourse. Men should be made aware that an HIV-positive woman who is menstruating with blood present is more likely to transmit the virus.

Unprotected Oral Receptive Intercourse. An HIV-negative person who performs unprotected fellatio (oral sex, blowjob, sucking dick) on an HIV-positive man is at medium risk for HIV transmission. If the HIV-positive man ejaculates, the risk is higher. A helpful caveat to teach clients is to "swallow or spit, don't let it sit," since the longer infected ejaculate is in the mouth, the greater the risk of infection. Some experts advise that strong mouthwashes, sodas, and alcoholic beverages should be avoided after performing oral sex on a male with HIV or a male of unknown status. Such beverages are considered to increase risk because they make the lining of the mouth vulnerable to penetration by the virus. It is best to rinse with water and not brush the teeth immediately afterward. There is minimal risk of HIV infection through the stomach (swallowing ejaculate) because the stomach acids immediately kill the virus. Research shows, however, that while the risk of HIV from swallowing semen is very low, unprotected oral sex with a person with HIV or an unknown HIV status should be discouraged (Scondras, 2000).

Unprotected Oral Insertive Intercourse. An HIV-negative man who is having unprotected fellatio (oral sex, blowjob, cock sucking) performed on him is at medium risk for infection by an HIV-positive person. The risk is higher if there are open sores in the mouth of the HIV-infected person (any gender).

Rimming. Rimming, which is also called anilingus (ass licking), is the oral sexual activity of licking around the anus. The CDC states that all oral sex, including fellatio, cunnilingus, and anilingus, is of lower risk than anal or vaginal sex (CDC, 2009). However, when there are mouth sores, anal warts (caused by human papilloma virus [HPV]), syphilis, gonorrhea, or hepatitis A, B, or C, the risks are much higher for HIV or other STD infection (McCarthy et al., 2010).

Blood Sports. Blood sports are sexual acts that involve bloodletting, which can include piercing, cutting, branding, shaving, or spanking with a wire brush. These acts vary in risk depending on the methods used. It is important to acknowledge that to prevent infection by HIV or any other virus or bacteria, anything inserted into the skin must be sterile, not merely clean. Needles, scalpels, and piercings must be disinfected. The area of the skin impacted should be wiped in expanding concentric circles with rubbing alcohol and a clean cotton ball prior to skin penetration (McCarthy et al., 2010). These activities may or may not be related to sex acts. If a person has his or her genitalia pierced, that person increases the risk of having a skin tear during sex play, which can create an opening for HIV infection or transmission.

Lower-Risk Sex Practices

Protected Vaginal or Anal Insertive or Receptive Intercourse. If vaginal or anal sex is performed with a latex or vinyl condom with a partner who is HIV positive or of unknown status, the risk of HIV infection is low. Male (penile condom) or female (vaginal condom) protection, if used carefully and consistently, is effective in reducing risk of HIV infection. Women can be counseled to feel empowered about requiring (not just asking for) the use of a condom. Female condoms can be used if the male partner is not prepared with a male condom or refuses to use one. Note, however, that female condoms can only be used for vaginal intercourse, not anal intercourse. Male condoms are usually made of latex, though vinyl male condoms are available for a higher price. Female condoms are made of vinyl. This distinction is relevant to clients who have latex allergies. Allergic skin reactions can make the skin more susceptible to infection. Social workers should tell clients that oil-based lubricants can quickly break down latex, causing a condom failure. Clients should use water-based lubricants with condoms.

Oral Sex Performed on a Female. Oral sex on a female (cunnilingus, eating out, going down on) is a lower-risk sex practice, and the risk can be lowered even more through the use of a dental dam, plastic food wrap, or other water-impervious barrier. A condom can be cut lengthwise to fashion a makeshift rubber dam to be placed over the female partner's vagina before oral contact. This practice also reduces the spread of other STDs.

Circumcision. Circumcision has been shown to reduce the risk of HIV infection for a male performing vaginal or anal insertive sex with an HIV-positive person (CDC, 2008).

Safer Sex Practices

Deep Kissing. Saliva does not contain the virus that causes HIV disease. However, if the practice causes abrasions in the mouth, the risk for transmission is increased.

Protected Sex with a Partner Who Recently Tested Negative for HIV. Vaginal, anal, or oral sex performed with a condom with a partner who proves he or she recently tested negative for HIV and other STDs is a safer sex practice.

Protected Sex with an HIV-Positive Partner Who Is on Successful ARV Therapy. In mid-2011, the results of HIV Prevention Trials Network (HPTN) Clinical Trial 052 were released, showing that if a person with HIV was started early on ARV medications, his or her risk of transmitting HIV was reduced by 96 percent (Cohen et al., 2011). Therefore, in sero-discordant couples (where one person is HIV positive and the other is HIV negative), it is now scientifically proven that early and uninterrupted treatment with ARVs (when CD4 count drops below 400 cells per milliliter) is part of effective HIV prevention.

Mutual Monogamy. Though one can never be entirely certain of the behaviors of a partner or partners, mutual monogamy (or sex with multiple partners who all agree to no sex outside of the group) is a safer practice. If the partners do not engage in any high-risk activities and avoid sexual contact with anyone else, the risk of introduction of HIV into the relationship is extremely low. The problem with reliance on monogamy for HIV protection is that one cannot determine if their partner(s) is being honest.

Mutual Masturbation. If an HIV-positive male engages with a partner or partners in mutual masturbation and ejaculates, the risk of HIV infection is very low because the ejaculate will not enter the partner's (partners') anus, vagina, or mouth, greatly reducing the risk of transmission. If an HIV-positive female engages in mutual masturbation with a partner, the risk of transmission is also low because the infected vaginal fluid will not enter the mouth, anus, or vagina. As long as HIV-infected semen, vaginal fluid, or blood does not come into contact with broken skin or a mucous membrane (like the eye, mouth, vagina, or rectum), there is very low risk for transmission. Unlike the cold virus, which can be spread by contact on outside surfaces, HIV becomes damaged when exposed to air (Cichocki, 2006). HIV needs a host to survive and replicate.

Use of Sex Toys. While open sharing of sex toys in a group carries a high risk of transmission of HIV and other STDs, using them monogamously carries a lower risk. Anything that has been in a person's anus (rectum) or vagina has a chance of transmitting infections of all kinds. Toys (such as dildos and vibrators) can be difficult to clean, but covering them with a condom prior to use can make them more hygienic. Sex toys used during solo masturbation should not be used on different parts of the same person's body. For example, a dildo used in the anus can transfer feces to the mouth or vagina if not thoroughly cleaned first. Medical cleaners, such as those that contain isopropanol and butyl cellosolve are better than use of hydrogen peroxide or household bleach (McCarthy et al., 2010). The person must thoroughly flush the cleaner from the device or body tissues could become inflamed to the point where the tissues are more susceptible to HIV or other infections. Leather toys (such as whips, floggers, or leather dildos) cannot be sterilized but should be cleaned as best as possible. If the leather has blood on it, it should not be shared. The main risk is not with regard to HIV infection, but to hepatitis infection.

Temperature Play. HIV and other STDs can be transmitted during hot and cold temperature play if there are cracks in the skin, open blisters, or inflammation caused by the high or low temperatures. If playing with ice, clients should know that sharp edges could cause cuts in skin and mucous membranes. Hot wax play can cause open burns and sores where HIV can be transmitted. The more responsible partners are when using hot and cold temperature play, so that the skin is not broken or inflamed, the lower the amount of HIV transmission risk.

Watersports. Watersports (golden showers) and other activities where urine is on the outside of intact skin pose very little risk for HIV transmission. Sex play that involves feces, a practice often called scat, does not pose risk if the skin is intact. Urine is relatively sterile, and therefore experts do not caution against drinking urine of a person potentially infected with HIV (Kull, 2002). Yet, urine, and especially feces, can contain blood, especially if passed though the urethra (urine), or rectum or anus (feces) when there was a tear or abrasion in the mucosal lining. Some have cautioned against drinking large quantities of urine from a person who is taking ARVs, as these and other recreational drugs and the ingested drug by-products can produce unintended consequences. Furthermore, urine can theoretically transmit hepatitis and other STDs (Gaul, 2010). Accidental or purposeful ingestion of feces can cause intestinal infections.

Safest Sex Practices

Masturbation. Self- or solo masturbation is considered completely safe from transmission of HIV. An exception is when the person introduces sex toys that have recently been used on another person.

Abstinence. Abstinence is often defined as not having any sexual intercourse or sex play with another partner. Therefore, self-masturbation can be considered an activity aligned with abstinence. Some people may choose to not engage in self-masturbation as part of their abstinence from sex. It is important to understand what a client means by the word when they identify themselves as abstinent. Some could mean that there is sex play with others, but no intercourse. And, as outlined above, there are many risky sexual activities that do not involve intercourse.

There are three important guidelines to convey to clients that transcend the HIV transmission risk continuum presented above. First, the more aggressive the sexual activities are, the more likely it is that an opportunity for HIV transmission will occur. Rough sex, such as sex acts that involve force that can cause bleeding or open cuts, will greatly increase the risks of HIV transmission, even if the person uses condoms. Second, lengthy sessions (for several hours, even six or eight hours) of sexual activity, especially with multiple partners, are likely to cause anal and vaginal linings to become more vulnerable to significant tearing, increasing the risk of HIV transmission. Furthermore, the more the tip of the penis is overused or abused, the more vulnerable the urethra is to providing access to the bloodstream, as is necessary for HIV infection or transmission. And third, there is an adage in HIV prevention work that "too much lubricant is not enough." The use of water-based lubricants designed for sexual activity greatly reduces the amount of irritation and abrasion of the vagina and anus or rectum during intercourse. Lubricants come in colors, scents, and flavors to enhance oral sex. Social workers interested in promotion of safe sex should always distribute individual packets of lubricants along with condoms. Use of a condom without lubricant is a riskier sex behavior than intercourse with a lubricant and a condom.

BDSM

BDSM is an acronym for a form of sexual expression that involves use of restraints. The broad term encompasses bondage and discipline, dominance and submission, and sadomasochism play (Connolly, 2006; Weiss, 2006). The BDSM community has been active for decades, but was recently popularized in films such as *Kill Bill* and *Secretary*, and on television shows such as *Buffy the Vampire Slayer* and in a few episodes of *Will and Grace* (Barker, Iantaffi, & Gupta, 2007). Participants in these group activities are either called tops (or dominants), because they exercise control over others, or bottoms (or submissives), meaning they are controlled. Individuals who alternate roles are called switches. In brief, the erotic sessions involve role-play of scenes involving the use of restraints and emergency signals to identify when someone needs to be released. There is a strict code of behavior, called SSC, for safe, sane and consensual, and there are preplay negotiations to discuss what activities and sexual behaviors are acceptable to each participant (Connolly, 2006). Because BDSM sexual activities can be very rough and practices involving blood are common, there can be a significant risk of transmission of HIV or other STDs. Like HIV, hepatitis is transmitted through blood-to-blood contact, but unlike HIV, it is a hardy virus that can survive outside the body for much longer than HIV. Therefore, devices and restraints used in BDSM activities should be carefully cleaned (McCarthy et al., 2010).

Questions about the Sexual Risk Behavior Continuum

1. Look at the list of sexual behaviors presented above. Which of these would you hesitate to discuss with clients?

2. Do you find any of the behaviors described above to be morally wrong? If so, why? And if so, would you be able to work with a client who reports these behaviors?

3. Some people may find it difficult to understand why a person would find a certain behavior described above to be sexually pleasurable. Is it necessary for a social worker to understand this in order to work effectively with a client?

4. Consider this case vignette: Porsha is a new HIV case manager at an AIDS service organization (ASO). She has worked as a medical social worker previously and believes she is comfortable talking about human sexuality. Porsha's supervisor asks her if she is ready to work with one of their most challenging clients, Baxter, who has come to the ASO saying he needs an emergency consultation. Baxter is a very outspoken male sex worker; the health department suspects him of spreading the virus to many men living in his zip code area. Porsha feels very confident that she can handle whatever Baxter wants to discuss. Baxter comes in, meets Porsha, and asks, "Can I give somebody HIV from watersports? I have this guy who is really into watersports and I got it all up in his ears and eyes. I'm not really that into it, but as long as it's at his place, then I don't care about the mess. But, is his eyes and ears a problem, Miss Porsha?" Porsha is not sure what he means by watersports, but she doesn't want to appear ignorant in front of this high-risk client that her supervisor has entrusted to her. She quickly thinks about waterskiing and jet skiing, but quickly rules these out, as it sounds like Baxter is referring to something that took place in a home. She thinks of a hot tub—and decides that sex in a hot tub must be what he means. She relaxes, since she knows that HIV can't be transmitted by bathing together. She learned about this on a documentary on AIDS in Africa. Therefore, she responds to Baxter by saying, "Thank you for your concern, Baxter, but bath water will not transmit HIV. So you can bathe safely with a partner, even if the water splashes in his or her eyes and ears." Baxter responds, "Taking a bath? Who's talking about taking a bath? I don't get paid to take a bath—don't I wish! This gentleman wants me to piss all over his head—he gets off on that BDSM dominance thing. Don't you know about sex work? Are you new here?" Baxter then gets up and storms out, shouting behind him about how he shouldn't expect someone not in "the business" to know what he's got to do.

- What do you think Porsha's next thought process will be like?

- How do you think Porsha's supervisor will respond to the news that Baxter stormed out of the agency?

- Do you think Baxter will return? If so, why? If not, why not?

- What should Porsha have done when Baxter raised his question about watersports and HIV transmission risk?

Condom Education

An important role for social workers in HIV prevention is to provide candid and thorough education to clients about how to protect themselves and their sex partners. This requires extensive knowledge about safe and safer sex practices and the ability to speak about these topics in a culturally tailored manner, meeting each client where he or she is. This section provides some detailed information on condom use. Social workers, especially those who have had little experience discussing sex, can use these tips to start conversations about safe sex with clients. A question-and-answer game using facts about condom use is one method for engaging a group in discussion about safe sex practices. Some of the following tips are from AVERT (2011).

- Most condoms are made of latex. People should not use oil-based lubricants such as Vaseline or mineral oil with latex condoms because the oils break down the latex, but they can use oil-based lubricants with vinyl condoms. They can use water-based lubricants with either type of condom. Natural (animal product) condoms do not prevent HIV and STDs; they are only for prevention of pregnancy. Sperm cannot penetrate the pores in the animal membrane, but viruses can penetrate the pores.

- Some condoms are lubricated. The advantage is that the lubricant helps prevent breakage (and therefore failure) of the condom. The disadvantage is that the lubricant can also cause slippage. Clients should not use condoms with a spermicide called Nonoxynol-9 for HIV prevention. While it was once thought to help with prevention of HIV transmission, it has been shown to cause irritation of the lining of the anus, increasing the risk of HIV transmission during anal sex.

- Condoms come in a variety of sizes, shapes, colors, scents, textures, and flavors. There are condom selection websites that are helpful for selecting the best type for each person.

- There is no age restriction on buying condoms. Therefore, sexually active youth without access to free condoms can purchase them from a convenience store, supermarket, drugstore, or online distributor.

- A person should use a new condom for each sexual experience and each partner. He or she should not rinse and reuse a condom because it may have become weakened or damaged.

- Many people are unaware of the correct way to apply a condom. The AVERT website contains a one-minute animated video demonstration that can be shown to clients (AVERT, 2011). Here are some of the main points to pass along to clients: Squeezing the tip of the condom while rolling the condom down the shaft of the penis prevents breakage by providing a space for ejaculate to be contained. Air bubbles can cause breakage. Carefully rolling the condom down a partially or fully erect penis will reduce air bubbles. If a lubricant is to be used, the person should apply it to the outside of the condom after it has been fully applied. If the condom will not easily roll, it may be on upside down. Since pre-ejaculate from the tip of the penis may be on the upside-down condom, the person should apply a new one, not simply turn it right side up.

- If vaginal intercourse is to follow anal intercourse, it is best to apply a new condom to reduce the risk of infection by introduction of fecal matter into the vagina.

- Condoms have expiration dates. They can dry out and become brittle.

- Condoms need to be stored in a cool, dry place. They should not be kept in a wallet because they can wear out from repeated pressure and body heat. Similarly, they should not be stored in a hot car.

- Condoms should not be doubled-up for extra protection. Use of two or more condoms at once can cause breakage and slippage.

- Condoms should be applied before any penetration. Pre-ejaculatory semen (pre-cum) contains not only active sperm, but also HIV virus.

- Many male clients express an unwillingness to use condoms during vaginal or anal intercourse and instead opt to take their chances. One way to encourage condom use for reduction of risk of HIV infection or transmission with this type of client is to suggest that they practice using condoms prior to use of them with a sex partner. For example, men who routinely masturbate with a condom express less discontent with their use during intercourse. The idea is that people are comfortable with what they are familiar with.

One of the most valuable interventions a social worker can provide for HIV prevention is thorough education about proper use of condoms. Therefore, HIV prevention social workers should become very comfortable in discussing these topics.

Condom Negotiation

One of the biggest barriers to consistent condom use is that some men and women report feeling unable to negotiate for use of condoms by their male partners. A valuable social work intervention is to empower both male and female clients through role-play on how to require, or at least ask for their partners to use condoms. It is important to acknowledge that use of condoms is subject to both cultural and religious restrictions. Culturally competent social workers will acknowledge these barriers and work with clients to find ways to defuse arguments against their use. It can be difficult for some clients to talk about using condoms. Still, workers should not let embarrassment become a health risk. Table 12.1 presents some dialogues to practice with clients of all genders and sexual orientations

Table 12.1. Condom Negotiation Excuses and Countering Responses

EXCUSE	ANSWER
Don't you trust me?	Trust isn't the point: people can have infections without realizing it.
It does not feel as good with a condom.	I'll feel more relaxed, and if I am more relaxed, I can make it feel better for you.
I don't stay hard when I put on a condom.	I'll help you put it on, and that will help you keep it hard.
I am afraid to ask him to use a condom. He'll think I don't trust him.	If you can't ask him, you probably don't trust him.
I can't feel a thing when I wear a condom.	Maybe that way you'll last even longer and that will make up for it.
I don't have a condom with me.	I do.
It's up to him … it's his decision.	It's your health. It should be your decision too!
I'm on the pill, you don't need a condom.	I'd like to use it anyway. It will help to protect us from infections we may not realize we have.
It just isn't as sensitive and I can't feel you.	Maybe that way you will last even longer and that will make up for it.
Putting it on interrupts everything.	Not if I help put it on.
I guess you don't really love me.	I do, but I am not risking my future to prove it.
I will pull out in time.	Women can get pregnant and get STDs from preejaculate.
But I love you.	Then you'll help us to protect ourselves.
Just this once.	Once is all it takes.

Source: www.plannedparenthood.org/health-topics/birth-control/condom-10187.htm and www.avert.org/condom.htm.

(AVERT, 2011). Common excuses for not using a condom are countered with responses, which negotiate for condom use.

HIV Risk Continuum for Injection Drug Use

According to the CDC, in 2009 injection drug use accounted for 12 percent of transmissions of HIV in the United States (CDC, 2011). Since the epidemic began, injection drug users have accounted for about one-third of all HIV transmissions. Sharing syringes and other equipment for drug injection is a well-known route of HIV transmission, but injection drug users are also at a higher risk for HIV infection through sexual transmission (CDC, 2007). Just like with sexual transmission behaviors, there is a continuum of risk with respect to injection drug use behaviors. Following is an HIV risk continuum presented, beginning with the most risky behaviors, which are most likely to result in HIV infection or transmission.

Riskiest Injection Drug Use Behaviors

Sharing uncleaned needles, syringes, and other injection paraphernalia (works), especially in shooting galleries where a large number of people may have used instruments, is high risk. HIV DNA has been found on cottons, cookers, and in wash water, even when they appeared clean (Shah et al., 1996).

Less-Risky Injection Drug Use Behaviors

Sharing cleaned needles, syringes, and works is less risky. Household bleach is effective but needles and syringes should be rinsed well with clean water after the use of bleach (NNAAPC, n.d.).

Drug paraphernalia reused repeatedly but by the same person is less risky. It is important to protect access to one's supplies, to make sure they are not infected with HIV or other viruses without one knowing.

Least-Risky Injection Drug Use Behaviors

Use of single-use needles and syringes is least risky because there is little risk of introduction of viruses. One must be very certain that the packaging for these items has not been previously opened.

Use of needle exchange programs that provide sterile needles in return for used ones is less risky. These programs have been shown to be effective at reducing HIV transmission and have not led to increased injection drug use as was feared (CDC, 2005).

Club Drug Use and HIV Risk

Non-injection drug use, such as crack cocaine, also contributes to the spread of HIV when users trade sex for drugs or money, or when they engage in risky behaviors that they might not engage in when sober (CDC, 2005). Furthermore, some club drugs are used to enhance sexual performance.

Club drugs are drugs that are used in dance clubs, circuit parties, or weekend-long rave parties (Mayer, Colfax, & Guzman, 2006). Club drug use is highest in the population groups at highest risk for HIV, including young MSM. Not only does the use of club drugs reduce inhibitions and increase sexual stamina, they have also been shown to have a negative impact on medication and treatment adherence for people living with HIV or AIDS. For these reasons, social workers interfacing with populations at risk for HIV infection, especially young MSM, should have a working knowledge of club drugs. This knowledge base is helpful for risk assessment of clients and development of risk reduction strategies.

Poppers. Research has shown that in a study of urban gay men, 20 percent reported using poppers in the six months prior to the study (Stall et al., 2001). Poppers are nitrites that are usually inhaled nasally. They are readily available on the internet and are sold legally as cleaning products. The popularity of poppers in sexual settings "is attributable to their orgasm-enhancing effects and to the belief that they relax the anal sphincter, making receptive anal sex more comfortable" (Mayer et al., 2006, p. 1465). The effect lasts a few minutes. Although they are very popular, the common practice of taking poppers with Viagra or another medication to enhance erections can cause cardiovascular collapse (Mayer et al., 2006).

MDMA. On the street, methylenedioxymethamphetamine is commonly called Ecstasy, XTC, X, or Lover's speed. It can produce both stimulant and psychedelic effects, similar to the hallucinogen mescaline (National Institute on Drug Abuse [NIDA], 2010). It is taken as a pill and is commonly used at dance clubs. It increases tactile sensations and is therefore seen as a pleasant accompaniment to sexual activity. A study of urban gay men showed that 12 percent reported using MDMA in the previous six months (Stall et al., 2001), and another study showed 19 percent of young MSM had used MDMA (Thiede et al., 2003).

Ketamine. Ketamine, or Special K, is a dissociative anesthetic that is frequently used in veterinary medicine. It is snorted, ingested, or injected and the effects can last from thirty to ninety minutes. The effects, sometimes called falling into a K-hole, are strong hallucinations and feelings of euphoria (Mayer et al., 2006). One study showed that 53 percent of young MSM reported ketamine use (Mansergh et al., 2001).

GHB. Gamma hydroxybutyrate is a drug that was approved in 2002 for the treatment of narcolepsy. Since then, GHB (G, Georgia homeboy, or grievous bodily harm) is popularly used by young people at dance clubs. It is ingested orally in liquid or powder form and is considered a date rape drug, due to its ability to incapacitate unsuspecting victims, preventing them from resisting a sexual assault (NIDA, 2010). It has an intoxicating effect. It is also used by bodybuilders to aid in fat reduction and muscle building. A study of MSM circuit party attendees showed that 25 percent used GHB (Mansergh et al., 2001).

Rohypnol. Flunitrazepam, or roofies, is the drug most commonly associated with date rape or acquaintance rape. Because Rohypnol and GHB are odorless, colorless, and tasteless, they can be used to secretly spike drinks. Therefore, dance club wisdom calls for people to keep control of their drink at all times, to prevent anyone from drugging them. Rohypnol is somewhat similar to Valium or Xanax.

Methamphetamine. Meth, speed, or crystal is a highly addictive stimulant that is closely related to amphetamine. Long-term consequences are weight loss, depression, severe dental disease, excessive teeth grinding (bruxism), and excessive picking and scratching of the skin (Mayer et al., 2006). A study of urban gay men showed 10 percent had used methamphetamine in the previous six months (Stall et al., 2001). Another study of young MSM showed 20 percent used amphetamines (Thiede et al., 2003).

It is difficult to ascertain if club drug use promotes sexual risk-taking behavior or if personal risk-taking tendencies promote both sexual risk-taking and club drug use. Nonetheless, data show that club drugs, including poppers, commonly accompany high-risk sexual activities. When a person is under the influence of drugs, he or she is less likely to use protection and adhere to other risk-reduction strategies, such as limiting the number of sex partners. Therefore, risk assessments and risk reduction strategies should address club drug and injection drug use. Additionally, the social worker should assess a client's use of alcohol, steroids (roids), and marijuana cigarettes laced with the drug PCP.

Case Example II

Ben opened the trunk of his state-owned car and placed his briefcase inside. As he walked to the front of the car, his supervisor, Evelyn, pulled up smoking a cigarette. Ben cringed when he saw her. He felt as if she was doing everything in her power to control him and not let him succeed at his job as a case manager with their HIV/AIDS agency.

Evelyn had been with the agency for more than a decade and was known for her management abilities in medical case management. Ben was a recent MSW (master of social work) graduate and a relatively new employee. Although he hadn't been working with HIV for long, he believed that medical case management did not take care of the whole person. He and Evelyn had been at odds for quite some time. That morning Ben had had a meeting with Evelyn, during which she told him that he was not discharging his clients soon enough. Ben argued that he believed that he needs to stay with his clients longer than the management plan of the HIV/AIDS agency prescribes in order to ensure that the clients follow the outlined care plan. Evelyn argued that the way they have been doing case management has worked for years and that he was not going to change that.

When Ben saw her as he was leaving, it brought back all of the emotions that he had felt that morning. He loved the work that he was doing, but had a sense of being trapped. He really believed that he was making a difference. However, if he were to work under the model that the HIV/AIDS agency has set up, he feels he would be doing a disservice to his clients by discharging them too soon.

He mustered up half of a smile and threw up his hand in a half-hearted wave. Evelyn quickly pulled into the parking space and motioned as if to say she wanted him to wait for a minute. He stood by the car thinking, "What now?"

Evelyn got out of her car and briskly walked over to Ben. "Are you headed to see a client?"

"Yes. I'm going to take a client to her first full medical appointment in years." Ben replied.

"Okay. Well I just wanted to let you know that I do think you are doing a great job. I also want you to get acquainted with how we do case management as well. It isn't personal because you do a great job."

Ben smiled and turned to get into the car. "Thanks. I appreciate it. I need to run."

"Okay, be careful." Evelyn returned to get her things from her car.

Ben drove off, feeling upset. "If I do such a good job, then why don't you let me do my job the way I do it!?," he thought. "Why do you think your way is better just because you have been doing it longer?" All of these thoughts ran through Ben's head as he drove to his client Linda's house. As he pulled up, he realized he needed to start thinking about her and her visit.

Linda is an African-American female client who is actively addicted to alcohol and crack cocaine. Ben met Linda five months prior when she was referred to him by the hospital. She was being discharged after having been admitted with pneumonia. She had a home to return to, but had told the hospital that she had known she was HIV positive for four years but not done anything about it. The hospital social worker called the HIV/AIDS agency, and Ben was assigned as her case manager.

This was Linda's third visit to the infectious disease clinic. On her first visit, she had lab work done. On the second visit, she spoke with the physician about the results of the lab tests and they agreed she should start on medication. On this visit, she is scheduled for a long session with the physician so he can conduct a physical and get her started on medications. For the last two appointments, Linda rode the bus to the appointments with bus passes provided by Ben. Ben wanted to attend the appointments with her, but he could not fit them in his schedule.

As Ben walked into the gate of Linda' duplex, he recalled that Linda has been in either really agreeable or disagreeable moods in the past. He hoped that today would be a good day with Linda. As he knocked on the door, he heard her yell, "Who is it?" in a more gruff tone than usual.

"Ben!" Ben replied, trying to match her harsh tone. He laughed at himself.

Linda came to the door and said, "Ben who?" as she swung open the door. "Ohhh! Social worker Ben. Hey. Give me one minute." She turned and went back into the house, leaving Ben standing on the porch. Ben chuckled to himself. "I wonder what other Bens she was expecting today." He looked around the porch of the duplex. Two broken plastic chairs. One had tape all around one of the legs, indicating failed attempts at fixing it. Many of the wooden planks on the porch were rotting away. Just as Ben began to wonder if it was safe for him to be standing on the porch, Linda came bounding out of the door with a big smile and the strong aroma of perfume. They both climbed into the state car and headed off for the clinic.

"So, when I knocked on your door, you said, 'Ben who?' Do you have other Bens in your life?" Ben joked with Linda.

Linda laughed back, "I have many men in my life, Mr. Ben! Don't play! You know we done talked about that before!"

Ben recalled quite vividly the times when Linda detailed her sexual history with him during her early visits. "Yes, Linda, I do recall. What did the doctor say when you told him?"

"Told him what? I didn't tell the doctor all my business like that!" Linda pulled down the visor looking for a mirror to put the finishing touches on her bangs.

Ben glanced over at Linda as he kept driving. "Wait, so the last time you were at the clinic you didn't tell the doctor about your male friends?"

"It didn't come up," Linda chuckled.

"So what did you two talk about last time?" Ben decided to find out what needed to be filled in on today's visit.

"We talked about them T-cells and virus cells like you talked about with me. We talked about my counts being bad so I needed to be on medicine. We talked about me not getting enough sleep and me stopping smoking. That was it." Linda would not make eye contact with Ben.

"So what about your substance abuse and sexual history? Did you talk about that with the doctor?" Ben recalled all the different details that Linda told him about, with respect to her sex work and her illegal drug use.

"So I'm supposed to be like, 'Hey, Dr. So-and-so. I'm Linda. I smoke an occasional crack rock and suck a dick from time to time." Linda looked over at Ben as they pulled to a stop light.

Ben looked right back over at Linda. "If that is your reality, then that is what you need to tell your doctor. He needs to understand your risk factors to help best mitigate them."

"Huh?" Linda blankly stared back at Ben.

"You and the doctor are on the same team fighting the opposing team together. The doctor needs to best understand what is going on with your body, and exactly how it is going on, so that he can best help you fight the HIV. If he doesn't know how much you are drinking, drugging, sexing, and so on, then he can't best help you." Ben's words were soft, but direct.

"So why he got to know how many dicks I'm sucking?" Linda giggled a little when she said this.

"So he knows what tests to administer for you, and how." Ben kept on driving. "Any other questions?"

"No."

"Okay. So in the past week, how many men have you had sex with?" Ben tried to look over at Linda's face as he kept driving toward the clinic.

"Oh, my heavens, Mr. Ben!" Linda screamed and laid her hands toward her neck as if she were offended. "I can't believe you would ask a lady like me a question like that. You know I am pure as . . . hell." They both laughed as she continued. "Seriously? Do you really want to know?"

Ben replied. "No, I really don't want to know. I do, however, want you to be able to honestly answer that question for the doctor when we get there. You know you can tell me because we have built trust between us. This time if you would like me to talk to the doctor for you, just to get you started, I can."

"No, no, I'm not ashamed." Linda interjected. "I just need to start thinking."

Ben added, "And think about how many drinks you have daily, how many cigarettes, how many drugs you do, what drugs, how many. . . ."

"Dang, Ben! You must want me to tell them my whole life story," Linda interrupted Ben. "Hell, last night I had this one dude and his friend. The one dude did me regular so he used a rubber but the other dude didn't."

Ben expected this conversation and kept going with it, knowing that the more information he has to help her share with the physician, the better. "Why did one of the guys wear a condom and the other one not?"

"Because he didn't do it regular."

"What is regular?" Ben was glad to come to a light so that he could look at Linda for this answer.

"You know. Regular means doing it regular and the other is the other." Linda pointed around her backside to her butt.

"Oh, so in your words, doing it regular is receiving sex vaginally. The other would be receiving sex anally?" Ben asked.

"Ewww, Ben! You sound so nasty talking about vaginal and anal. You make it sound so gross." Linda laughed out of discomfort.

"Well, is that what you are referring to?" Ben asked with a patient smile.

"Yeah, I guess so." Linda said, with a big blushing grin. "But me and the doctor already talked about all that."

"Oh, really?"

"Mmm, hmm!"

"When did you talk with the doctor about your sexual activities?"

"Last visit."

"And you told him that you have sex for money and how you have sex?" Ben asked directly and looked over at her to try to make eye contact.

"What do you mean how I have sex?" Linda laughed and began to get fidgety.

"Anally, orally, or vaginally. Mutual masturbation or solo. Did you talk with the doctor about how you have sex?" Ben smiled. "Remember how you told me that I was not ready to hear about your sex life that day in my office? Then you proceeded to tell me all kinds of things that you said would 'make me blush?' Well, you need to tell the doctor all those things."

Linda tried to hide her face like she was embarrassed. "Really, Ben? I have to tell him all that? He'll judge me."

"I won't say if he will or won't judge you. I will say that he needs to know all of that in order to create the best care plan for you. So, can I count on you to be honest today? I'll be right there with you."

"I guess." Linda said with a half-hearted smile. "You'll be there with me, right?"

"Yes. I can even bring the subjects back up if you would like me to."

"No, I got this. I'll talk with the doctor and tell him everything. I'm used to talking to mens about sex. But when he shocked, don't say I didn't tell you so!"

Ben and Linda laughed as they parked at the clinic. As she swung her legs out of the front seat of the state car, Linda pulled down on her skirt hem and up on her neckline.

References

AVERT. (2011). Using condoms, condom types and sizes. Retrieved from http://www.avert.org/condom.htm

Barker, M., Iantaffi, A., & Gupta, C. (2007). Kinky clients, kinky counseling? The challenges and potentials of BDSM. In L. Moon (Ed.), *Feeling queer or queer feelings: Radical approaches to counseling sex, sexualities and genders* (pp. 106–124). London, UK: Routledge.

California STD/HIV Prevention Training Center. (2006). A guide to sexual history taking with men who have sex with men. Chlamydia Care Quality Improvement Toolbox. Conference handout.

Centers for Disease Control and Prevention (CDC). (2005). Update: Syringe exchange programs—United States, 2002. *Morbidity and Mortality Weekly Report, 54*(27), 673–676.

Centers for Disease Control and Prevention (CDC). (2007). Drug-associated HIV transmission continues in the United States. Fact Sheet. Retrieved from http://www.cdc.gov/hiv/resources/factsheets/idu.htm

Centers for Disease Control and Prevention (CDC). (2008). CDC HIV/AIDS Science Facts: Male circumcision and risk for HIV transmission and other health conditions: Implications for the United States. Retrieved from http://www.cdc.gov/hiv/resources/factsheets/PDF/circumcision.pdf

Centers for Disease Control and Prevention (CDC). (2009). Oral sex and HIV risk. Retrieved from http://www.cdc.gov/hiv/resources/factsheets/pdf/oralsex.pdf

Centers for Disease Control and Prevention (CDC). (2011). HIV/AIDS statistics and surveillance. Retrieved from http://www.cdc.gov/hiv/topics/surveillance/basic.htm#hivaidsexposure

Cichocki, M. (2006). HIV/AIDS: How long does HIV live outside the body? About.com. Retrieved from http://aids.about.com/b/2006/11/07/faq-how-long-does-hiv-live-outside-the-body.htm

Cohen, M., Chen, Y., McCauley, M., Gamble, T., Hosseinipour, M., Kumarasamy, N., . . . , Fleming, T. for the HTPN 052 Study team. (2011). Prevention of HIV-1 infection with early-antiretroviral therapy. *The New England Journal of Medicine, 365*, 493–505.

Connolly, P. (2006). Psychological functioning of Bondage/Domination/Sado-Masochism (BDSM) practitioners. *Journal of Psychology & Human Sexuality, 18*(1), 79–120.

Dabrowska, B., & Lauer, S. (2011). *There's no biz like pozbiz: An HIV-positive escort goes deep into Berlin's bareback scene.* Vice Beta. Retrieved from http://www.vice.com/read/there-s-no-biz-like-pozbiz-714-v18n2

Furman, R., Rowan, D., & Bender, K. (2009). *An experiential approach to group work.* Chicago: Lyceum Books.

Gaul, S. (2010). Golden showers from a health perspective. EmpowHER. Retrieved from http://www.empowher.com/sexually-transmitted-diseases/content/golden-showers-health-perspective

Grov, C., & Parsons, J. T. (2006). Bug chasing and gift giving: The potential for HIV transmission among barebackers on the internet. *AIDS Education & Prevention, 18*(6), 490–503.

Halkitis, P. N., & Parsons, J. T. (2003). Intentional unsafe sex (barebacking) among HIV-positive gay men who seek sexual partners on the internet. *AIDS Care, 15*(3), 376–378.

Kinnell, A. M. (2002). Soliciting client questions in HIV prevention and test counseling. *Research on Language and Social Interaction, 35*(3), 367–393.

Kull, R. (2002). *Ask the experts about safe sex and HIV prevention: Watersports for HIV+ people.* The Body: The complete HIV/AIDS resource. Retrieved from http://www.thebody.com/Forums/AIDS/SafeSex/Q134792.html

Mansergh, G., Colfax, G., Marks, G., Rader, M., Guzman, R., & Buchbinder, S. (2001). The Circuit Party Men's Health Survey: Findings and implications for gay and bisexual men. *American Journal of Public Health, 91*(6), 953–958.

Maurice, W. L., & Bowman, M. (1999). Talking about sexual issues: History-taking and interviewing. In W. Maurice & M. Bowman, *Sexual medicine in primary care* (pp. 1–25). St. Louis, MO: Mosby.

Mayer, K. H., Colfax, G., & Guzman, R. (2006). Club drugs and HIV infection: A review. *Clinical Infectious Diseases, 42*(10), 1463–1469.

McCarthy, D., Wagner, J., & Jacques, T. H. (2010). *BDSM: Safer kinky sex.* The AIDS Committee of Toronto. Safer BDSM Education Project. Retrieved from http://www.actoronto.org/home.nsf/pages/bdsm

Minnesota AIDS Project. (2012). HIV risk reduction: Sexual transmission risk reduction. Retrieved from http://www.mnaidsproject.org/education/educate-yourself/hiv-risk-reduction.php

National Institute on Drug Abuse (NIDA). (2010). Drugs of abuse. Retrieved from http://www.drugabuse.gov/drugs-abuse

National Native American AIDS Prevention Center (NNAAPC). (n.d.) Sexual-risk reduction fact sheet. Retrieved from http://www.nnaapc.org/pdf/Fact-Sheets/Fact-sheet-Sexual.pdf

Pisani, E. (2010, February). *Sex, drugs and HIV—Let's get rational.* TED Talks: Ideas worth sharing. Retrieved from http://www.ted.com/talks/elizabeth_pisani_sex_drugs_and_hiv_let_s_get_rational_1.html

Scondras, D. (2000). *Search for a cure: Don't swallow: A look at the risks of oral sex.* The Body: The complete HIV/AIDS resources. Retrieved from http://www.thebody.com/content/art32502.html?ic=2004

Shah, S., Shapshak, P., Rivers, J., Stewart, R., Weatherby, N., Xin, K. Q., Page, J.B., . . . , McCoy, C. B. (1996). Detection of HIV-1 DNA in needle/syringes, para-phernalia, and washes from shooting galleries in Miami: A preliminary labo-ratory report. *Journal of Acquired Immune Deficiency Syndromes & Human Retrovirology, 11*(3), 301–306.

Stall, R., Paul, J. P., Greenwood, G., Pollack, L. M., Bein, E., Crosby, G. M., Millis, T.C., . . . , Catania, J. A. (2001). Alcohol use, drug use and alcohol-related problems among men who have sex with men: The Urban Men's Health Study. *Addiction, 96*(11), 1589–1601.

Substance Abuse and Mental Health Services Administration (SAMHSA). (2000). *Substance abuse treatment for persons with HIV/AIDS.* Treatment Improve-ment Protocol (TIP) Series, No. 37. Rockville, MD: Author.

Thiede, H., Valleroy, L. A., MacKellar, D. A., Celentano, D. D., Ford, W. L., Hagan, H., . . . , and for the Young Men's Study Group. (2003). Regional patterns and correlates of substance use among young men who have sex with men in 7 US urban cities. *American Journal of Public Health*, *93*(11), 1915–1921.

Tomlinson, J. (1998). ABC of sexual health: Taking a sexual history. *British Medical Journal*, *317*(7172), 1573–1576.

Weiss, M. (2006). Mainstreaming kink: The politics of BDSM representations in the U.S. popular media. *Journal of Homosexuality*, *50*(2/3), 103–130.

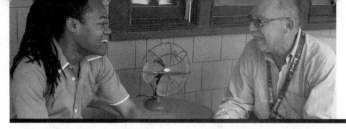

13

The Adherence Conundrum

Lisa Cox

King Louis XIV: You have a physician. What does he do?

French Playwright Molière: Sire, we converse. He gives me advice which I do not follow, and I get better.

—W. Treue, *Doctor at Court* (1958, p. 41)

Historical Significance of Medication Adherence

Prior to the 1981 discovery of the human immunodeficiency virus (HIV), health-care providers, including social workers, practiced in a world without HIV and the acquired immune deficiency syndrome (AIDS). In 1981, as epidemiologists and physicians were watching people die from pneumocystis carinii pneumonia (PCP), Kaposi sarcoma (KS), and toxoplasmosis, there were no medication protocols to which to adhere. Only in 1987 was the first antiretroviral (ARV) medication, named AZT (azidothymidine; also known as zidovudine, or brand name Retrovir), approved for prescription purposes. These early doses of AZT were typically prescribed at 1,200 milligrams, a dosage that caused extreme side effects. Approximately three years later, the AZT dose was cut in half. Consequently, people living with AIDS (PLWA) experienced side effects that were less devastating, and saved money from not having to fill their prescriptions so frequently.

With HIV/AIDS medications available in 1987 clinical drug trials could be implemented and evaluated. AIDS became a chronic manageable disease, generating optimism and hope about the future for HIV-infected people and their loved ones. Spanning the years between 1990 and 2000, when opportunistic infections such as mycobacterium avium complex, cryptococcal meningitis, and cancers were prevalent, numerous HIV-infected people were recruited into both hospital- and community-based AIDS clinical trials. These methodological assessments helped answer scientific questions regarding the safety and efficacy of new treatments and of new methods for administering existing treatments, and depended on study participants' continuing committed participation. AIDS clinical trial researchers judged the validity of drug studies conducted by the industry (e.g., pharmaceutical companies) and the National Institutes of Health (NIH) on the ability of those studies to recruit and retain adherent study participants.

Consequently, adherence—the commonly used term for medication compliance, or concordance, as some Australians say—has become part of the everyday lexicon of scientists, social workers, and researchers who help HIV-infected people adjust to a lifetime of taking prescriptions. As HIV disease has morphed from an acute illness to a chronic illness, adherence has evolved as a major and minor lifestyle issue for people living with HIV and AIDS. Some authorities have called treatment adherence the most serious problem facing medical practice. Both simple and complex definitions of adherence abound. In health care, perhaps the most widely accepted definition of adherence is the extent to which a person's behavior (in terms of taking medications, following diets, or executing lifestyle changes) coincides with medical or health advice. This definition emphasizes aspects of dosage and pill taking, both of them aspects of medication adherence. Despite these definitions, what seems most important is what adherence means to the person infected with HIV disease.

In reality, people living with HIV and people living with AIDS must grapple with medication adherence issues amidst the normal stressors of daily living. When health-care providers, including social workers, encourage patients to adhere to strict medication regimen schedules, those patients are often required to make lifestyle changes. For example, vacations require careful forethought because prescriptions must be filled in advance, some medications require refrigeration, and others are affected by the ingestion of grapefruit and some anti-anxiety medications.

Existing literature on adherence is voluminous, sometimes inconclusive, and often controversial. Nevertheless, medical clinicians have been aware of the need for patient adherence for centuries. Haynes (1979) wryly noted that the "first recorded instance of noncompliance took place in the Garden of Eden" (p. 3). An ancient

Greek treatise on physician decorum, attributed to Hippocrates, gives the following advice: "Keep watch also on the faults of patients which makes them lie about the taking of things prescribed" (Jones, 1923, p. 297).

Goals of Medication Adherence for People Living with HIV Disease or Advanced AIDS

Health-care providers often tell their HIV-infected patients that there are at least five good reasons why excellent adherence to their treatment regimen is important. The goals of medication adherence are to decrease viral load, prevent opportunistic infections, enhance the immune system, improve quality of life, and maximize longevity. Professionals who prescribe HIV medications and counsel HIV/AIDS patients about making healthy lifestyle choices realize the importance of education, coaching, and monitoring. Patients must understand the life cycle of HIV and the potential side effects and drug resistance issues that are associated with highly active antiretroviral therapy (HAART). HAART consists of approximately thirty medications for which there is FDA approval. The thirty HAART medications (as of 2012) fall into several drug classifications: nucleotide reverse transcriptase inhibitors (NRTI), nonnucleoside reverse transcriptase inhibitors (NNRTI), protease inhibitors, fusion inhibitors, and entry inhibitors.

Adherence and HIV Outcomes

The human factor is as crucial as the pharmacologic factor in determining therapeutic outcomes. The most potent treatments are useless in the face of poor adherence. In the field of HIV/AIDS, high levels of adherence to ARV therapy have been shown to have significant effects on viral load, immune reconstitution, and mortality. Suboptimal adherence can lead to ARV resistance because of ongoing viral replication in the presence of the selective environmental pressure of ARV medications. So how much adherence is enough?

Health-care providers would like to see their patients achieve perfect adherence to their prescribed medications and lifestyle recommendations, regarding diet and exercise. People living with HIV and people living with AIDS on the other hand, find strict adherence to be challenging, yet most try their best to adhere to their HAART regimen. Realistically, however, people do forget doses or take "drug holidays." When people miss doses of HIV medications, viral replication and drug resistance may occur, and HIV may be more readily spread throughout the community.

Genotype and phenotype tests both provide baseline data and help clinicians and patients better understand how HIV is currently acting in the body. A genotypic analysis indicates a given HIV's genetic resistance to a given drug, and a phenotypic analysis is a virus-culture drug assay. Phenotypic results are easier to interpret than genotypic results because they do not require the expert interpretation of complex mutation patterns. Phenotype testing is very expensive—approximately $1,000 per test. So oftentimes, patients rely on the cheaper and faster (one-week) genotypic testing that costs about $500. Furthermore, most third-party payers do not cover these tests. Specifically, the genotype is the sequences of nucleotide bases that constitute a gene, whereas the phenotype refers to a defined behavior, especially drug susceptibility related to HIV drug resistance. The more advanced phenosense genotype test is also a helpful tool in a clinician's armamentarium.

Health-care providers have endeavored to manage the challenge of patient adherence for centuries. The medical literature reveals how difficult it is for patients to stick to even the simplest treatment regimens. Factors associated with poor compliance include perceived need of medication, unstable housing, mental illness, and major life crises. Also creating adherence problems are pill burden, pill size, frequency and timing of dose, dietary or water requirements or restrictions, liquid formulations, unpleasant drug taste, adverse events, storage requirements, number of prescriptions, and other factors such as the number of co-payments, refills, and medication bottles (Stine, 2010, p. 97).

Adherence to a drug regimen means taking all the prescribed anti-HIV drugs at the scheduled times and not missing any doses. Whenever people are asked to alter or maintain new behaviors to treat an existing condition or to prevent a threatened one, there is a possibility that they will not comply consistently and correctly with the prescribed activities.

An interesting exercise to highlight the challenges of adherence with HAART might involve the following class adherence experiment. Virologist and textbook author Gerald Stine (2012, p. 95) conceptualized this assignment, and used it with his students at the University of North Florida. Teachers and students should try this so all can better relate to what it must be like for HIV-infected people who must be compliant with their powerfully potent medications.

> **Box 13.1. Class Adherence Experiment**
>
> For the next four days, you will need to take four different-colored M & M candies at three specified times per day between 6:00 a.m. and 12:00 midnight. Keep your M & M candies in a safe place and record your compliance on a dosing schedule sheet.
>
> (One week later, in class) Let's look at our dosing schedule sheets and discuss how compliant we were. Did anyone comply at the 100 percent level? 90 percent level? 80 percent level? 70 percent level? 0 percent level? Do you think the results would be much different for other students? For HIV-infected people?

Theories, Measures, and Models to Understand Adherence

Why do patients miss doses? Do they miss doses because they forgot, they are depressed, they ran out, they are away from home, or because there is a change in their daily routine? Are there other reasons? Most literature reports that adherence rates decline over time. The "pill fatigue" phenomenon is prominent even in the most adherent patients. A clinical research drug trial, known as SMART found evidence that drug holidays are a bad idea for HIV-infected people who are prescribed a complex regimen (Stine, 2009).

What is a complex regimen? Generally, dosing more than two times a day, a large number of pills that require swallowing, food and fluid restrictions, or special medication storage requirements like refrigeration constitute a complex regimen. Fortunately, a wide range of HIV-infected people living in 2012 may have a regimen that requires only three or four pills once a day, or in some cases just one pill a day. Ideally, health-care providers would like to see their patients continue for many years on the first regimen that they prescribe. This is because every regimen after the first one is typically not simple.

Vignettes later in this chapter illustrate the variability and the formidable challenge that both one-pill prescriptions and complex medication regimens have for newly diagnosed HIV-infected patients and those who have been living with HIV/AIDS for some time. Patients' ability to maintain excellent medication adherence is often challenged when they start on a once-a-day formulation, but because of noncompliance need to move to a more complex regimen.

Clinical trial researchers, community-based research physicians, nurses, and other health-care providers have learned lessons from other chronic illnesses as to why some people comply with their physician's advice and others do not. Researchers have learned that a simple regimen will likely increase adherence behavior and rates. For example, data have shown that 90 percent of people can comply with a simple one-time-a-day treatment regimen. For optimal virologic suppression, clinicians advise that patients with HIV be 95 percent adherent. This means that they cannot miss a dose more than once a month.

Unreliable predictors of adherence have consistently included age, education level, socioeconomic status, sex, race, gender, and previous substance use. To date, no clinical trials specifically related to substance abuse, adherence, and HIV have been done in the United States. Of interest, the drug Sustiva (Efavirenz) typically causes 50 percent of people who take it to have side effects that include very vivid dreams. Patients' dreams may be erotic or give the sensation that they are being pursued. Therefore, health-care providers must counsel and talk patients through potential side effects. Savvy and experienced health-care providers state that they never start their patients on new medications unless the timeframe is such that the patient may contact the provider if problems ensue. Predictors of adherence can involve positive or negative factors.

Negative predictors of adherence include

- Unstable housing

- Mental illness

- Major life crises (e.g., new HIV diagnosis, marriage)

- Active substance use (especially crack cocaine)

- Significant side effects

Positive predictors of adherence include

- Client's belief in ARV regimen

- Experienced medical provider

- Existence of social support

- Clients that are adherent with office visits

- Clients that are employed

Other associated factors are

- Perceived need of medication

- Pill burden and pill size

- Frequency and timing of dose

- Dietary or water requirements or restrictions

- Liquid formulations

- Unpleasant drug taste

- Adverse events

- Storage requirements

- Number of prescriptions

- Number of copayments, refills, and medication bottles

These realities are illustrated by imagining the practice of a community nurse practitioner. She has shared with staff that she wants to see newer or sicker patients once a month. Patients need to come in to see her, to see a case-manager or mental health therapist, or to obtain bus tickets so that they can become disciplined, habituate, and keep their appointments. She has found that this consistency of contact promotes adherence, thereby measurably reducing the development of drug resistance. She knows skipping only a few pills can trigger the emergence of drug-resistant strains of HIV, which could be worse than the initial infection. Then, the situation might be overwhelming to the person taking ARV and anyone else to whom he or she has transmitted the virus.

Social workers in some infectious disease clinic settings are also using innovative strategies to increase adherence with appointments and medications. The utility of social workers' involvement in nonbillable intake interviews is under study.

Measures of adherence vary. Patient self-reports, provider estimation, pill counts, smart pill bottles (called MEMS caps, or medication event monitoring systems, used in some clinical trials), pharmacy records, and directly observed therapy (such as in methadone maintenance clinics) are examples of measures. Adherence measures are linked to the dosing frequency and pill quantity of the prescribed HIV medications, as well as the monetary and economic resources at the patient's disposal. Some physicians have been willing to confidentially bill patients so they can pay out of pocket rather than submitting insurance paperwork to their current employers and insurance companies. Medicaid typically gives patients a thirty-day supply of drugs at a time, but private insurers may approve drug prescriptions for as much as sixty days.

Adherence behaviors are also indirectly linked to death rates. An important and significant statistic was reported in the 1997 National Vital Statistics Report with regard to death rates. This report documented for the first time that deaths related to HIV disease dropped from 11.1 deaths per 100,000 in 1996 to 5.9 deaths per 100,000 in 1997. In addition, this statistic also showed a significant decrease in the presence of opportunistic infections for people with HIV. Such statistical data elucidate the role of HIV medications in reducing opportunistic infections and, consequently, in reducing the number of deaths associated with HIV disease or advanced AIDS.

Financial Realities of Medication Adherence

The Gay Men's Health Crisis, a nonprofit group in New York City, states that the per patient cost of drugs to fight HIV/AIDS, excluding a protease inhibitor, amounts to about $19,000 a year. This amount does not include physician visits or routine blood tests. A *New York Times* article estimated that drugs for someone with symptomatic AIDS cost about $70,000 a year. Others have reported yearly costs that range from $84,000 to $150,000 if they are using protease inhibitors. With such exorbitant costs, people with HIV may sometimes forgo rent payments or food purchases in order to afford medicine. Some have even turned to the desperate practice of cashing in life insurance policies or to viatical settlements, where a portion of another person's policy is bought or sold.

Existing Resources, Interventions, and Strategies to Enhance Adherence

Because HAART is so expensive, patients require resources to access their medications and support their lifestyle and well-being. Existing resources such as AIDS Drug Assistance Programs (ADAP) represent a vital mechanism for HIV-infected patients to obtain HAART. In some northern states like New Jersey, a single person can qualify for ADAP medications on the state formulary if they earn less than $57,000 a year. ADAP also covers hepatitis C and diabetes drugs through the federal Ryan White CARE Act. By contrast, some southern states such as North Carolina often have long waiting lists: residents of these states who are living with HIV may have serious problems readily accessing HIV medications. Social workers and health-care providers must know about the resource that is the Ryan White CARE Act, initially passed and funded in 1990 with its multiple parts (formerly called titles). This Act routinely undergoes Congressional reauthorization and covers care, treatment services, testing, and prevention services in large metropolitan areas where the HIV epidemic is most severe. Since HIV is a name-reportable disease, it behooves states to have an accurate reporting of cases through county health departments for funding purposes. If people living with HIV or AIDS have insurance or access to Ryan White funding, they can access HAART. Therefore, sustained dependence on HAART requires strict adherence strategies for patients and health-care providers alike.

Health-care providers, whether primary care physicians, clinical trial physician investigators or research nurses, or experienced health social workers, should inform HIV-infected patients about the importance of avoiding drug reactions, and the advantages of joining clinical drug trials in an adherent manner. To facilitate adherence health-care providers, in collaboration with their patients, need to:

- Inform client and anticipate side effects

- Simplify food requirements

- Avoid adverse drug reactions

- Reduce dose frequency and overall number of pills

- Make prescription refills accessible

To maximize adherence, social workers of patients or clients with HIV, in collaboration with their physician, need to be responsible for following strategies, such as:

- Establish client readiness to take prescriptions before first prescription is written

- Treat substance abuse and depression before starting medications

- Negotiate treatment plans that the patient understands and commits to

- Take time and multiple encounters to educate and explain therapy goals and need for adherence

- Recruit family and friends to support the treatment plan (e.g., buddies, med coaches)

- Develop concrete plans for specific regimen; relate those plans to meals, daily schedules, and side effects

- Provide written schedules and pictures of medications, daily or weekly pillboxes, and alarm clocks

- Develop adherence support groups, or add adherence issues to regular agenda of support groups

- Consider pill trials

Adherence strategies that are essentially the responsibility of the health-care providers are:

- Establish trust

- Educate, inform, support, and monitor on an ongoing basis

- Provide access between visits for questions and problems

- Listen to patient(s)

- Monitor adherence

- Use positive reinforcement: share CD4 cell counts and viral load

- Use entire health-care team, including the front desk staff

- Consider impact of new diagnosis on adherence, depression, liver disease, wasting, and chemical dependency

Health-care-team-related strategies include the following:

- Provide training

- Discern why patient is not adhering to medications: Did patient forget? Is he or she drug intolerant? Are there too many pills?

Health Social Work Practice Involving AIDS and Adherence

The context of how medical care is delivered in the United States has implications for how social workers need to interface with people with HIV. Clients need support for HIV medication adherence, appointment keeping, and lifestyle adjustments. Social workers are often required to advocate for people living with HIV and people living with AIDS so that stigma is decreased and education and access to resources, including medications, is increased. In the United States, HIV disease has disproportionately affected socially oppressed groups such as gay men, people of color, and intravenous drug users. In many ways, in the field of health care, the constantly changing challenge of HIV/AIDS has affected the shape of social work practice with these groups. For example, social work practitioners do prevention work with people at risk for HIV infection, and they work with people infected with HIV at all stages of the illness, including diagnosis, asymptomatic status, symptomatic status, advanced AIDS, and death (Linsk & Marder, 1992). Social workers affiliated with AIDS clinical trials often work with HIV-infected clients in assessing social support needs, participating in intake processes, helping to obtain medication, and encouraging subsequent adherence.

Historically, medical social work practice was based in the community and primarily addressed public health concerns like syphilis, tuberculosis, and polio. As hospitals became strategic centers of medical practice, the micro and macro system roles of medical social workers evolved. Physicians hired social workers as community liaisons and medication compliance educators to augment physicians' work. With the advent of HIV disease, social workers were employed in both in-patient and out-patient settings, and had to stay abreast of issues related to economic concerns, demographic trends, family issues, rapidly changing medication therapies, and adherence (Lynch, Lloyd, & Fimbres, 1993; Mancoske, 1996).

Patient compliance is increasingly much researched. By 1984, only 154 articles, letters, and editorials were listed under the title heading for patient compliance in *Index Medicus*, the publication physicians frequently consult during literature searches. Throughout the 1990s, articles on adherence tripled those published up to 1984 (Lloyd, 1996). Therefore, little research on the personal and environmental variables that affected treatment adherence or adaptive coping strategies for HIV-infected people existed before the late 1990s. The public does not realize that the first rigorous research concerning adherence levels appeared in 1943. From 1943 to 1953, effective new medications appeared in the form of broad spectrum antibiotics, anti-tuberculosis drugs, such as streptomycin and isoniazid, and the phenothiazine tranquilizers for treatment of schizophrenia. Before the 1940s, medical practitioners typically regarded noncompliance as a moral issue, thereby shifting the onus of responsibility onto the patient. This cohort of health-care providers saw no indication that noncompliance might be an intriguing pattern of behavior that deserved wider exploration (Cox, 1997).

Throughout the 1970s and 1980s, many adherence study results appeared in the *Journal of Compliance in Health Care.* A literature search on the topic of medication compliance today yields seventy to one hundred new articles each month, thus illustrating the emphasis medical practitioners currently place on adherence. However, social work researchers were slow to conduct and publish empirical research on adherence, especially in the field of HIV/AIDS.

In the twenty-first century, both medical and social work practitioners have conducted and published research on adherence with HAART and adherence behavior research continues to be presented at International AIDS conference venues that now occur every other year. Typically, literature has measured adherence behaviors by looking at assessment of biological effects, monitoring of attendance at appointments, clinical judgments, measures of drug levels, patient reactivity, patient self-reports, and pill counts.

Linkage of Social Support to Adherence

Empirical studies also have linked features of social support to adherence. For example, a 1996 longitudinal observational study of forty-six HIV-infected men evaluated the prevalence of and variables associated with ARV therapy adherence (Singh, Squier, Sivek, & Wagener, 1996). The findings revealed that depression, psychological stress, mood disturbance, and poor stress management were predictive of poor medication adherence.

Morse and colleagues (1991) studied adherence and social support in an experimental anti-HIV drug protocol that sampled forty asymptomatic HIV seropositive persons who consented to participate in a double-blind, placebo-controlled trial of the effectiveness of AZT. Study participants were surveyed at six-month intervals using a self-report instrument and nurse ratings. Morse and colleagues (1991) learned that more adherent subjects or study participants reported that they found it easier to talk to their assigned study nurse and saw the study nurse as supportive, informative, and caring. This study concluded participants identified as "more compliant are better able to elicit and receive support from both personal and clinical relationships" (p. 1163).

Cox (1997, 2002, 2009) studied the relative influence of social support on compliance and reported on data from a compliance study embedded into both prevention and treatment HIV study protocols. She found that in the 179 HIV-infected study participants, emotional support and being employed emerged as important discriminant variables.

An entire published volume of *The Journal of HIV and Social Services* was devoted to HIV adherence issues (2007, volume 6). Additional figures extracted from conference handouts over the past decade visualize the importance of adherence issues with regard to HIV/AIDS. For example, table 13.1 shows a selection of determinants of successful adherence.

Table 13.1. Determinants of Successful Adherence

Access/Resources	Social Support	Adherence Technique
Consistent access to medication and other treatment services	Personal support	Provider/capability building
Access to support services	Support for caregivers	Engaging client
Access to mental health and substance abuse treatment	Relationship with health-care provider	Maintaining the relationship
Stable economic resources, including housing	Social care: Case management, psychotherapy	Ensuring client understands implications of adherence
	Support groups	Empowering client role in selecting therapies
	Clients' cultural and health beliefs and practices	

Source: Linsk & Bonik (2000).

Figure 13.1 reveals how social workers and peer counselors can effectively assist HIV-infected clients be more adherent.

Figure 13.1. Adherence Interventions

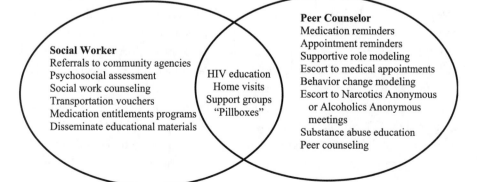

Table 13.2 illustrates the multiple challenges to medication adherence, across disease factors, treatment regimen, and individual and family context.

Table 13.2. Challenges to Medication Adherence

Disease Factors	Treatment Regimen	Individual and Family Context
Chronicity of illness	Frequency of dosing	Client cultural and health beliefs
Presence of symptoms	Convenience or inconvenience	Client–provider relationship
Changes in symptoms	Complexity or difficulty	Mental health or substance abuse history
	Number of medications prescribed	Life stressors
	Side effects	
	Perceived efficacy of drugs	

The ADHERE model is part of the trainer curriculum developed by and available through the Spectrum: Mental Health Training and Education of Social Workers Project (Tomaszewski, 2005):

Assess client knowledge and readiness

Dialogue about health beliefs

Holistic approach including environment and culture

Empower client to implement action plan

Reinforce strategies and revise as needed

Evaluate progress and resources

Evidence-Based Social Work Practice

Personal Challenges for Social Workers and Their HIV-Infected Clients. The role of the HIV/AIDS social worker who works in health settings, such as a clinical trial consortium, AIDS Service Organization (ASO), or an infectious disease (sometimes referred to as ID) clinic in a hospital or private practice is rather specialized. Infectious disease clinic social workers conduct intake assessments, advocate for clients who must have prescriptions filled, and negotiate complicated paperwork associated with insurance and drug companies and entitlement program systems. Clients present across the entire spectrum of HIV disease. Social workers counsel the newly diagnosed, those who are asymptomatic, and those who suffer with symptoms in the form of cancers, opportunistic infections, dementia, or accompanying mental health diagnoses. Clients are mothers, fathers, children, and grandparents. Client demographics cut across all races, ethnicities, and religious beliefs. These clients have contracted HIV through blood, breast milk, or bodily fluids. These clients may be wealthy, employed, homeless, or poor. Real-life stories about how people with HIV disease manage adherence issues may best be appreciated by reading and thinking about case vignettes of people living with HIV and AIDS. Such vignettes are presented later in this chapter.

Cultural Diversity Issues

Giddens, Ka'opua, Kaplan, and Linsk (2009), in conjunction with a RAND Corporation and Oregon State University survey, developed education and training materials related to cultural competence. Using some of their conclusions, the HIV/AIDS Spectrum Project at the National Association of Social Workers (NASW) in Washington, DC, has suggested that in order to be culturally competent social workers should discuss the following with HIV-infected clients:

- Primary cultural beliefs and values

  - Individualism versus collectivism

  - Concept of time

- Their view or conceptualization of disease

  - Their cultural beliefs about the cause and treatment of disease

- A historical context of culture and health care (that may lead to mistrust)

  - For example: Tuskegee syphilis study or refusal of blood banks to accept blood from MSM (men who have sex with men)

  - Belief (e.g., conspiracy theory) that U.S. government created AIDS to eradicate or control African Americans

According to Poindexter (2010, p. 56), in her *Handbook of HIV and Social Work*, "cultural competence—values, awareness, knowledge, and skills—is complex, difficult to contextualize, and even more difficult to realize in practice." No one person holds the definitive knowledge of facts about a particular cultural group, or can fully understand the effect of cultural beliefs, values, and experiences on others. Stigma, shame, oppression, social injustice, and resource inequity are closely related to the experiences of many people living with HIV disease and have altered their life course and viewpoints. The Health Resources and Services Administration (HRSA, a division of the U.S. Department of Health and Human Services, or DHHS) and the National Center for Cultural Competence offer a conceptual model of cultural competence in HIV (Poindexter, 2010, p. 47). The main concepts of this model suggest that practitioners will need to help people living with HIV disease across four interlocking systems: the (1) individual, (2) family, (3) organization(s), and (4) society and community.

HRSA's (2001) framework offers nine domains to consider in assessing cultural competence: (1) values and attitudes, (2) cultural sensitivity, (3) communication, (4) policies and procedures, (5) training and staff development, (6) facility characteristics, (7) intervention and treatment model features, (8) family and community participation, and (9) monitoring, evaluation, and research. HIV medication adherence as it relates to clear communication between client and worker during social work interventions warrants special consideration.

Cultural sensitivity with respect to stigma across cultures requires special attention. Stigma, defined as a "token of disgrace, dishonor, or infamy," is a powerful deterrent of individual freedom and self-determination. According to Poindexter (2010, p. 49), "Stigma is experienced as fear, anxiety, shame, disenfranchisement, hostility, ostracism, and a threat to survival, and it is influenced by sociocultural experiences and norms that influence disclosure, self-protection, coping behaviors, and acceptance. Stigma is perceived or experienced not only because of a person's HIV status, but is further complicated by related issues of accepting one's own self (sexuality, membership in an oppressed group, level of acculturation), feeling guilty about a specific lifestyle (drugs, sex work), and the need to conform for safety and support."

Case Examples

Vignette #1 (Jim): HIV Positive, Insured, Employed, Yet Financially Challenged to Adhere

One of the biggest struggles HIV/AIDS social workers experience is helping insured clients manage hefty, cumulative copays. For example, a social worker employed at an infectious disease clinic in Virginia shared how she and two additional social workers spent a lot of their time working with Jim, an employed HIV-infected male client who had ample insurance. However, although Jim had a co-insurance for his high-priced HIV medications, due to his other bills he could not afford his medications on a regular basis.

Unfortunately, Jim's income made him ineligible for Ryan White funds or any other financial resources to assist with ongoing co-pays. In response to this insured patient's quandary, multiple social workers spent much time and extra effort making copious phone calls on his behalf. As a result, the social workers discovered that Jim could access a drug savings card through his insurance company. It was a little-known resource that any employee at his workplace was eligible to use. Also, the infectious disease clinic social workers were able to get the sum of his co-insurance fees reduced considerably, so Jim could now afford it. Jim's copay costs eventually dropped from several thousand dollars to $600 to $700 a month, and eventually to less than $200 a month. So, while the couple hundred dollars a month was still a burden for him with his other expenses, with his income Jim was eventually able to afford his monthly prescribed HIV medications, enabling him to be as adherent and healthy as possible.

Side Story. While the social workers made phone calls to research available options, assess the resources, and broker and advocate for the client, Jim's physician's assistant, another health-care team member, changed Jim's medications to a regimen he thought would be less expensive for the client. Actually, this new prescribed regimen was not cheaper. Serendipitously, this new medication turned out to be a drug that Jim could better tolerate. The lesson learned is that finances can still greatly affect an HIV-infected person's level of adherence, even if he has medical insurance coverage.

Questions for Reflection

1. How would you assess Jim's initial perceptions of his health status, efficacy of treatment, and ability to adhere? How about his current perceptions?

2. How might you work with Jim regarding his financial resources?

3. How could you help Jim develop an action plan to prepare for the unexpected?

Assessment:

Skills:

Resources:

Vignette #2 (Dorothy): New HIV-Positive Diagnosis and Readiness to Adhere

Dorothy is a forty-year-old Caucasian woman, newly diagnosed with HIV disease, who was recently admitted to the hospital. Before being hospitalized for community-acquired pneumonia, Dorothy had been very healthy. She was mentally eager to obtain medical care at the infectious disease clinic, but had difficulty in physically crossing the threshold of the clinic door. Eventually, Dorothy kept her two initial clinic appointments and the social workers coached her with encouragement and provided extensive answers to her many questions about HIV. Consequently, Dorothy has remained very compliant keeping appointments and she continues to educate herself about HIV/AIDS. Fortunately, she has insurance, remains employed, and she is doing remarkably well in adhering to her HIV regimen.

Side Story. Dorothy, an example of a recently diagnosed, White, non-drug-using heterosexual client, presented with above-average fear and a lot of shame about being told she has a stigmatizing HIV disease. With proper education and time, she became a relatively low-maintenance and compliant patient after her initial drug regimen was established. The lesson learned is that clients have to be ready to comply not only with prescribed medicines, but also with medical appointments and concomitant lifestyle changes.

Questions for Reflection

1. How would you assess Dorothy's understanding of drug therapy?

2. How would you be client centered with Dorothy in order to help reduce anxiety?

3. How might you help her appreciate the need for excellent medication adherence and appointment keeping?

4. Taking into consideration the high level of stigma Dorothy is experiencing, what does she need to consider with regard to privacy issues?

Assessment:

Skills:

Resources:

Vignette #3 (Frances): New HIV-Positive Diagnosis

Frances is a highly educated forty-year-old heterosexual Caucasian (White) woman who was recently diagnosed with HIV infection. She currently works as a bookkeeper in an accounting firm. She was formerly married and has a grown daughter and a grandchild. Her family is what appears to keep her motivated. Frances believes she contracted HIV from her former boyfriend. Currently, her CD4 cell count hovers around 756. Her viral load was at 6,000 the last time she was examined. These results mean that Frances is doing well and is not currently a candidate for HIV-related medications.

Upon initial assessment, the clinic health-care team learned that Frances had a history of depression. Prior to her diagnosis with HIV, her primary care physician had prescribed her some antidepressants. Fortunately, Frances has been regularly seeing a therapist for counseling and she is doing very well with antidepressants. Frances stays up to date on her immunizations, gets an annual flu shot, and complies with well woman exams, such as mammograms and Pap smears.

Side Story. As an educated White woman, Frances is an outlier in some general HIV/AIDS clinic populations, where much larger numbers of gay men and African-American men, who are either homosexual or bisexual (down low), receive care. Frances' story is also a good example of how a stably employed client who believes in her ARV regimen, has an experienced HIV care provider, and strong social supports will likely be adherent. Frances was compliant not only with taking her meds, but also with keeping up with mental health care, attending infectious disease clinic visits, and getting her prescriptions refilled promptly. The lesson learned is that patients like Frances, when presented with consistently encouraging clinical lab results, will generally tend to be adherent with monthly appointments and health-care recommendations.

Questions for Reflection

1. Will your biopsychosocial assessment address culturally based beliefs? How so? If not, why?

2. How might you help Frances create goals that involve her, her health-care provider(s), her family, and her friends?

3. How could you help Frances identify cues or reminders to help her be adherent? (e.g., trigger the memory with meals, television programs, exercise, etc.)?

Assessment:

Skills:

Resources:

Vignette #4 (Christopher): Long-time HIV-Positive Black Gay Man Who Takes Drug Holidays

Christopher is a fifty-seven-year-old Black gay man who has never married and has been coming to the infectious disease clinic for a long time. Soon after his diagnosis, a male social worker named Mel worked with him with respect to adherence issues, when he first was put on medications. Christopher worked with Mel to address many complex issues. At first, he struggled with medication adherence, but he finally did become compliant and did well. Christopher was one of those clients who believed that his CD4 count was high enough where he could take breaks from his daily pills. He also was part of a clinical drug trial study after he was initially diagnosed. This particular clinical study allowed him to come off HIV medications once his CD4 cell count exceeded a certain point, approximately 800 cells per cubic millimeter of blood. He's now been off medications for about five years. The infectious disease clinic has followed Chris for nearly twelve years. Now he is back on meds, however, because he became sick. Christopher's CD4 count is low, and his viral load has been increasing. He is still working and therefore has medical insurance coverage.

Even though Christopher had been through the medication scenario before taking a drug holiday, he seems to be dragging his feet about starting his medication regimen again. For example, he has not called his insurance company to learn what his medication copays will be. He does not yet know if he can afford the medications the physician has selected for him. Therefore, he does not know if he needs help with securing financial assistance for his copays.

It has taken Chris several months to finally take his financial information to the infectious disease clinic social workers. He repeatedly verbalizes some reluctance to get back on meds. The social worker who sees Christopher doesn't think he wants to face what the news that his HIV disease is progressing means for him. There is an underlying understanding that he has to take medications, otherwise "his numbers will keep dropping" and he will potentially become quite ill.

The clinic staff responded to his reticence by connecting Christopher with an advocate, or adherence coach. The social workers are concerned that Chris will now suffer medication side effects because he has been on a drug holiday for so long. Additionally, restarting a medical protocol is a painful reminder to Christopher that he is HIV positive, even though he tried to forget.

Side Story. Christopher's situation brings up many of his old feelings and fears again, as well as mental health and coping issues. Chris knows he is HIV positive but as long as he was not taking pills, he did not have a constant reminder that he had a dangerous virus lying latent inside him.

In the past decade or two, much has changed on the HIV/AIDS medication front. In the late 1980s, infectious disease health-care providers only had one drug to prescribe: AZT. The next ARV to be used was DDI (didanosine, brand name Videx) followed by combination therapy (AIDS cocktail), and now HAART and many new drug classifications. The lesson learned in Chris' scenario is that there are many factors that determine when people are started on HIV medication regimens, and on which medications they start. Routinely having one's CD4 count, viral load, and genotype tested is a lot for an HIV-infected patient to think about.

Questions for Reflection

1. How would you outline possible consequences of non-adherence with Christopher?

2. How could you help Christopher see that he, and no one else, is in charge of his medication adherence? How could you use a contract?

3. How helpful might it be to ask Christopher specific questions about adherence and non-adherence? (e.g., "How many doses did you miss in the past day, two days, or week?")

Assessment:

Skills:

Resources:

Vignette #5 (Mehari and Senayit): Married Couple from Ethiopia

A married couple from Ethiopia, a country in northeastern Africa, has sought services from a social worker in an HIV/AIDS clinic. Their case raises the need for practicing with cultural sensitivity and willingness to adapt interventions based on specific needs of the case. Mehari and Senayit are both HIV-positive. They started on a drug regimen when they were in their home country of Ethiopia, prior to coming to the United States as refugees. After they escaped from duress in Africa, they initiated contact with an infectious disease physician in the United States so they could keep up their drug regimen. The physician who worked with them thought they had been put on a very interesting and peculiar regimen. He decided to change the regimen. Senayit was of childbearing age and expressed to the physician that she wanted to have children. Her new regimen would need to include only medications that would not be harmful to a developing pregnancy. Keeping this in mind, and also in an effort to help the couple stay as compliant as possible, the physician constructed a regimen that they both could be on. Because they would both take the same drugs at the same time, they could support each other and provide extra accountability.

Side Story. There are many factors to consider if a woman with HIV wants to get pregnant. Many couples who are both positive (sero-concordant), or couples where one is positive and one is negative (sero-discordant), successfully give birth to HIV-negative babies. This possibility is not reached without effort, including planning, counseling, and special drug regimens. In some instances where finances are available, sperm washing is practiced if the man is HIV-positive. The lesson learned in working with this Ethiopian couple is that, despite one's country of origin, patients' values must be considered and communication must occur about the desire for building a family, despite being diagnosed with the now chronic condition of HIV disease. In 2010, transmission rates from mother to child were greatly reduced through prescription of nevirapine. Currently in the United States, a very small percentage of babies acquire HIV during birth or become HIV-positive through breast feeding by an HIV-positive mother (or other woman, like a wet nurse). While medical professionals in the United States encourage that babies born to HIV-positive mothers be exclusively formula fed, social workers should be aware that due to cultural factors or cost, mothers may insist on short- or long-term breast-feeding, or combination feeding.

Questions for Reflection

1. How can you incorporate ideas from Giddens and colleagues (2009) cultural competency research to assess how this couple is coping with the medication regimen?

2. How can you let the couple know you are there to support them, not judge them? How can you implement the ADHERE model (p. 368)?

3. How can you actively create an environment that encourages the development of cooperative strategies and skill building?

Assessment:

Skills:

Resources:

Vignette# 6 (Joyce): Pregnant Woman Does Not Know Her HIV-Positive Status

Joyce was first seen by health professionals at a point very late in her pregnancy. It was not until this point that she learned she was HIV-positive. She went into labor before she could be started on a medication protocol that included nevirapine. When the baby was born, he was put on triple-drug therapy. This is not typical, but in this case, there was a higher-than-usual risk of transmission. During the delivery, there was a lot of blood present, due to torn membranes. Usually, HIV-positive pregnant women who seek medical help for their pregnancies are put on meds early, to keep their viral load suppressed. Many of the women who comply with their treatment manage to keep their viral loads suppressed so that they can have vaginal deliveries of HIV-negative babies. When born, the newborns are also given medication for a period. Testing is required to make sure they remain HIV negative.

The aforementioned patients captured in each of the vignettes illustrate an array of adherence issues and treatment strategies that depend on both the clients' stage of HIV infection and their available health insurance benefits and insurance realities. Multiple patient, provider, and contextual factors dictate the type of medications that health-care providers such as physicians prescribe to patients with HIV and how adherent their patients are upon consistent face-to-face or phone monitoring by advocates, research study nurses, or social work case managers. Physicians prescribe medicines, yet a supportive team of health-care providers, such as nurses, social workers, and AIDS service organization advocates/buddies/coaches, provide ongoing adherence monitoring.

Assessment:

Skills:

Resources:

Typical Prescriptions Today

As of 2012, physicians can choose from multiple classifications of drugs. For example, Atripla is dosed as one pill, once a day. When the patient disrupts this simple regimen and misses doses, he or she becomes drug resistant. Atripla is usually only given to populations that have proven to be responsible in other aspects of their life. There is an expectation that patients with a track record of continual work or a high level of education will be more adherent. It would not be suitable for a homeless patient to be on this medication, since the likelihood of adherence is low. Unfortunately, a homeless patient would be best prescribed a regimen that is less simple than one pill a day. In addition to Atripla, another frequently prescribed HIV medication is called Truvada, which is also a combination therapy drug. Once-a-day combinations create regimens that patients can easily remember; the future development of HIV/AIDS clinical trials definitely consider this reality.

Future of HIV and Adherence

To truly appreciate the intricacies of medication adherence, one must understand some basic immunology and virology as it applies to the life cycle of the HIV. A retrovirus includes a single strand of RNA that is inserted into a host cell in order to replicate. From a biological standpoint, HIV is classified as a retrovirus. It is one of only three retroviruses that are known to infect humans. Human hosts are required for HIV to replicate, and HIV does so quite differently from other viruses. HIV effectively hijacks people's immune systems in order to replicate itself.

Sero-conversion is the term used to indicate the development of antibodies in the blood serum as a result of an infection (or immunization). With respect to HIV, sero-conversion is the term used to describe when the person became HIV positive. If a person of average health is infected with HIV and does not take any ARV medications, he or she can likely live another seven to eleven years after HIV sero-conversion. Clinical manifestations of HIV-related symptoms and illnesses (opportunistic infections, cancers) will continue to emerge and require blood work and monitoring through diagnostic markers such as viral load and CD4 cell counts. Protocols governing when a person should start HIV medications are often amended over time and will likely continue to be an area for debate. The adage, "Hit early, hit hard," has been challenged and health-care providers must, in concert with their HIV-positive patients, make careful decisions. The regimen of drugs constructed for each patient is dependent on whether they are asymptomatic, are HIV symptomatic, have advanced AIDS, and have other health-related factors.

There are more than thirty FDA-approved HIV ARV medications, classified as nukes (NRTIs), nonnukes (NNRTIs), or protease inhibitors. Researchers continue to study other classes of medication, such as the previously mentioned entry inhibitors, integrase inhibitors, and maturation inhibitors. No matter the drug classification, side effects are inevitable. Physicians should seriously consider prescribing them because they have been shown to have a high impact on a person's level of adherence. While most people can adapt to short-term side effects, highly adverse events or long-term side effects require serious scrutiny.

Advancements in drug formulations have minimized the number of pills people must take, yet poor medication adherence continues to be a widespread problem. Health-care providers and social workers still need to study and observe multiple biopsychosocial factors that predict medication adherence, such as "socioeconomic status, race, gender, psychiatric conditions and cognitive functioning, family and social support networks, attitudes toward treatment, physician-patient relationships and rapport, and the complexity of treatment regimens" (Poindexter, 2010, p. 20).

Social workers can best help their HIV-infected clients be adherent to medications by being informed, supportive, and real. Clients must realize that they need to take their drugs on time, every time. Missing just a few pills can trigger drug-resistant strains of HIV to emerge, which could create a condition worse than the initial infection. And last, but not least, social workers need to stay current with community resources across federal, state, and local levels.

Web Resources

For Social Work Professionals

NASW: www.socialworkers.org

NASW HIV/AIDS Spectrum Project: http://www.socialworkers.org/practice/
hiv_aids/default.asp

For HIV/AIDS Treatment Information

AMFAR: The American Foundation for AIDS Research: 1-800-39AMFAR
(392-6237)

AIDS Treatment Data Network: 1-800-734-7104

AIDS Treatment News: 1-800-TREAT 1-2 (873-2812)

National HIV Treatment: 1-800-822-7422

For information about HIV/AIDS clinical trials conducted by NIH and the Food
and Drug Administration (FDA)–approved efficacy trials, call National AIDS
Clinical Trials Information Service (ACTIS): 1-800-TRIALS-A (874-2572).

For information about National HIV/AIDS resources, call AIDS Action Council
(1-202-547-3101).

Gay Men's Health Crisis (1-212-807-6655)

Mothers of AIDS Patients (1-619-234-3432)

National AIDS Information Clearinghouse (1-301-762-5111)

National AIDS Network (1-202-546-2424)

Project Inform (Alternative AIDS info) (1-800-822-7422)

Public Health Service Hotline (1-800-342-2437)

Centers for Disease Control and Prevention (1-404-639-2070)

American Red Cross (1-202-639-3223)

Guide to Social Security and Supplemental Security Income (SSI) Disability
(1-800-772-1213)

References

Cox, L. E. (1997). Dissertation: *The relative influence of social support on the medication compliance of people with HIV infection.* Richmond, VA: Virginia Commonwealth University (Copyrighted).

Cox, L. E. (2002). Social support, medication compliance and HIV/AIDS. *Social Work Health and Mental Health-Practice, Research and Programs.* Guest editors: A. C. Jackson, and S. P. Segal. Binghamton, NY: Haworth Press.

Cox, L. E. (2009). Predictors of medication adherence in an AIDS clinical trial: Patient and clinician perceptions. *Health & Social Work, 34*(4), 257–264. (Special Issue: HIV/AIDS among People of Color.)

Giddens, B., Ka'opua, L., Kaplan, L., & Linsk, N. (2009). The role of social work in medication treatment adherence: HIV/AIDS as a case study. In E. Tomaszewski (Ed.), *NASW HIV/AIDS Spectrum: Mental Health Training and Education of Social Workers Project.* Washington, DC: National Association of Social Workers (NASW).

Haynes, R. B. (1979). Introduction. In R. B. Hayes, D. W. Taylor, & D. L. Sackett (Eds.), *Compliance in health care* (pp. 11–22). Baltimore, MD: Johns Hopkins University Press.

Health Resources and Services Administration (HRSA). (2001). *Transforming the face of health professions through cultural and linguistic competence: The role of the HRSA Centers of Excellence.* U.S. Department of Health and Human Services. Retrieved from http://www.hrsa.gov/culturalcompetence/cultcompedu.pdf

Jones, W. H. (1923). *On decorum.* In E. Capps, T. E. Page, & W. H. D. Rouse (Eds.), *Hippocrates* (pp. 269–301). Loeb Classical Library (Vol. 2, p. 297). London: William Heinemann; New York: G. P. Putnam.

Linsk, N. C., & Marder, R. E. (1992). Medical social work long term care referrals for people with HIV infection. *Health & Social Work, 17*(2), 105–115.

Linsk, N.C., & Bonik (2000). *Handout.* Received at HIV & Social Work conference workshop venue, San Diego, CA.

Lloyd, G. (1996). *HIV infection and AIDS: Annotated bibliography of social work literature 1981–1995.* New Orleans: Tulane Institute for Research and Training in HIV/AIDS counseling. School of Social Work.

Lynch, V. J., Lloyd, G. A., & Fimbres, M. F. (Eds.). (1993). *The expanding face of AIDS: Implications for social work practice.* Westport, CT: Auburn House.

Mancoske, R. J. (1996). HIV/AIDS and suicide: Further precautions. *Social Work, 41*(3), 325–326.

Morse, E. V., Simon, P. M., Coburn, M., Hyslop, N., Greenspan, D., & Balson, P. M. (1991). Determinants of subject compliance within an experimental anti-HIV drug protocol. *Social Science and Medicine, 32*(10), 1161–1167.

Poindexter, C. (2010). *Handbook of HIV and social work.* Hoboken, NJ: John Wiley & Sons.

Singh, N., Squier, C., Sivek, C., & Wagener, M. (1996). Determinants of compliance with antiretroviral therapy in patients with human immunodeficiency virus: Prospective assessment with implications for enhancing compliance. *AIDS Care, 8*(3), 261–269.

Stine, G. J. (2009). *AIDS Update 2009.* New York: McGraw Hill Company.

Stine, G. J. (2010). *AIDS Update 2010.* New York: McGraw Hill Company.

Stine, G. J. (2012). *AIDS Update 2012.* New York: McGraw Hill Company.

Tomaszewski, E. (Ed.). (2005). *The role of social work in medication treatment adherence: HIV/AIDS as a case study.* NASW HIV/AIDS Spectrum: Mental Health Training and Education of Social Workers Project. Washington, DC: Developed under contract with the Center for Mental Health Services (CMHS) of the Substance Abuse and Mental Health Services Administration. U.S. Department of Health and Human Services (DHHS), Rockville, MD. Contract #280-01-8055 (update Contract # 280-09-0202)

Treue, W. (1958). *Doctor at court.* London: Wiedgeld and Nicolson.

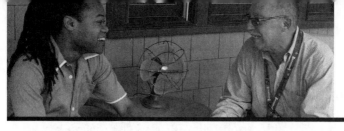

14

Spirituality and People Living with HIV

Mary Boudreau and Susan Grettenberger

We should consider ourselves spirits having a human experience rather than humans having an occasional spiritual experience.

—Anonymous

Why Address Spirituality and Religion?

Many social workers seem to be uncomfortable when working with clients in the arenas of spirituality and religion. Somehow these may seem unprofessional, perhaps not sufficiently evidence based. There are concerns, particularly for social workers who are themselves religious, about spiritual and religious work with clients. Discussing a client's spirituality and religion may feel like an ethically gray area, given the perceived risk of imposing one's own beliefs on a client. Yet, there is increasing recognition in the profession that social workers should assess and address client spirituality and religion as part of holistic work with clients. For persons facing a chronic or life-threatening illness such as HIV/AIDS (human immunodeficiency virus and acquired immune deficiency syndrome), these matters are often especially important.

During the early days of the HIV/AIDS epidemic, effective medical treatments to slow the disease's progression were not available. Far too many people were dying because of HIV-related complications. Social workers functioned much like hospice social workers, primarily responding to immediate daily living concerns and meeting end-of-life needs, such as palliative care, emotional and spiritual preparation for death, and healing within personal relationships. Then, in the mid-1990s, intensive medical research on HIV led to the advent of effective treatment regimens. Consequently, the role of social workers expanded considerably as most people with HIV embraced the opportunity to live longer, or, in some cases, had to reorient to the idea that they would live at all after preparing to die. Yet, many spiritual and religious concerns remained for persons living with HIV (PLWH).

As the advent of medication treatments for HIV and AIDS developed, so did the state of social work with persons with HIV. How do social workers help people with HIV cope with the challenges of living many years with this disease? In order to live a longer, healthier life a person with HIV must find ways to balance the physical, emotional, social, and spiritual aspects of their lives. Many clients struggle with spiritual issues as they face a life of living with HIV. Social workers must be prepared to assist them with those issues, lest client needs go unmet.

This chapter provides a framework for considering the spiritual and religious needs of clients, and suggests practice principles for effectively addressing those needs with persons living with HIV. The chapter opens with a discussion of the concepts of spirituality and religion. Practice principles are suggested to effectively address the needs of persons living with HIV.

Spirituality and Religion

Spirituality and religion are often thought of as synonymous. They are certainly closely related, yet are different concepts. At the onset, it is useful to understand them as distinct but related. Table 14.1 presents some of the differences between these concepts. Understanding and defining spirituality can happen from various perspectives. For many people, spirituality reflects an individual's beliefs about life's purpose and meaning as it relates to the sacred. Van Hook, Hugen, and Aguilar (2001) summarize the most prominent attempts in social work literature to define spirituality, suggesting it encompasses purposes or concepts such as seeking transcendence, searching for meaning in life, finding purpose, and framing one's values. They further suggest that all the definitions from social work authors lead to an understanding of spirituality as a factor permeating the lives of those who experience it or as being an organizing part of one's whole existence. At the core of all of these definitions is the idea that spirituality offers meaning in life, providing people with an understanding of how their lives fit into the whole of humanity and, even, into the whole of time. Others, however, focus more on the process of spirituality. For example, Mbali Creezzo, a South African healer, suggests that "*spirituality*, for me [is] . . . , defined as connection to all the worlds: inner, outer, other, and natural" (Walker, 2009, p. 225; emphasis in original). Spirituality influences how one handles major life transitions such as birth, death, health problems, and relationships. Spirituality may be experienced through purposeful presence in nature, or perhaps through serendipity of experiences. Some actively seek spirituality in rituals such as prayer, meditation, sacred ceremonies, religious services, and music. Spirituality may encompass practices encouraged by religious traditions, such as fasting, pilgrimage, and service to others through time or material contributions (Foster, 1998). Spirituality is typically experiential and can be quite private, even when individuals are with groups of other people. Some might describe a spiritual experience as experiencing a sense of peace or perhaps having a sense of connection with something greater than or beyond self. Yet in spite of the individuality of much spiritual experience, communal spirituality is at the root of nearly all religions.

Table 14.1. Spirituality and Religion: A Comparison

Spirituality	Religion
Spirituality is based in personal experience.	Religion is institutional.
Spirituality may be experienced within a group setting, but often is experienced alone.	Religion frequently involves a group experience.
Spirituality does not necessarily include a particular understanding of a higher power or deity.	Religion typically includes specific understanding of the role of a higher power or deity.
Rituals may be part of spirituality, typically created and defined by the person.	Religion has specific rituals or traditions, or both, shared by adherents of the religion.
If there are shared spiritual experiences, they are less formal.	Religion contains shared experiences, traditions, and beliefs, often defined by the religion.
Spirituality is an individual experience that may have no other context.	Religion provides a context for understanding the world and the place of humans in that world. This context includes the history and story of the start of the religion.
Spirituality does not require adherence to a religion.	Religion provides interpretations of spiritual experiences.
Some people describe spirituality as transformative.	Religion provides guidance for living, including rules about behavior and morality.
It is possible to be spiritual but not religious.	It is possible to be religious but not spiritual.

For many people, spirituality and religion intersect. At that intersection, the person's spirituality influences and is embedded in the religious context. A religious context may also influence how people define spiritual experiences.

Religion, on the other hand, is a group expression or shared interpretation of these experiences. It often involves specific doctrines and belief statements. Religion is typically an expression of beliefs held in common by many people and it is often institutionalized (Hopcke, 2004). Van Hook and colleagues (2001, p. 13) define "a person as religious if he or she belongs to or identifies with a specific religious group; accepts most or all of the beliefs, values, and doctrines of that religious group; and participates in required practices, ceremonies and rituals of that group." These beliefs may include a prescription of what is moral or immoral. Such codes of conduct are part of many religions. For example, although this oversimplifies the concept, Christians refer to violations of moral expectations as sins. Learning the particulars of specific religions is important, as each tradition is different. Furthermore, there are variations within religions, just as one might find within any group. So while one can assume there are expectations and rules within religions, one should always check the validity of those assumptions for any one individual or religious congregation. This is an essential and important social work practice point.

In contrast to spirituality, which tends to be more rooted in the individual, religions usually have organizational structures. This may include anything from a sacred space or a physical structure, such as a building, to a worldwide organization of millions of people who meet with or belong to local groups. Religions include common practices or rituals, many of which have been handed down through centuries. Shared rituals such as communion (Christian), Ramadan (Muslim), and Passover (Jewish) are followed at specific times and have prescribed meanings in addition to spiritual purposes. These rituals provide shared experiences for members of the religion, uniting them and forming a group identity. Many religions also have writings through which common understandings of the history and basic principles of the religion are communicated across generations. Such writings serve to teach newcomers about the religion and its traditions as well as to provide guidance in how its adherents should behave. The *Bible* (Christian), *Torah* (Jewish), and *Koran* (Islam) are all sacred writings. Even spiritually based Alcoholics Anonymous, which members will assure you is not a religion, has several core writings such as *The Big Book*, shared rituals and purposes, along with a formal, international organization. It is helpful for social workers to become familiar with the teachings of major religions and other spiritually based organizations to be responsive to clients.

Box 14.1. Self-Reflection I

Check what you know about religion:

- Name all the religions you can think of. You have two minutes.

- Compare your list with someone else in class. Did you arrive at a similar list?

- Which religion do you know the most about?

- Are there any about which you know nothing?

- How might you learn more about other religions?

The Interface between Spirituality and Religion

It is often presumed by adherents of religions or people of faith that the purpose of a religion is to support spiritual experience, yet many people do not lay claim to both religion and spirituality. For example, some people find their religious congregation or institution to be a place for social support and comfort, but find little spirituality in their involvement in the religion. Others might engage in a variety of spiritual practices, while having little use for a formal religion. People may have been raised in a religious tradition that they no longer practice. Others may have no experience with organized religion. Finally, while some people may experience only one or the other, others may merge spirituality and religion. As always, social workers need to start where the client is in order to provide effective intervention. Remember, people are influenced not only by present behaviors, but also by experiences in their past with respect to religion and spirituality. A person educated in a Catholic high school and raised in the church will still be influenced by those experiences years later, even if she no longer identifies as Catholic. Table 14.1 captures some of the points of contrast between spirituality and religion. While the chart is helpful to organize observations of clients, remember that generalizations do not apply to every situation.

Benefits of Religion

Participation in religion offers at least three potential contributions to persons living with HIV. One is to provide a community of support through a religious congregation. Because religious communities nearly always include people of different generations, different economic statuses, and varied social situations, they can be the source of a variety of supports for members. The second contribution of belonging to an organized religious community is that it offers ways for its members to find meaning in life. This can happen through formal religious studies, informal interactions with others, rituals, and social activities. Finally, helping others is vital to enhancing one's sense of self-worth and opportunities to do so abound through religious congregations. Religious groups often sponsor services to specific populations, such as persons in poverty, people in recovery, people who are homeless, persons who are deaf, or children experiencing problems at school.

Recognition of the power and importance of service is reflected in a variety of institutions such as in the principles of major religions, the twelve steps of Alcoholics Anonymous, and requirements of various secular service programs, which often have their roots in religious traditions. Nearly all of the major religions emphasize service to others as an important aspect of meeting religious obligations. This explains, in part, the multitude of religiously affiliated social service organizations, hospitals, emergency relief organizations, shelters, and food pantries found across the United States. Note, too, that many 12-step programs such as Alcoholics Anonymous are held in the buildings of religious congregations.

Religious congregations may also explicitly provide support to those with HIV. Many participate in collaborative efforts to help people with HIV, guided by religious leadership and clergy in groups such as the AIDS Interfaith Council. Some religious groups incorporate HIV prevention into their work, while others serve people with HIV in conjunction with other health efforts. In the African-American faith community, programs that are particularly successful include "teaching proactive coping skills and addressing ways to improve overall quality of life, spiritually based health programs delivered in the church could be an effective mechanism of health promotion" (Braxton, Lang, Sales, Wingood, & DiClemente, 2007, p. 24). Boxes 14.2 and 14.3 provide examples of such ministries.

Box 14.2. The Balm in Gilead

The Balm in Gilead is an organization whose mission is "to prevent diseases and to improve the health status of people of the African Diaspora by providing support to faith institutions" (Balm in Gilead, n.d.). Among its ministries is the Tanzania HIV/AIDS Interfaith Partnership, an outreach to the Christian and Muslim populations of Tanzania, in East Africa.

> **Box 14.3. Hollywood United Methodist Church**
>
> Hollywood United Methodist Church's HIV/AIDS ministry began in the1980s. Its activities now include delivering meals to patients waiting for care at the University of Southern California Clinic, ongoing work on the AIDS quilt, and sponsorship of spiritual retreats for persons living with HIV and AIDS and their families. As a sign to all of its support, the church's tower sports a twenty-foot red ribbon.

Benefits of Spirituality

Spirituality, which may or may not be linked to religion, is potentially a better starting point for social work interventions than religion. Though it may be more abstract and elusive, it is worth the effort to address spirituality with clients for the benefit of the client. Studies empirically establish these benefits, and there is little to suggest harm as a result of addressing spirituality with a client. Tsevat (2006) found that about half of people living with HIV reported that their sense of spirituality improved following their diagnosis, and that this increase in spirituality, or religiosity, had a positive effect on their physical health. Spiritual development can have other benefits, including increases in self-discipline, inner peace, transformation, and connectedness to the divine (Foster, 1998). These benefits often lead to improved relationships with others. Despite the challenges of incorporating spirituality into a client's biopsychosocial assessment and treatment plan, it is vital for the social worker to do so. Van Hook and Aguilar (2001) provide an excellent discussion of the benefits of religion and spirituality, particularly as it relates to health outcomes.

Spirituality and Religion: Can They Have Negative Impacts?

There is little known about negative effects of spirituality on people, including those living with HIV. Although some gain strength from religion, however, others do not. The disappointing reality is that religion does not provide the inner healing and wholeness for everyone. For many individuals, there is a disconnection between religion and their lives, whether resultant from negative experiences in their younger years or from perceived judgments related to the behaviors that led to their infection. As discussed at the start of this chapter, one function of religions can be to offer moral judgments of people's behavior. People with HIV are often associated with highly stigmatized behaviors such as injection drug use or same-gender sexual activity, so they have often experienced overt condemnation or have internalized a sense of being "bad people." Experiences of religiously motivated condemnation and rejection are common among people who identify as lesbian, gay, bisexual, or transgendered (LGBT). Sexual minorities have often been hurt directly or indirectly by institutional religion. Churches and similar institutions are sometimes run by religious extremists. The ubiquitous antigay religious demonstrations at gay events often include signs such as, "God hates faggots." Some religious groups define HIV as God's punishment for misbehavior.

The organized efforts of various powerful religious organizations assert that LGBT people are sinful or evil, which has had a negative impact on the rights and sense of self-worth of LGBT persons, even if a given individual has not experienced direct discrimination or judgment. Public displays of such antigay sentiment within religious institutions include, for example, the eight-year boycott of Disney theme parks by the Southern Baptist Convention. The boycott, which began in 1997, was intended to convey displeasure with Disney's domestic partner benefits and "gay days" at its theme parks. While there are increasing numbers of individual religious communities committed to acceptance of LGBT persons, the affirming presence of those individual religious communities is not enough to bridge the hurt, guilt, shame, and rejection that some LGBT people have experienced from religion at large. In response, many of these people have separated themselves entirely from organized religion.

Similarly, religious persons or institutions often condemn persons with substance abuse problems as sinners. Within many religious traditions, drinking any alcohol is seen as a sin or a violation of God's expectations. For some believers, excessive drinking of alcohol or use of illicit drugs is viewed as a sign of demonic possession or a failure of spirit rather than a problem with physiological or psychological roots. These judgments can become even more difficult for individuals to handle if they are using alcohol or other drugs as a way of coping with feelings about their sexual orientation. Rather than support people in their quest for health and sobriety, religious congregations may press people to deal with their sin of substance abuse in ways that imply judgment. Ironically, as noted above, congregations of some of these same traditions may provide free space to supportive services such as Alcoholics Anonymous and Narcotics Anonymous.

When religion conjures up pain and hurt rather than affirmation and growth, an effective social worker must understand the personal ways in which religion has affected their clients. Taking this stance allows the worker to help clients resolve points of pain and conflict and, potentially, to develop a spiritual expression or religious experience that is affirming and growth oriented. It is essential for the social worker be self-aware, carefully examining his or her own point of reference regarding religion. Whether positive or negative, the social worker's own experience must be very carefully self-monitored, lest it inappropriately influence work with the client.

Box 14.4. Self-Reflection II

Self-reflection: What do you bring to the interaction with a client?

- What parts of your religious experience have been helpful to you?

- What parts have been hurtful or confusing as you make life decisions?

- Have you experienced a situation that was free of the harms you just identified? Identify one way the helpful or hurtful experiences could influence your interactions with clients.

Illness

Because religion and spirituality often surface when people are facing a serious or life-changing chronic illness, they become very relevant when dealing with HIV and AIDS. For millennia, religion and spirituality have provided a strong sense of hope and security when people have faced personal tragedies, including terminal illness and death. Depending on the particular situation and people's spiritual backgrounds, they may feel a sense of hope that a miracle cure will save them from their illness or provide relief from symptoms such as pain. Conversely, depending on the person's beliefs, he or she may perceive having HIV as divine punishment for moral failings. When an individual is faced with HIV infection, past behaviors, such as having had sex out of wedlock, engaging in same-sex behaviors, or being addicted to drugs, may lead to feelings of HIV being punishment. It is common for humans to wonder what will follow their death; diagnosis of a potentially terminal illness often intensifies such questions. Possible responses may be influenced by one's religious beliefs, potentially leading to either a sense of hope or a sense of foreboding. Being diagnosed with HIV may increase a person's participation in religious practices such as prayer. When facing an awareness of personal and potentially imminent mortality, spirituality may be considered by many as the "only hope," as Obi Wan Kenobi was to the Jedi in the first *Star Wars* film.

Stages of Loss: A Model for Understanding the Evolving Impact of Spirituality. Of particular relevance in understanding the spiritual aspects of a chronic or terminal illness is the work of Dr. Elisabeth Kübler-Ross. Although her work is no longer seen as the primary model for understanding the process of loss and grief, it still provides points of reflection that can be useful here.

Loss is a large part of dealing with serious illness. Having HIV involves a number of potential losses. Among these are possible loss of health, threats to one's relationships, loss of status in society, loss of one's sense of invulnerability, loss of trust in people one loves, and, of course, the ultimate loss: the loss of one's life. Facing one's mortality nearly inevitably raises concerns of a more spiritual nature. Understanding the stages of grief and loss provides additional understanding of spiritual issues faced by persons living with HIV. Often thought of as psychological stages, each of Kübler-Ross' five classic stages also includes spiritual dimensions. In her pioneering book, *On Death and Dying*, Kübler-Ross (1969) articulated multiple stages of grief that provide a helpful paradigm for understanding and working with clients as they face life-changing events and significant losses, such as those of chronic illness. These stages—denial, anger, bargaining, depression, and acceptance—provide insight into what clients with HIV often experience, and offer clues about intervention. Each stage illuminates unique challenges of negotiating significant losses. The presence or absence of hope is woven through each stage, as hope is often seen as an outgrowth of spirituality. As Kübler-Ross (1969, p. 148) acknowledges,

> We were always impressed that even the most accepting, the most realistic patients left the possibility open for some cure, for the discovery of a new drug. . . . It is this glimpse of hope which maintains them through days, weeks, or months of suffering. It is the feeling that all this must have some meaning, will pay off eventually if they can only endure it for a little while longer: It is the hope that occasionally sneaks in. . . . It gives the terminally ill a sense of a special mission in life which helps them maintain their spirits.

Understanding Kübler-Ross' stages can provide context for holistic work, including spiritual dimensions, with any client experiencing loss. Exploring the stages from a spirituality perspective gives insight into the client's specific situation, allowing the social worker to plan personalized and, hopefully, a more helpful intervention. The discussion of stages that follows is presented in a typical order of progression. The real life progression, as with any human response, is not necessarily so neatly ordered. Stages may come in different orders, and they may not all occur. A person may move in and out of a stage, moving forward, then back, then forward more. The best-case outcome is for a person to eventually move through all the stages to acceptance, but unfortunately not all people come to terms with their losses. The role of the social worker is to provide support for the client as they negotiate loss, coming to a point of acceptance that allows one to live in a healthy and meaningful way, albeit with HIV.

Denial

The first stage typically faced upon learning of a significant loss is denial. Sometimes the person simply cannot comprehend that the news given to them is true. Denial "functions as a buffer after unexpected shocking news, allows the patient to collect himself, and with time, mobilize other, less radical defenses" (Kübler-Ross, 1989, p. 52). She suggested that denial also is reflected in the way society initially dealt with the entire HIV epidemic, as she said early in the epidemic, "[It] has become quite obvious that we also attempt to deny AIDS, to pretend it is none of our business!" (Kübler-Ross, 1989, p. 5). For some, denial even precedes receiving a diagnosis, as a person may recognize personal risk but avoid seeking care. Despite guidelines encouraging universal testing for all adults and aggressive counseling and testing outreach in the populations whose behavior puts them most at risk, the Centers for Disease Control and Prevention (CDC) estimate that 25 percent of people living with HIV are undiagnosed (CDC, 2010). Others seek out testing, perhaps anonymously, yet do not return for test results or simply disappear after learning their HIV diagnosis.

As Kübler-Ross suggested, denial can be an important protective mechanism when people first learn their diagnosis, keeping them from being overwhelmed. The duration of denial aspects of coping will vary by individual, often recurring even as it gradually subsides. The worker must be sensitive to the specific needs of an individual. Sustained denial, on the other hand, is problematic. As they refuse to face a serious health threat, people fail to secure important health care and continue to engage in high-risk behaviors, infecting others. Denial can be exacerbated by spiritual issues or religious training. For example, John learned he was HIV positive through testing at the local jail. He was diagnosed with pneumocystis carinii pneumonia (PCP), the rare and preventable form of pneumonia frequently associated with HIV. While in jail, he was in detox treatment from alcohol and cocaine use. Upon learning of his diagnosis, he suffered an immediate spiritual crisis as he was faced with the threat of the end of his life. He considered suicide, but his Catholic upbringing led him to a belief that suicide, which the Catholic Church considers to be a sin, would result in even more divine punishment. With the exception of HIV counselors and nurses who visited him at the jail, he had no social or spiritual support, and he was overwhelmed with guilt, fear, and shame. He disappeared immediately after release from jail, presumably to return to his life of addiction and denial.

Anger

The next stage of loss is often anger. People become angry that they are being subjected to the anticipated losses associated with having HIV. They are angry about what may be viewed as an injustice. They may be angry that they will not experience things they had hoped to experience in life or about the adjustments they will need to make in their lives. For some, anger also externalizes or locates responsibility—or sometimes blame—for their situation, outside themselves. Others may focus anger internally as they realize their situation is partially the result of decisions they have made.

Anger is not necessarily viewed by helpers as a spiritual crisis, yet it can be just that. Many people direct the anger they feel at God, or a higher power or creator, for making them vulnerable to such a horrific disease. Their belief systems may not allow them to explain how this could happen, other than that their deity is punishing them. They may feel that whatever their perceived misbehavior, they do not merit this punishment. At the same time, people may feel conflicted and guilty for blaming God. All of this may cause a person to turn away from their religious grounding or spiritual self, because they feel betrayed.

Anger can impact other relationships as well, as people face fear and self-loathing, or even anger at those they have loved and trusted the most. For example, this anger can be directed at the person who infected them. Barb was furious when she learned her husband's severe illness was due to HIV-related complications. Her anger intensified when she learned that she was also infected with HIV. Years later, she admitted to her support group, "I was so angry, I wanted to kill him, and I was even angry when he died before I had a chance to kill him myself." After reconnecting with her Native American spiritual roots and practicing healing rituals, she was able to turn her anger into action by becoming an advocate for women with HIV.

Bargaining

Bargaining is a stage in which a person tries to find a way out of his or her situation by offering trade-offs. By its very nature, the bargaining stage has a religious or spiritual nature, as one is bargaining with a higher power. Persons who have not been especially religious often turn to God through bargaining. Perhaps they perceive that having HIV is the result of misbehavior, and attempt to make up for their perceived bad behavior. It can be expressed through promises to God or a higher power that the person will do specific things and be a better person. Many people with HIV who have long been away from their childhood spiritual practices find themselves falling back on their childhood traditions and beliefs as they bargain. HIV test counselors, when informing someone they have tested positive for HIV, frequently hear such pledges. Promises made during bargaining tend to be somewhat desperate and unrealistic. "If I can only be healed of this, I will go back to God and never have sex again!" "I will go to mass every day for the rest of my life if I am retested and it's negative." Typically, the result sought by the individual does not occur. One of the challenges for social workers helping someone who is or has engaged in serious bargaining is helping them to resolve whatever feelings they may have when the desired negotiation fails.

Box 14.5. Experiencing Our Own Losses

Have you ever experienced a loss, such as a break-up or the threat of someone dying, and found yourself bargaining? What promises did you make? Then what happened? What might have helped you at the time?

Depression

One possible response of someone who begins to recognize that bargaining will not or has not changed his or her health situation is to slip into depression. The social worker needs to take depression seriously with any client, as the consequences of clinical depression can be quite profound. Because depressive symptoms can be indicative of a major mood disorder, the social worker should ensure appropriate assessment and diagnosis, as well as psychiatric treatment when indicated, for any client demonstrating symptoms of depression.

Depression can be addressed as part of or as the cause of a spiritual crisis. The spiritual impact of depression can be withdrawal from life-enhancing spiritual practices, numbing feelings of well-being, and general lack of energy for healing and wholeness. On the flip side, spiritual growth and wellness can successfully lead a person through depression due to a loss. As with all the stages, it is possible to get stuck in one stage, so it is critical for the social worker to assist a person during depression. Furthermore, the social worker must pay appropriate attention to the risk of suicide during depression, even acute depression triggered by a loss. Since depression can be a reflection of a spiritual crisis, addressing the spiritual dimensions can be a key to moving through this stage.

Some people refuse such help that has a spiritual focus. For example, Sara has been HIV positive for more than fifteen years. She also experiences severe bouts of depression. She and her husband, who is also HIV positive, moved to a small community in order to be near his family, yet she feels isolated and exhausted most of the time. She cries often, has no appetite, and smokes cigarettes and drinks coffee throughout the day. She does not have any goals or plans for the future. She states, "God must have left me here on earth for a reason," but she expresses that she has no idea what that reason is. Despite encouragement, she refuses support groups, counseling, spiritual counseling, antidepressants, or other treatments for her depression, but often asks her physician for help obtaining anti-anxiety medications and medicinal marijuana, both of which can have future depressant effects. Sara is caught in a cycle of depression that is not being addressed by her current spiritual, social, and treatment plan.

Acceptance

Acceptance is the ultimate goal in the process of coping with loss. With acceptance, one is able to deal with loss through understanding the reality of the situation, recognition of the challenges, willingness to live with the loss, and hope for the future. Acceptance brings the resolution of and healthy response to the loss. Achieving this stage allows the individual to move beyond facing the implications of the loss to living life with the loss. With HIV, this means acceptance of limitations and the loss of freedoms that will continue for the rest of one's life. As with many chronic diseases, the individual is tied to a structured drug regimen that requires daily attentiveness. HIV-related illness or medication-related side effects may impair functioning. Choosing to avoid the risk of passing the infection to others is another limitation for persons in intimate relationships. Acceptance of the uncertainties that come with the disease is also important. For some, acceptance comes through the spiritual realm. Spiritually driven acceptance may result from renewal, such as arriving at a new understanding of the meaning or purpose of one's life. For some individuals, this process may come from new-found spirituality.

Acceptance is not simply a destination: it is a process with many steps. For example, one significant step may mean finding the courage to tell another person one is HIV positive. It may evolve into participating in an AIDS walk, leading a support group, or even being interviewed on television. For many people, coming out as HIV positive to spiritual leaders may be one of the most difficult hurdles to over-come as they evolve toward acceptance. The role of the social worker is to facilitate the ability of the person to find a way through each of these stages in order to live with acceptance of having HIV. Remember, though, that the stages are not fixed. Even when a person finds acceptance, there may be times of anger about or depres-sion related to having HIV. Therefore, there may continue to be points of spiritual crisis or questioning that require support from a social worker or others. The example below demonstrates the potential of spirituality and religion in helping people negotiate their HIV disease.

Case Example I

Betty had a long journey toward acceptance after receiving her HIV diagno-sis. A widow in her late sixties, she learned she was HIV positive during a hos-pitalization for an acute illness. Her husband, her only sexual partner, had died suddenly several years before. Although she was unsure how she had been exposed, she recalled she had received blood transfusions in the 1980s, a time when there was risk of infection from the blood supply. Betty was a very reli-gious person, with little knowledge about HIV disease. At the time of her diag-nosis, she was living with one of her adult children and served as a caregiver for her grandchildren. Her life focused on her traditional role within her fam-ily. At the time of her diagnosis, out of fear of what others would think of her HIV diagnosis, she withdrew from the few activities connected to her religious congregation in which she participated. Her stress peaked the morning her son-in-law told her he was going to send her home to get help "because we don't want you here!" In one of those unexplainable coincidences of timing, her new case manager made an unplanned stop at Betty's home that morn-ing on the way into work. When she arrived, Betty was standing by the front door with her bags packed, crying. The worker's timely arrival led Betty to get the help she needed to restart her life, help that included spiritual renewal.

Addressing Betty's emotional and spiritual states was significant to making progress with her tangible needs such as housing, finances, education and training, and access to health care. At first, Betty was simply too frozen by her religious beliefs and shame to make meaningful strides toward her concrete goals, but her case manager encouraged her to continue her spiritual practices and to connect to a congregation. The relationships she formed and the acceptance she experienced helped her to overcome some of the barriers she faced. With the help of a scholarship from her church, she even returned to school to finish her degree. Betty often spoke of her case manager as "my angel," reflecting her deeply spiritual perspective. Her case manager, also a spiritual person, agreed that divine prompting had led her to stop and check on Betty on that fateful day, early in their relationship. Betty was able to grow into acceptance of having HIV, later becoming a source of support for many younger women who had HIV.

Summary of Kübler-Ross

People living with HIV have distinct and changing spiritual needs that may be enhanced by understanding Kübler-Ross' stages. The way one views life experiences has a profound impact as well, particularly around the search for meaning following an HIV diagnosis. As Kübler-Ross explains, "[The] belief has long died that suffering here on earth will be rewarded in heaven. Suffering has lost its meaning . . . if we take part in church activities in order to socialize . . . then we are deprived of the church's former purpose, namely, to give hope, a purpose in tragedies here on earth, and an attempt to understand and bring meaning to otherwise inacceptable painful occurrences of our life" (Kübler-Ross, 1969, p. 29). Finding meaning, hope, and comprehension in collaboration with our clients remains an important challenge for social workers. Finding a community of support, which often occurs within a religious congregation, is also important. Being a support in these areas can be a valuable point of intervention as clients resolve complex feelings about their HIV disease.

Question for Reflection

1. Think of a death of a loved one that you have experienced, or another significant incidence of loss. Can you identify having experienced the stages of grief and loss? Which one(s)? What does this and other experiences with grief and

loss teach you that is useful to your work with clients dealing with loss associated with HIV and AIDS?

Effective Social Work Practice and Developing Spiritual Competence

Effective practice in the areas of religion and spirituality can be rewarding for both the client and social worker. It calls for a range of generalist social work knowledge, skills, and values, including competency in and commitment to

- Assessment of client's religious and spiritual needs;

- Planning;

- Respect for and knowledge of the client's religious traditions;

- Problem solving;

- Referral to religiously appropriate resources;

- Knowledge of possible conflicts between religious rules and norms and HIV care;

- Facilitation between medical provider and client on religious issues;

- Support for client, as well as brokering and advocacy, to secure religiously appropriate services to meet client goals;

- Solid knowledge of social work ethics in which to ground one's practice;

- Effective evaluation of client outcomes; and

- Empowerment.

Assessment

Despite the challenges, using religion and spirituality in work with people with HIV can be very rewarding. Social work practice with any client system begins with engagement and assessment. Assessment requires intentionality on the part of the social worker, as intake instruments at agencies may include only one question about the client's religion and entirely lack questions related to spirituality. The purpose of assessment is to learn the extent to which religion and spirituality are a part of the person's life, to determine the potential ways in which these might help or be barriers for people, and to understand what meaning they have for a person. The extent of supports available through religious communities with which the person identifies are also important.

As in all assessments, the use of open-ended questions is helpful. Asking for elaboration after the initial reply from the client is often productive in providing useful details. Questions might include some of the following:

- Do you consider yourself to be a religious person? Explain what being religious means to you.

- Do you belong to a religious congregation or were you raised in a particular tradition?

- What effects has that experience had on you?

- How have or do your beliefs impact your life?

- Talk about any specific practices that are especially helpful to you.

- How has your HIV status affected what you believe?

- What are your thoughts on the meaning of your life?

- Tell me about any times when you had an experience that you felt was spiritual.

- If there has been a time when you felt a spiritual connection, what was it?

- What are your beliefs about life after death? (Use this question with caution. It may be more appropriate if the client has initiated a discussion of death or dying.)

These questions serve a number of purposes, including encouraging clients to explore their beliefs and resources, as well as increasing the depth of the helping relationship. In addition, they can help to identify areas that the client experiences as gaps in their lives, providing information about how the client and social worker, working together, can fill these gaps.

Question for Reflection

1. What ideas do you have for other nonjudgmental and open-ended questions that encourage disclosure of additional information from a client about his or her spirituality and religious background?

Finding Resources

If sensitive to the client's needs, a social worker can be a great resource for developing strategies to meet these needs. A social worker should develop resources and connections with local groups from a variety of religious and spiritual belief systems. Although larger cities may have more resources available, if people are interested and committed, small groups can be developed in rural areas. If one is cautious in assessing their openness, churches can be a resource in these communities. The internet also provides wonderful resources, but one should be cautious here as well, given the nature of some online resources that may impose a message of condemnation. Given the social worker's duty to do no harm, it is imperative for workers to find spiritual and religious resources that focus on health and well-being in an affirming way. Effective social workers should do their homework and thoroughly examine web pages before recommending them to clients.

Negotiating Religious Needs and HIV Care

The need to understand the religious traditions and rituals of clients cannot be overstated. Various circumstances related to religion can pop up in unexpected ways. In order to be effective and responsive, the social worker must become conversant around the specific religious traditions of each client. As with all needs, once one has spent some time learning from individuals, it becomes easier to figure out what issues might emerge. This lessens the surprise factor and increases the likelihood of being able to fully respond to the client's needs as they emerge. A complete assessment early in the relationship and openness on the part of the social worker to learn about the client's religious needs improves the likelihood of the social worker understanding important needs before they have to be addressed. Communicating an attitude of acceptance and affirmation of all religious traditions creates a helpful tone for practice with respect to people's religious needs.

Box 14.6. Working with Client Religious Practices

Ramadan is an Islamic ritual time of sacrifice and purification. Throughout Ramadan, most Muslims refrain from eating, drinking, and certain other activities during daylight hours. These prohibitions can be a real challenge to an HIV-positive person with a strict regimen of medications. A social worker could work with the client and physician in anticipation of Ramadan, and assist in creating a medication schedule that would meet the religious restrictions. For example, people may gradually adjust their dosing times so they take the meds before sunrise and after sunset.

Advocacy and Brokering with People Living with AIDS. When clients' religious needs are not being met, the social worker can provide a bridge to meeting these needs. Sometimes religious needs are not fully met when an individual is from a minority culture, or is new to an area, such as is the case with displaced refugees. Social workers can accomplish a great deal by educating other professionals about the client's cultural and religious needs. The social worker may be in a position of advocating for the client with insurance companies and medical providers. Since some religious beliefs may involve higher costs, such as burial rather than cremation, the social worker may be in a position to find ways of funding these costs, such as working with the individual's religious organization, if there is one. The client situation in Box 14.7 illustrates the type of situation that could occur and would be unfamiliar to a non-Hindu social worker. A more common need might be finding funding for the burial of an indigent client, in which case a local church might have cemetery plots donated by members for such use.

Box 14.7. Assisting with Religious Practices

One client, a thirty-five-year-old Hindu man, had been born in India. Upon his death, the family wished to arrange for his ashes to be scattered on the Ganges River, in keeping with Hindu tradition. The social worker assisted the family in securing needed permissions and resources to successfully return his ashes to India as the family and he desired.

Enhancing Spiritual Strengths

Another strategy that can be useful is for the social worker to work directly with the client to develop new spiritual practices or enhance existing religious practices. A thorough spiritual assessment provides an understanding of what rituals and practices already have meaning to the client. While evidence-based practice is important in social work, creativity also plays an important role in the practice of most social workers. Here, creativity can help the social worker to collaborate with the client in developing meaningful rituals or in revitalizing practices that have been helpful in the past.

Rituals assist people in becoming centered. Social workers often find that their clients are involved with 12-step programs. All practitioners should learn about the spiritual meaning of the twelve steps in order to support clients as they work through them. Encouraging clients to figure out new rituals or new meanings for old rituals, including religious rituals, often assists them in finding a focus, which enhances their well-being. Indeed, many rituals and practices are essential to religions, yet they need not be religiously based in order to be helpful. The following are some suggestions of practices that have been useful, yet need not be exercised in a religious context:

- Meditation is an ancient practice. This practice, while not commonly part of corporate practices of many religions, can be easily taught and is very accessible for individuals to practice within their own homes or personal space. Music often can be used to enhance meditation, and workers may be effective in guiding meditation if they themselves practice it.

- Giving is widely believed to move people from a focus on self to a focus on others. One can give of time or financial resources. Cami Walker (2009), diagnosed as a young woman with multiple sclerosis, experienced a dramatic change in her health and mental state when she shifted her focus from herself to giving to others. While giving is not a cure for chronic illness, it can be spiritually energizing, which improves well-being.

- Sacred space is a key element of spiritual experience and ritual. Many people exist in cluttered or difficult spaces in most aspects of their lives. Yet, sacred space can be created or identified, providing clients with a place of retreat for quiet and centering. Sacred space is not restricted to designated religious places, although those can be very meaningful for people. Places in nature, such as near flowing water or woods, are sacred for some people. While a social worker can assist the client in thinking about what spaces might serve this purpose, ultimately the client will need to discover what spaces have meaning for him or her.

- Objects can enhance sacred space or rituals. In particular, water and fire have long held deep meaning that seems almost imprinted in the human psyche. Perhaps the importance of water and fire in human survival contributes to this. Fire, whether from candles, fireplaces, or outside pits, can be a symbol of renewal or can be used by clients to symbolically rid themselves of unwanted memories or thoughts. Water may symbolize renewal and new life. Within religious traditions, water is used symbolically to signal personal transformation.

- Walking a labyrinth is another ancient spiritual practice increasingly accessible in the United States, whether in churches, hospitals, or even public parks. For many, journeying through a labyrinth is a metaphor of the journey inward. A labyrinth walk provides opportunities for reflection and centering. Many resources are available on the internet related to the meaning of the labyrinth and ways to use this walk.

- Creation of symbols with clients is often helpful. Symbols can help clients remember lessons they have learned or deepen their spiritual experiences. Any concrete object or written materials can become a symbol if a person agrees to the new meaning given. Here again, the social worker can assist the client in identifying what symbols might be helpful to him or her.

Working with Faith-Based Organizations

This chapter devotes considerable attention to the religious and spiritual needs of clients. Much of what makes social workers effective is their ability to assist clients in locating and securing services from the variety of organizations, which typically includes both secular and faith-based organizations. The faith-based group usually comprises both nonprofit organizations and religious congregations. Faith-based organizations have long been a resource to which social workers turn for assistance with concrete needs such as food, shelter, clothing, and emergency funding. Cultivating and maintaining relationships with these organizations is considered to be an important part of good social work practice. There can be, however, challenges when serving persons with HIV. A problem could arise with something as simple as entering a congregation's building. For example, a client may simply find it too difficult to go to a religious congregation's food pantry. Yet, in many places, faith-based organizations provide the bulk of tangible services to people with HIV. There can be significant contradictions and tensions within religious groups. For example, the Roman Catholic Church funds more than 25 percent of the services globally available for persons living with HIV (Barragan, 2006). At the same time, the Catholic Church has purposely taken actions that create barriers to effective risk reduction and is seen as an opponent of what many professionals view as sound public health policies. For example, even early in the epidemic, "the prominent concerns in the AIDS prevention arena are the Vatican's opposition to condoms and its ability to sway national and international policies that subsequently impact on HIV/AIDS prevention strategies and services" (Watts, 2006, p. 46).

Working with faith-based organizations requires a conscious assessment by the social worker of the beliefs of the individual organization and its staff. Recognizing the ways in which people have felt judged and mistreated by faith communities puts the social worker in a position of needing to screen organizations for practices and policies that may be inappropriate. An example would be anti-gay or anti-lesbian rhetoric being espoused at a soup kitchen or a food pantry.

An additional challenge social workers face is negotiating the rules and regulations in some faith-based agencies and settings. In many locations, faith-based organizations are essentially the only game in town, and provide vital services. At the same time, these organizations may have policies that conflict with social work ethics and values. A social worker may appropriately wonder, "Is it ethical to allow an agency's regulations to interfere with a client's needs being met?" Such restrictions may include prohibitions on access to condoms or other forms of birth control or disease barriers, constraints on discussing abortion, or opposition to affirming the lives of LGBT people. Ethically, social workers must weigh the cost of limiting services with the benefits of the advocacy they can do within a particular agency. There are no easy answers for social workers. It can be a helpful resource for the social worker to find the support and understanding of other workers facing similar dilemmas, as well as to obtain the support of professional organizations such as the National Association of Social Workers (NASW). Conferences such as the annual National Conference on Social Work and HIV/AIDS offer considerable support from peers and opportunities to address all areas of social work practice, including social work ethics and the spiritual concerns of clients.

Social workers can help people with HIV gain support from religious organizations in a number of ways. It is crucial for social workers to be familiar with local religious communities and their levels of acceptance of persons living with HIV, as well as their acceptance of persons with addiction issues, people who have been sex workers, and people who are LGBT. It is essential for the social worker to identify which religious congregations will be supportive and welcoming, given the harm that might be done should one inadvertently send a client to a place where he or she will be judged or, even worse, condemned. Once the worker has identified supportive faith communities, those communities can become a consistent resource.

Many congregations hold healing services and social workers can advocate that HIV be directly addressed at these services. Inviting religious leaders from many faiths to participate in community awareness events such as World AIDS Day services and National HIV Testing Week can encourage understanding and fellowship. Encouraging church groups to raise money for local HIV food pantries and to participate in AIDS walks can create new connections and deepen understanding. Providing books and flyers to local religious groups can also encourage development of deeper understanding. Many nonprofit agencies, including religious groups, face limited resources. Sharing resources such as facilities for meetings and groups can help bridge understanding.

Case Example II

This example is a composite of the situation of several clients, and it reflects some of the challenges of providing spiritual support to people living with HIV. As you read this story, consider the following areas:

Assessment

- What is the client's spiritual and religious background, and how do these influence her life?

- What beliefs does she have that provide her with resources and strength?

- What beliefs does she have that create challenges for her?

- What questions would you have for her? For her family?

Intervention

- What are some ways you would try to enhance this support?

- What are some ways the social worker provided spiritual support?

- How could a social worker enhance her spiritual experiences?

- What are some ways the social worker learned more about Tenneh's spiritual practices?

- Are there some resources in your community that would or would not be appropriate? Consider what qualities you would look for in a program or religious congregation when making a referral for spiritual or religious support.

Cultural/Diversity

- Identify some challenges in cross-religious social work.

- What cultural or other issues might challenge you in working with Tenneh?

Self-Issues

As you read this, consider what feelings you might have with respect to Tenneh. Identify what they are and what you know about why you might feel that way. Be as honest as possible, as self-reflection yields growth.

Tenneh is a woman in her early forties who came to the United States as a refugee from a war-torn country in Africa. She is a well-educated woman who had a professional position in her home country before the civil war broke out. Tenneh, like too many others, ran for her life with her family. They became separated, and, tragically, her husband, her parents, and several of her children were killed. She carried her remaining son to a refugee camp in another country, where she was raped by mercenaries. She soon learned that as a result of the rape she was both pregnant and infected with HIV.

Tenneh's middle-class world was turned upside down by her experiences and losses. She considered suicide. Her Christian religious background stopped her, as she believed suicide is a sin. Tenneh reflects back on how at that point in her life she looked into her toddler son's eyes and knew she had to live, so that he would live. She began the long process of applying for asylum in the United States. During the long wait for her paperwork to be approved, her second son was born in a crowded refugee camp. She called her son "Merci à Dieu" (thanks to God) because she wanted his life to be marked with gratitude, not resentment. Though it took several years of concerted effort, eventually she and her children emigrated to the United States. They arrived alone, speaking no English. In spite of all she had suffered, Tenneh brought with her a great deal of hope, hope that was rooted in large measure in her faith and in her belief that God would help her to raise her sons.

First assigned to a refugee resettlement agency, Tenneh eventually connected with a social work agency for people with HIV. At first, her social worker focused on addressing her practical needs by securing emergency housing, enrolling her children in schools, linking her with medical care, and helping her secure employment. However, as the worker–client relationship deepened, it became evident that Tenneh's emotional and spiritual needs were being neglected. Although her resilience and faith had helped to sustain her through her initial ordeal, depression and other mental health symptoms were evident in her exhaustion, feelings of mistrust and isolation, difficulty with goal setting, and even her high blood pressure. Her lack of spiritual support and connections to a religious community had weakened her resilience.

There were several barriers between the social worker and Tenneh, including cultural and language differences, along with Tenneh's mistrust of most others due to all of her traumatic experiences. The social worker struggled to communicate with Tenneh, using the bit of high school French she knew. As often happens with recent immigrants, the available interpreters were from the small local enclave of people from her country of origin. Not wanting them to know her HIV status, Tenneh refused interpreters at the agency and physician's office. Eventually, she and her worker developed a trusting relationship within which Tenneh began the long process of healing. A crucial moment came when they sat together on a beach, watching the children play in the water. Tenneh finally shared the story of her rape and the deaths of her family members. She was finally able to cry, beginning to grieve the harm she had suffered, and sharing stories about the faith that had sustained her. With support and encouragement from her social worker, Tenneh expressed how her religious and spiritual foundations had been sustaining for her. Her faith, quite literally, had kept her alive in very difficult circumstances. Tenneh blended practices from several faith traditions, and combined her own Christianity with the traditional cultural beliefs of her people, and her late husband's Muslim religion. For example, she and her children do not eat pork, a Muslim, not a Christian practice.

This story illustrates several challenges in addressing spiritual issues with people with HIV. Often, the spiritual dilemmas they are facing are initiated by far more than their HIV status. They may be related to family history, life crises, and past behaviors that have initiated shame or guilt, or fears about the future, both in life and death. Spiritual beliefs for many people are not a pure faith, but a hybridization of many belief systems that reflect our culture, our education and intellectual practices, the people who touch our lives, and our experiences of a higher power. Therefore, one should hesitate to make assumptions based on what we see or even read on an intake form. As always, it is vital for social workers to ask pertinent questions, and to be open to the fact that these realities may change.

Ethical Issues in Working with Clients about Spirituality and Religion

For social workers, understanding one's own reactions and orientations is a fundamental competency. For some, working in spirituality and religion is the area that will most challenge them. Because so much of spirituality and religion is personal and subjective, working in these areas requires considerable care to engage with clients in ethically appropriate ways. Here, two sample ethical issues and attendant social work obligations are considered.

One ethical obligation familiar to all social workers is section 1.05 of the NASW Code of Ethics: Cultural Competence and Social Diversity. The essence of the three specifics found in this section are (a) understanding culture from a strengths perspective; (b) having adequate knowledge about and competence in working with their clients' cultures; and (c) understanding the nature of social diversity and oppression with respect to many characteristics, including religion. In other words, it is the obligation of the social worker to competently meet people where they are in their spiritual and religious journeys, no matter what the client's or social worker's traditions are. This can be a daunting task, given the variety of religious traditions, yet it is what is expected of social workers. Simply using one's own experience for a point of reference is not enough. One must explore each person's religious background with care and in an accepting way, through listening and, if necessary, outside research. Fortunately, the internet provides ready access to considerable objective information about nearly all religious traditions. As always, use of the internet requires careful screening for accuracy and freedom from bias.

Section 1.02 of the NASW Code of Ethics asserts that social workers respect and promote the right of clients to self-determination and assist clients in their efforts to identify and clarify their goals. This is an area in which personal beliefs and religious orientation must be carefully monitored. A social worker who strongly believes in the power of prayer may be tempted to press a client to accept prayer or may even simply say, "I will be praying for you." Conversely, a nonbelieving social worker may find it difficult to work with a client who has religious convictions, perhaps ignoring the religious aspects of the client's needs. Both of these examples are a form of imposing one's beliefs and experiences on clients, which is never acceptable. Figuring out one's own interests and beliefs is an excellent beginning point in ensuring that one is engaged in work that is ethical.

Case Example III

> Mike works with a thirty-six-year-old HIV-positive man, Tom. Tom was raised Catholic and attends mass regularly. He has had sexual relationships with a number of men and no women. He states that he is not gay and is trying to stop seeing men because it is a sin. He seems to have a great deal of guilt about his behavior and his denial is leading him to engage in sometimes

unsafe sexual behaviors. Mike, also Catholic, sees Tom's efforts to deal with his sexual behavior as a positive step toward living in a more authentic, personally healthy way.

- What ethical considerations are there in this situation?

- What issues does this situation raise for you, given your own religious orientation, if you have one?

- What might you do in this situation? What is the basis for that decision?

Personal Challenges for Social Workers

Social workers, along with their clients, face challenges in addressing spirituality. Social workers often face their own grief and sense of powerlessness in dealing with HIV. Some may have HIV themselves. Most, if they have worked in the field for any length of time, have experienced deaths of multiple clients. Religion and spirituality may provide comfort and hope. On the other hand, one's personal faith or beliefs may be challenged by the realities and inequities of a disease like HIV. Still, other social workers may not have a religious orientation. All will, at times, struggle to reconcile the circumstances of their clients with their own understanding of the world. On a slightly different theme, many professionals have had their own painful or difficult personal experiences with religion, sometimes in the form of discrimination and rejection. Clients may perpetuate this hurt, such as by saying, "Gay people are going to hell" to a social worker who is gay. Yet in spite of any negative feelings social workers may have toward organized religion, it is essential for them to work with religious congregations. Too often, resources in a community are limited, and those limited resources are situated only in local religious congregations. Finding a way to resolve one's own personal challenges in a way that allows the social worker to work cooperatively with relevant religious organizations is imperative to providing good services.

Questions for Reflection

1. How would you define or explain spirituality?

2. How would you define or explain religion?

3. How do spirituality and religion interface?

4. Are you comfortable working with others about religion and spirituality? Why or why not?

5. What are ways that religion may have caused pain for people living with HIV?

6. How might religion and spirituality have been helpful to people living with HIV?

7. How do you expect your own religious beliefs or lack of religious beliefs will affect your work with clients, particularly people living with HIV?

8. In what ways do you find religion a source of healing, especially around the issue of HIV?

9. In what ways do you find religion a source of hurtfulness, especially around the issue of HIV?

10. How can a social worker be supportive of a client's beliefs, even when they conflict with his or her own (e.g., a client who has a strong religious viewpoint against homosexuality)?

11. What is the impact of stigma on the lives of people living with HIV?

12. Discuss the life cycle challenge hope versus despair in the lives of people living with HIV.

Web Resources

Some of these are specific to a particular religion. Others are HIV websites with pages about religion.

Soulforce: http://www.soulforce.org.

Higher Ground: www.hghiv.org. This site offers an example of an organization focused on holistic healing.

The Body: http://www.thebody.com/index/religion.html.

AIDS Action Committee of Massachusetts, Spirituality and HIV: http://www.aac.org/.

References

Balm in Gilead. n.d. http://www.balmingilead.org/index.php/about/mission.html

Barragan, J. (2006). The Catholic Church helps fight AIDS. In M. Wilson (Ed.). *World Religion: Opposing Viewpoints Series* (pp. 33–39). Detroit: Greenhaven Press.

Braxton, N., Lang, D. L., Sales, J. M., Wingood, G. M., & DiClemente, R. J. (2007). The role of spirituality in sustaining the psychological well-being of HIV-positive Black women. *Women and Health, 46*(2), 113–130.

Centers for Disease Control and Prevention (CDC). (2010). Retrieved from http://www.cdc.gov/hiv/topics/surveillance/resources/reports/index.htm# surveillance

Foster, R. (1998). *Celebration of discipline: The path of spiritual growth.* New York: Harper Collins.

Hopcke, R. (2004, May). The place of religion and spirituality in HIV counseling. *Focus: A Guide of AIDS Research and Counseling, 19*(5):1–5.

Kübler-Ross, E. (1969). *On death and dying: What the dying have to teach doctors, nurses, clergy, and their own families.* New York: Touchstone.

Kübler-Ross, E. (1989). *AIDS: The ultimate challenge.* New York: Collier Books.

Tsevat, J. (2006) Spirituality/religion and quality of life in patients with HIV/AIDS. *Journal of General Internal Medicine, 21*(S5), S1–S2.

Van Hook, M., Hugen, L., & Aguilar, M. (Eds.) (2001). *Spirituality within religious traditions in social work practice.* Pacific Grove, CA: Brooks/Cole.

Van Hook, M., & Aguilar, M. (2001). Health, religion and spirituality. In M. Van Hook, L. Hugen, & M. Aguilar (Eds.), *Spirituality within religious traditions in social work practice* (pp. 273–286). Pacific Grove, CA: Brooks/Cole.

Walker, C. (2009). *29 Gifts: How a month of giving can change your life.* Philadelphia: De Capo.

Watts, C. (2006). The Catholic Church undermines AIDS prevention efforts. In M. Wilson (Ed.), *World Religion: Opposing Viewpoints Series* (pp. 40–46). Detroit: Greenhaven Press.

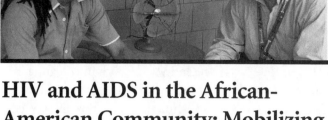

15

HIV and AIDS in the African-American Community: Mobilizing the Black Faith Community

Diana Rowan and Ayana Simon

Our lives begin to end the day we become silent about things that matter.

—**Dr. Martin Luther King Jr.**

Introduction

At all stages of the HIV/AIDS (human immunodeficiency virus and acquired immune deficiency syndrome) continuum, from a positive HIV diagnosis to the end stage of AIDS, African Americans are disproportionately affected (Francis & Liverpool, 2009). According to the Centers for Disease Control and Prevention (CDC, 2010), although Blacks represent only about 12 percent of the U.S. population, in 2007 they accounted for 46 percent of those known to be living with HIV. In 2006, 45 percent of new HIV infections were in Blacks. The rate of new infection for Black women was nearly fifteen times as high as that for White women, and nearly four times that for Hispanic or Latina women. The rate of infection for Black men was six times as high as that for White men, nearly three times that for Hispanic or Latino men, and twice that for Black women. The CDC (2010) predicts that one in sixteen Black men will be diagnosed with HIV during his lifetime, as will one in thirty Black women. Black men who have sex with men (MSM) contract more than 60 percent of the new infections among Black men, with most new infections occurring in Black young men who have sex with men (young MSM) (aged thirteen to twenty-nine).

The inequity in the epidemiologic trends is not new. In 1998, leaders of the U.S. Congressional Black Caucus referred to the HIV/AIDS epidemic as a state of emergency in the Black community, urging heightened mobilization of education and prevention efforts in communities of color, particularly African-American communities (Baker, 1999; Hicks, Allen, & Wright, 2005). In response, President Clinton targeted federal funds to Black and Hispanic communities to develop culturally sensitive HIV-prevention programs and to increase access to the latest treatments (Baker, 1999). More recently, with continuing high rates of infection in the African-American community, the CDC has encouraged broader participation by faith leaders and African-American churches in HIV education and prevention efforts (Lindley, Coleman, Gaddist, & White, 2010).

It is essential for African-American faith communities to engage in the fight against HIV for a number of reasons. Social constructionists have noted that being ill is considered to be outside of social norms and thus sickness has often been linked to sin (Harris, 2010; Lorber, 1997). The connection of sickness to sin constructed throughout society in turn affects diseases such as HIV/AIDS (Conrad & Schneider, 1992). To deconstruct the linkage of AIDS to sin requires a vocal stance by the faith community. Furthermore, Black churches have a long legacy of advancing social justice for African Americans. And finally, the mandate of the faith community to relieve suffering in the community is in line with the missions of AIDS service organizations (ASOs). Although many Black churches have been slow to respond to the AIDS pandemic, momentum is now building and efforts are becoming more coordinated. This chapter examines the role of Black faith communities in efforts to prevent the spread of HIV in the Black community and in the care of those living with HIV and AIDS. The chapter looks at barriers to effective AIDS advocacy by the Black church as well as opportunities for success. The chapter describes various types of interventions in different regions of the country, and presents recommendations for successful collaboration between the African-American faith community and community-based organizations (CBOs), especially ASOs. Finally, a case example illustrates the themes presented in the chapter.

The Role of the Black Church

Religion is an important element of African-American culture, and the Black church is one of the most stable institutions in the African-American community (Hatcher, Burley, & Lee-Ouga, 2008). Douglas and Hopson (2001, p. 96) described the Black church as "a multitudinous community of churches, which are diversified by origin, denomination, doctrine, worshipping culture, spiritual expression, class, size, and other less obvious factors . . . they share a special history, culture and role in Black life, all of which attest to their collective identity as the Black church." The Black church is made up of seven Black American Protestant denominations that had their origins in slavery and emancipation (Harris, 2010).

Box 15.1. Seven Black Christian Denominations

African Methodist Episcopal Church (AME)

African Methodist Episcopal Zion Church (AMEZ)

Christian Methodist Episcopal Church (CME)

National Baptist Convention USA, Incorporated (NBC)

National Baptist Convention of America, Unincorporated (NBCA)

Progressive National Baptist Convention (PNBC)

Church of God in Christ (COGIC)

Black churches range in size from small congregations meeting in homes or a rented space to mega-churches with thousands of members. New denominations of Christian churches with Black leadership continue to develop, and these new houses of worship tend to model themselves after traditional Black churches (Harris, 2010).

As early as 1903 intellectual leader W. E. B. Du Bois wrote about the dominant role of the church in Black culture, as did sociological scholar E. Franklin Frazier during the civil rights movement in 1964 (Harris, 2010). Since the time of slavery, churches have provided the African-American community a foundation for spiritual growth, political and civic activity, and social cohesion (Lindley et al., 2010). The church has historically fought for equality for Blacks and has played a key role in promoting racial awareness, well-being, and social service provision (Harris, 2010). It is often the first place where comfort is sought (Swartz, 2002).

The African-American church possesses many strengths that have allowed it to maintain its influence in the community. One strength is the diversity of the parishioners, who come from all age ranges and social strata. Another strength is a high level of stability in many Black churches; parishioners are often longstanding members. Furthermore, church members attend services frequently, and often participate in outreach activities to the larger African-American community (Berkley-Patton et al., 2010). These assets position the Black church to extend the reach of HIV prevention and care services to parts of the community that would otherwise go under or unserved (Berkley-Patton et al., 2010).

The African-American pastor or priest serves the community as a teacher, preacher, politician, and, increasingly, as a change agent for health (Francis, Lam, Cance, & Hogan, 2009). Given the importance of the Black church in the community, however, it has the potential to play a much larger role in health promotion and disease prevention than it has played to date (Smith, Simmons, & Mayer, 2005). African-American ministers are in a unique position to "affect knowledge, attitudes, beliefs, and behaviors within their congregations. Through their personal linkages to community members, clergy are often able to get their message across without encountering the resistance that other . . . [community workers] might experience" (Swartz, 2002, p. 3). Community members often view church leaders as reliable sources of information and support; these leaders also have close contact with disenfranchised groups.

Any discussion including the concept of "the Black Church" would be incomplete without acknowledging that it is a dishonest notion to suggest that in all ways "the Black Church" is a single entity. There is great diversity within the African-American faith community and African-American churches. There are scores of new denominations, worship houses, mosques, and other types of places to gather to practice one's faith. There are Black Catholics, Episcopalians, Mormons, Pentecostals, Jews, Muslims, Quakers, Methodists, Inter-denominationalists, nondenominationalists, and the Nation of Islam (Gant, in review). And, there is diversity in venues, from small rural churches, to mega-churches, and African-American televangelist ministries. Still, African-American faith communities have generally been unified in their support of issues of social justice and are therefore important considerations for inclusion in efforts to stem the tide of destruction caused by HIV in Black communities.

The Black Churches and HIV

One of the reasons cited for the high rates of HIV in the Black community is the community's slow response in addressing the virus (Harris, 2010). Scholars have noted that Black churches did not immediately respond on a broad scale to the AIDS pandemic because the Black community did not consider AIDS an issue that required a response. Harris (2010, p. 24) has cited research demonstrating that "sensitive issues of sex, sexuality, and drug use were difficult for many Blacks—particularly religious leaders—to discuss openly." In the 1980s and 1990s, most Black churches, as well as churches and houses of faith in other parts of the broader community, either ignored or actively condemned those who were HIV positive or living with AIDS (Harris, 2010). Nevertheless, some African Americans mobilized early in the pandemic, although their efforts were not large or coordinated, compared to the efforts of the gay and lesbian communities. In the early days of AIDS, a small number of African-American churches, synagogues, and other Black religious institutions organized clothing drives, food pantries, and even housing for those suffering from AIDS. However, to date the Black response has lacked the large-scale mobilizations by the NAACP (National Association for the Advancement of Colored People) seen during the civil rights movement. Nevertheless, a leader in the United Methodist Church and an expert on the relationship between religion and health has called the current rate of HIV disease a threat to civil rights. He notes that high HIV rates mandate Black churches to act as a liberating institution on a level consistent with its civil rights movement history (Hatcher et al., 2008).

> ### Box 15.2. Speaking about HIV/AIDS
>
> Those of us who understand that God has called us to serve and not judge see this as an opportunity to serve our community and help people in need, regardless of their individual circumstances. When the church speaks, people listen, and when the church speaks about HIV/AIDS, permission is given to Christians to address this growing concern.
>
> —Bishop T. D. Jakes, 2007, pastor of the Potter's House,
> a Black megachurch in Dallas, Texas (in Sagle, 2007, p. 17)

Since HIV is spread though behaviors that some religious leaders consider to be immoral, people living with HIV or AIDS (PLWHA) are sometimes thought of as "deserving what they get" or "receiving their punishment from God" (Harris, 2010, p. 25). In 1992, early in the second decade of the pandemic, a survey of Black clergy found that 35 percent of respondents believed HIV/AIDS was a curse from God (Hatcher et al., 2008). However, less than a decade later, in 2000, a survey of ministers found that a majority of respondents believed HIV/AIDS was among the top issues in which the Black church should be involved (Hatcher et al., 2008). Still, conservative beliefs about HIV risk factors continue to permeate Black culture, leading individual church members who may desire to engage in HIV health promotion to experience conflict between their wish to help out and their concern about potential stigmatization (Hatcher et al., 2008). Some may also have internal conflicts over theology and "WWJD: What Would Jesus Do."

Barriers to Involvement of the Black Church in HIV/AIDS Education and Services: The Biblical Position on Homosexuality

---

Box 15.3. Marvin McMickle on HIV/AIDS

Does the fact that some people may have contracted HIV/AIDS through homosexual acts constitute a sufficient reason for the Black church, or any faith community for that matter, to refuse to respond to this issue with anything other than judgment and condemnation? Does the fact that people with HIV/AIDS may have engaged in behaviors that some church people may find objectionable at best and immoral at worst serve as sufficient reason to turn away from those people and ignore this problem? At the moment, the answer to that question seems to be yes. Many in the church, including many who stand behind the pulpit, seem to be saying that if you contract this deadly disease because you engaged in "sinful behavior," then "you reap what you sow."

—McMickle (2008, p. 67)

A 2010 survey by Harris of a sample of twenty-eight Black church leaders in New York City found that they initially had trouble confronting AIDS in the Black community because they were unable to confront homosexuality and sexual issues. A local AIDS activist said, "I think most people—most churches did not respond in the early days because they did not know what . . . HIV was. The national public media, public health put it out there that it was a gay disease, a gay White disease, . . . and the Church, historically, has not been homosexual affirming so that was a turnoff right there" (Harris, 2010, p. 31).

Two respondents in the Harris study held steadfast to the claim that homosexuality is a sin. The Biblical passages that most religious leaders refer to in justifying their condemnation of homosexuality are from the Old Testament book of Leviticus: "Thou shalt not lie with mankind, as with womankind; it is an abomination" (Leviticus 18:22); and "If a man also lie with mankind, as he lieth with a woman, both of them have committed an abomination: they shall surely be put to death; their blood shall be upon them" (Leviticus 20:13).

One Harris study respondent provided a quote that illustrates the adage, "Love the sinner, but hate the sin." He distinguished being "welcoming of" from being "affirming of" gay members in their African-American church: "We hold very firm to the Bible. Now we are not going to beat somebody over the head with it.

We are a church. . . . We are welcoming to everybody that comes to the church. However, we are not going to yield on our Biblical foundation and what the Bible says. I would say that if a person comes to our church [who] is gay or lesbian, they will be welcomed into the congregation. . . . There is not going to be affirming of that lifestyle. . . . But we are welcoming of whoever comes here" (Harris, 2010, p. 32).

Still, heterosexist attitudes continue to predominate in the Black church, as illustrated by this quote from an African-American AIDS activist in New York City: "[Churches] still associate HIV with homosexuality. They believe that homosexuality causes AIDS. They believe that myth, that fact, that lie. And they hate homosexuals. They just absolutely hate homosexuals, so they connect their hatred of a group of people to this dreaded disease and of course they are misguided. . . . Folks cannot get past their theological position on homosexuality, and if you can't get past that, you can't address HIV because HIV has nothing to do with homosexuality" (Harris, 2010, p. 32).

Box 15.4. Definitions

Homophobia is the irrational fear of or aversion to homosexuality (same-sex sexuality) or homosexuals (gay men and lesbians). For example, verbal or physical gay-bashing is homophobia.

Heterosexism is the belief that any nonheterosexual form of behavior, identity, or relationship is not normal and should be stigmatized. For example, support for a ban on gay marriage is heterosexism.

Sexual prejudice is a new term used to reflect antigay attitudes and behaviors. The term does not assume that antigay attitudes are irrational or evil, but they are a specific type of prejudice, such as that involving race or age.

Discomfort with Sexual Deviance

It seems that it is not AIDS as an illness that some people struggle to address, but rather issues related to sexuality. Research suggests that some within the Black community perceive same-sex sexuality to be White deviant behavior that has infiltrated the Black community (Griffin, 2006). Some argue that much of the homophobia in the Black community rests in the belief that homosexuality is a result of European influences during slavery. Some contend that Black lesbian and gay church members have to remain closeted because any notion of sexual deviance must be denied or silenced. Although the Black church is not unique in its opposition to free expression of sexuality, the reasons for the opposition may be unique. Studies suggest that opposition to free expression of sexuality originated with the dehumanization of Blacks during slavery, when a great deal of focus was placed on Black sexuality and the Black body (Douglas, 2003). Blacks were portrayed as hypersexed, without intellect, morals, or decency (Harris, 2010). There is a contention that postslavery, to distance itself from the negative stereotypes of Black sexuality, the Black community embraced a very conservative stance toward sex and "deviant" sexuality, including premarital sex, extramarital sex, pregnancies outside of marriage, and especially same-sex sexuality. Douglas (2003) argues that the Black church criticized all forms of sexual depravity as a way of freeing the Black community from the White oppressors and proving that Blacks and their sexuality were legitimate. Furthermore, in continuing efforts to gain self-respect through "proper conduct," Black churches have tried to separate themselves from all deviant behavior, including alcohol consumption, drug use, and, at one time, even dancing (Harris, 2010).

Lack of Acknowledgement of High-Risk Community Members.   Another apparent barrier to engagement of the Black church in HIV/AIDS–related work is lack of awareness of high-risk members in churches. A 2005 survey of eighteen African-American ministers in Rhode Island found that the ministers as a whole did not report serving a high-risk congregation, nor did they acknowledge the significant numbers of intravenous drug users and men who have sex with men (MSM) among their membership (Smith et al., 2005). Only three of the eighteen reported having any MSM members, and only two reported having any intravenous drug users in their congregations. When asked about the need for HIV-prevention services in their church's neighborhood, 78 percent of the ministers believed there was a need, but only 11 percent reported providing or helping in some way to facilitate the provision of HIV-related services in their community.

Lack of Financial Resources for HIV/AIDS Ministries or Programs

Harris (2010) has noted that financial strain appears to be the "largest obstacle to true AIDS awareness and education within Black communities and churches" (p. 38). Similarly, Smith and colleagues (2005, p. 1684) found that the reasons why the Black church leaders that participated in their study did not offer HIV/AIDS services were linked to scarce financial resources rather than issues of morality: "While some churches cited opposition to homosexuality and promiscuity as reasons for not offering HIV/AIDS prevention programming, these did not emerge as the dominant reasons for not offering HIV/AIDS services."

Multiplicity of "Isms"

African-American church congregations must deal with multiple "isms," such as racism, classism, and elitism, as well as unemployment, poverty, and limited access to health care. These interlocking systems of oppression are contributors to the practice of risky HIV-related behaviors such as unprotected sex, substance or alcohol use, and injection drug use (Hicks et al., 2005). In the face of so many systems of oppression, the fight against HIV/AIDS can get lost. Church leaders may assume that if they speak against the multiple systems of oppression they do not need to address HIV specifically. Focusing energy on a single health-related threat may even be considered an unaffordable luxury. Thus, the church's response may be holistic, but can seem to ignore the major issue of HIV prevention and care.

AIDS-Related Stigma

The CDC has defined AIDS-related stigma as prejudice, discounting, discrediting, and discrimination against people perceived to have HIV/AIDS, particularly gay men and injection drug users. This stigma has long been a significant impediment to HIV-prevention efforts, especially in the African-American community. The stigma has been a barrier not only to HIV testing for African Americans, but also for those who know they are HIV positive. The stigma is a barrier to disclosure of HIV status, seeking medical treatment, and adhering to their antiretroviral (ARV) treatments (Lindley et al., 2010). Widespread AIDS-related stigma can also validate a pattern of "victim blaming," which is the belief that infected individuals are responsible for their illness and therefore do not deserve help. Religious institutions can reinforce this belief.

Box 15.5. Self-Test: Do You Stigmatize People with AIDS?

- Suppose you had a young child who was attending school with a child who has been diagnosed with AIDS. How comfortable would you be? Would you encourage your child to befriend the other child?

- Suppose you worked at an office where a man working closely with you developed AIDS. How comfortable would you be continuing to work with him?

- Suppose you knew the deli clerk at your local grocery store had AIDS. Would you allow that clerk to cut your deli meats?

- Suppose a friend gave you a beautiful sweater that was nearly new. You loved to wear it, then later found out it had once belonged to a person who died of AIDS. How would you feel about wearing the sweater?

- Have you ever wondered if you could get HIV from a public toilet? From a drinking glass?

- Do you think it would be helpful if local health departments published a list of names of people who have tested HIV positive?

- Suppose you learned that your minister was HIV positive. Would this impact your opinion of the person?

- Suppose a friend said that he believed that if people get AIDS from sex or drug use they get what they deserve. How would you respond?

- Do you think the ban on immigrants with HIV should be reinstated?

- Suppose someone you know saw you taking an HIV quick-test at an HIV-prevention event. Would you be embarrassed?

- Would you date a person who has HIV?

Visit www.AIDSstigma.net. There you will find a complete list of AIDS stigma survey items. The website also contains information that is helpful in combating AIDS stigma in yourself and those you know.

Types of HIV/AIDS-Related Interventions Facilitated by the Black Church

While the involvement of African-American churches in HIV/AIDS is far from ideal, progress is being made. The African-American faith community reports a number of long-standing initiatives to work on HIV prevention and risk reduction, and to care for people living with HIV/AIDS, as well as numerous newer initiatives.

These initiatives vary from programs that focus on individuals and small groups, to education programs that are church wide and community wide, as well as advocacy efforts. Some well-known and some less-publicized approaches are briefly described below to illustrate the variety of avenues available for intervention.

The Balm in Gilead

The Balm in Gilead, Inc., is a leader in the education of African-American clergy across the nation; this organization focuses on increasing clergy's involvement in HIV prevention and education in their churches and neighborhoods (Hatcher et al., 2008). Founded twenty years ago, The Balm in Gilead is an international non-governmental organization with offices in Richmond, Virginia, and Dar es Salaam, Tanzania. The organization's mission is to "prevent disease and improve the health status of people of the African Diaspora by providing support to faith institutions in the areas of program design, implementation and evaluation which strengthens their capacity to deliver programs and services that contribute to the elimination of health disparities" (The Balm in Gilead, 2010). The organization's efforts focus on elimination of HIV/AIDS, but they also address cervical cancer, diabetes, and other health conditions disproportionately affecting African Americans. In a 2005 interview, CEO and founder Pernessa C. Seele explained the impetus for starting the organization: "In 1989, the [African American] church was being devastated by HIV. . . . People were saying the church didn't want to deal with it—the church didn't know how to deal with it. Putting AIDS education into a context of prayer, into a context of something that was culturally and spiritually appropriate, opened the door for the faith community to start addressing HIV and AIDS" (McKnight, 2005, p. 72).

> **Box 15.6. National Black HIV/AIDS Awareness Day**
>
> National Black HIV/AIDS Awareness Day is held on February 7 of every year. Visit www.blackaidsday.org for information on events in your area.

Seele notes that the major problem of AIDS is stigma, and at the core of this is the belief that AIDS comes from sin. She believes that the stigma of AIDS "stops people from getting information, getting treatment, and giving or getting care" (McKnight, 2005, p. 72). She believes the need to dismantle the stigma is the fundamental reason for getting the faith community involved.

The Balm in Gilead offers a wide range of programs. In 2005, the organization started the Denominational Leadership Health Initiative, which works with three historical Black Methodist denominations. The program provides ongoing training and technical support to health coordinators at various levels of the denominations, to ensure that they are fully engaged and providing quality health education and disease prevention to congregations and communities (The Balm in Gilead, 2010).

The organization also offers the HealthShare website to congregations that affiliate; this is an interactive faith- and health-focused website offering on-line training, discussion boards, and webinars. A study by Hicks and colleagues in 2005 concluded that a major barrier to providing HIV/AIDS–related education and services is that the pastors are not equipped to speak on these issues. One pastor interviewed in the Hicks and colleagues (2005, p. 194) study said, "The Black preacher/priest does not know it all. Because we have this title does not mean that we have the answers to all these issues. Many [churches] will have to bring in experts who are more informed about specific issues so that the community is better educated, including the pastor or faith leader." The HealthShare website is a cost-effective and convenient way to deliver expert health advice and training for African-American church leaders, volunteers, and congregants.

A major focus of The Balm in Gilead is to use the power of prayer to effect change in the HIV/AIDS rate in the African-American community. Beginning with the Harlem Week of Prayer, Pernessa Seele has engaged Harlem's Christian, Muslim, Jewish, and other faith communities in attracting national attention to the urgent need to enlist the African-American faith community in the fight against HIV/AIDS. The Balm in Gilead now organizes the National Week of Prayer for the Healing of HIV/AIDS each March. President Barack Obama has recognized the event, affirming, "Although we have made great strides in the fight against HIV/AIDS, our battle is far from over" (The Balm in Gilead, 2010). The organization also has available "E-worship books" that include prayers for healing of HIV and acceptance and understanding of those suffering with AIDS. For example, one prayer goes as follows:

O God, we confess our sin in the midst of HIV and AIDS. . . . We have silenced those who live with AIDS and HIV. And when their ailments become visible, we have removed them from our midst to hospitals, to hospices and to the streets.

How many more people have to be stricken before we get it that HIV/AIDS is not going to go away just because we ignore them? How many more must die? How many more orphans and widows? . . . Interrupt our silences with your Spirit. Our denial ends so that we can become part of the solution instead of part of the problem.

A special prayer is included for the gay Christian:

God, I am tired of always being hidden, of our rights being disregarded. You may know me and love me but the church is hiding the truth. God, you know . . . that I'm gay, but the church doesn't want to admit it, and I'm tired of waiting.

The Balm in Gilead offers advice on their website on how to develop sermons on HIV and AIDS. Written by Reverend Dr. James Forbes, Jr., of the Riverside Church in New York City, the site advises that preachers consider using the following Biblical passages: Luke 10:25–37 (the good Samaritan); Matthew 7:7–12 (the golden rule); John 9:1–7 (sin and blame); and John 13:31–35 (love one another).

The Balm in Gilead also coordinates Our Church Lights the Way: The National Faith-Based HIV Testing Campaign, which is designed to mobilize Christian leaders, especially those serving African Americans, to "speak loudly from their pulpits" and encourage every person in their congregation to get tested for HIV. The organization encourages churches to coordinate with the local health department or ASO to hold an on-site testing event.

The Balm in Gilead is a national advocacy group that provides a wide variety of resources and guidance to faith communities so that they can tailor interventions to the needs of their congregation and community. The interventions described below represent approaches that are more localized.

Project F.A.I.T.H.

In January 2006, "Project F.A.I.T.H. (Fostering AIDS Initiatives That Heal) was established to reduce the stigma of HIV and AIDS among African Americans in South Carolina. The project funded churches with the goal of providing HIV-related programs and services to both their congregations and communities. In the project's first year, twenty-two churches received funds" (Lindley et al., 2010, p. 12). The aims of Project F.A.I.T.H. are to reduce stigmatizing attitudes among church members, and to provide needed services to those at risk.

Gospel Against AIDS

Since 1997, Gospel Against AIDS has operated with a mission to "empower religious leaders to become change agents in their communities of faith by equipping them to provide on-site preventive education, technical assistance and outreach support to those infected and affected by HIV/AIDS" (Gospel Against AIDS, 2003). The nonprofit organization is based in Detroit, Michigan, but has a service area that covers the major cities of the state and region. They provide "HIV 101" training and technical assistance for groups with a desire to start programs focused on HIV prevention from a faith-based perspective. They have interfaced with a wide variety of groups and communities, including schools, universities, hospitals, correctional facilities, sororities and fraternities, and for-profit businesses. They have translated their curriculum into multiple languages and distributed it internationally.

Black Church Outreach Project

In Austin, Texas, the Black Church Outreach Project is working to increase awareness of the continued spread of HIV/AIDS in the African-American community. The program has been successful in reaching a population that is "historically inaccessible, unreceptive, and unresponsive to current prevention efforts" (Runnels, 2011, Overview). The approaches that this program uses include community forums, educational workshops, and invited speakers.

Metropolitan Community Foundation

In 1997, the Metropolitan Community Church of San Francisco, located in the primarily gay community of The Castro, established the Metropolitan Community Foundation as a secular, 501(c) 3 nonprofit CBO to address the AIDS epidemic. As an epicenter of the AIDS pandemic, San Francisco experienced the "profound and tragic effects" of AIDS beginning as early as 1983. The first known death of a church member from AIDS occurred in 1983, and it is estimated that at least 500 more members of this church have died in the decades since. During the peak of the crisis, it was not uncommon to see "three or four funerals on each day of the weekend, and rapid growth in church membership could barely keep pace with the rate of deaths." In the 1980s, "even in the midst of this virtually unbearable period, the church persevered, with fellow members supporting one another during the most painful times" (Metropolitan Community Church of San Francisco, 2012). The Metropolitan Community Church's saying, "We are the body of Christ, and we have AIDS," still motivates people living with HIV and AIDS; the congregation and the associated foundation continue to be recognized as the vanguard of advocacy efforts for people with HIV and AIDS, not only for the primarily gay community in The Castro of San Francisco, but for the gay community nationwide. This faith-based example of proactive AIDS advocacy and outreach is not part of the African-American church, but shows how other faith communities have been and continue to be instrumental in a community-level (and broader) response.

Recommendations for Practice

The following are tips offered in the literature and by the authors for developing and carrying out interventions on behalf of or in collaboration with African American or other faith-based organizations.

Recognize the Church's Level of Readiness

The social work adage of "meet them where they are" holds true when approaching a faith-based organization about partnering to reach members of the African-American community with messages and services related to HIV/AIDS. Berkley-Patton and colleagues (2010, p. 233) recommend "meeting churches at their level of readiness." Those authors note that a safe environment should be fostered where people can discuss their Biblical and personal beliefs about condom use, sex outside of marriage, abstinence for youth, homosexuality, and other controversial topics. Griffith, Campbell, Ober Allen, Robinson, and Kretman Stewart (2010) suggest that rather than excluding churches and ministers who are seen as conservative, social workers should make efforts to find and cultivate areas of agreement. Trust that eventually community awareness will lead to community action, though it may not happen overnight.

Be Culturally Competent

The study by Hicks and colleagues (2005) quoted a Black pastor in Washington, DC, as criticizing local ASOs for not aligning their message and programs with non-White communities. ASOs are already fighting the myth that AIDS is a gay White man's disease. And social workers responsible for programming should make concerted efforts to ensure that programs are relevant to the communities where new infections are occurring, whether these are Black, Hispanic, or other types of communities. If a faith-based organization is reaching out to people in same-sex relationships, the organization should let these people know they will not be judged if they seek services. A respondent in the Hicks and colleagues (2005) study said that since LGBTQ (lesbian, gay, bisexual, transgender, and questioning) is not a common term used in communities of color, the CDC uses the terms MSM and WSW (women who have sex with women) to describe behaviors, rather than identifying people based on labels. Hicks et al. (2005, p. 193) suggest the term "same gender loving people" (Hicks et al., 2005, p. 193) as more accepting.

Ministers interested in being culturally competent should acknowledge that "preaching hellfire and damnation" is not the way to win converts or teach them about HIV (Swartz, 2002, p. 2). Likewise, if staff at ASOs and other CBOs want to engage with members of the faith community—ministers and congregants alike—they must learn their language and not offend with positions that demean or do not acknowledge the importance of faith and spirituality. Much has been written about cultural competence in practicing social work with African Americans. Much less has been written about being sensitive to faith and religion, yet resources are available for social workers to increase their competence.

Characterize HIV and AIDS Outreach as Ministry

People of faith are united in a common desire to serve. The lack of engagement of many Black congregations in HIV and AIDS prevention, education, and outreach may be in part due to the fact that these activities have not been recognized as a legitimate form of service "unto the Lord." A Black pastor in Washington, DC, was quoted (Hicks et al., 2005, p. 194) as saying that "There is a general fear . . . and people don't want to be associated with 'sinners', which further expands the community's silence around [HIV, AIDS, and sexuality]." The Black church follows a Christian doctrine based on Biblical principles. Christianity can be seen as focusing on a message of following Jesus' example of service and love. Rather than focusing on institutional rules or taboos, the ministry of service calls for followers to ask themselves, "What would Jesus do?" Jesus often performed unpopular tasks and communicated with and served unpopular people of his time (Hicks et al., 2005). Some have called AIDS the modern day leprosy. Jesus did not avoid outreach to those whose behaviors or ailments were seen as outside of the mainstream. Framing the call for mobilization of the African-American faith community to fight HIV in the Black community as a part of crucial ministry and service may help to engage a larger number of churches.

Approach Churches with a Broad-Based Tool Bag

Interventions all along the micro-, mezzo-, and macro-level spectrum have been shown to be effective in engaging the faith community in HIV and AIDS education and outreach. It is advisable for social workers who cultivate the involvement of the faith community to have a long list of options. If one avenue is blocked, the social worker can suggest another immediately. Different houses of faith may present different barriers to involvement in the fight against AIDS. Below are ways that a church can become involved. Suggesting multiple options increases the chances that one option will be acceptable to the church decision-makers.

- Have HIV-prevention and education materials available at the church.

- Distribute condoms and lubricants at the church, or if not at the church, have the church use its influence in the community to arrange for distribution at other key sites in the community.

- Hold a prayer service for those lost to AIDS, for the many needs of those living with AIDS and HIV, and for prayers of protection so that others will not be infected or affected.

- Have the pastor mention AIDS and HIV from the pulpit, but not only in relation to Africa.

- Have the pastor preach a message about safe sex, same-sex sexuality, and openness about sexual issues.

- Ask the church to advertise AIDS-related services or ASO fundraisers in the materials distributed at services.

- Ask the pastoral staff to reach out to other ministers in the community and build a coalition of churches united in the fight against AIDS.

- Host an HIV testing event at the church.

- Help to infuse AIDS awareness in the list of goals for the ministerial alliance in the community, if one exists.

- Allocate a portion of the church's mission budget to local HIV/AIDS services.

- Conduct a food drive or establish a permanent food pantry for people with HIV or AIDS.

- Be open and nonjudgmental during pastoral counseling sessions and listen to church members discuss HIV/AIDS or other topics related to sexuality.

- Hold support groups for special populations, such as those living with HIV, those living with AIDS, and those affected by HIV/AIDS (friends, family, caregivers).

- Become an affiliate of the nonprofit organization The Balm in Gilead, or participate in their National Week of Prayer for the Healing of HIV/AIDS each March.

- Recognize February 7 as National Black HIV/AIDS Awareness Day.

- Form a program targeting youth to teach about sexuality, safe sex, HIV/STD prevention, and reduction of high-risk behaviors.

- Infuse HIV-related material into the women's ministry, with an emphasis on how the pandemic is affecting African-American women.

- Infuse sexual risk and HIV-related material into the seniors' ministry, citing examples of how seniors are at risk because of lack of experience with safe sex practices and lack of recognition of risky behaviors.

- Use the pastor's relationships with local political stakeholders to educate policymakers and legislators about epidemiological trends in HIV and AIDS in the region, pointing out which groups are disproportionately affected.

- Enlist the help of the wife of the pastor (the "first lady," in a traditional Black church) to influence and educate community leaders.

- Form a speakers bureau of people with first-hand experiences to speak about the impacts of HIV and AIDS in the Black and larger communities.

- Organize an AIDS walk, or walk as a group in an established community AIDS walk.

- Develop a comprehensive program for meeting the needs of people with HIV or AIDS in the church and local community.

- Support the legislative efforts of the National Black Leadership Commission on AIDS.

- Ask the pastoral team to brainstorm about ideas on how they can be a part of the solution to the AIDS crisis in the Black community.

- If barriers exist to all of the above, as a first step, ask the pastoral staff to pray for people with HIV or AIDS in the community and to be open at a later date to infusing an HIV/AIDS theme into their ministries.

Box 15.7. National Black Leadership Commission on AIDS

The National Black Leadership Commission on AIDS, founded in 1987, is a nonprofit organization with a mission to "educate, organize, and empower Black leaders, including clergy, elected officials, medical practitioners, business professionals, social policy experts, and the media, to meet the challenge of fighting HIV/AIDS and other health disparities in their local communities." The signature legislative proposal of NBLCA is The National Black Clergy for the Elimination of HIV/AIDS Act of 2009, which is a comprehensive proposal for fighting AIDS in the Black community. National Black Leadership Commission on AIDS is actively seeking more co-sponsors for the bill, which are needed to get a legislative hearing and send it to the floors of the House and Senate.

The highlights of initiatives called for in the bill are these (Globe-Newswire, 2010, para. 8):

✓ Calls for voluntary, routine HIV testing as part of all health exams, including those in emergency rooms, clinics, and private physician offices;

✓ Calls upon the President to declare HIV/AIDS an epidemic in the Black community;

✓ Directs the U.S. Department of Health and Human Services to make grants to public health agencies and faith-based organizations to conduct outreach programs for HIV/AIDS testing and prevention;

✓ Directs the U.S. Health and Human Services Department to expand and intensify educational activities targeting Black women, youth and men having sex with men;

✓ Mandates a national media outreach program to urge testing for HIV and AIDS; and

✓ Requires a study of biological and behavioral factors that lead to higher rates of HIV and AIDS among Black Americans.

As always, remember to set achievable goals and to celebrate small steps of progress. Social work practice is based on the importance and primacy of human relationships. Work toward cultivating long-term alliances with persons of influence in key churches in the community. As the number of key supporters in the African-American faith community grows, the larger community will become more aware of opportunities to address the AIDS crisis. As momentum grows, community awareness leads to community action.

Lessons from Africa

To do nothing can lead to destruction. To wait for help from the larger community may bring help too late. What has happened in Sub-Saharan Africa teaches the lesson that the leadership in the community must quickly address AIDS or that community will be ravaged by the disease. Consider Uganda. This was one of the first countries in Sub-Saharan Africa to be hit hard by the pandemic of what was called "slim disease." Rather than wait for help from the West, the president of Uganda authorized a major HIV-prevention campaign. At the same time, a grassroots organization called The AIDS Support Organization, or TASO (www.tasouganda.org), developed a comprehensive and timely response. The goal was to educate the public about how to avoid becoming infected, promoting the ABC (Abstain, Be faithful, use Condoms) model. While other regions of the continent were denying the problem, as early as 1987 Uganda was active with the ABC prevention message, though they were not giving much attention to care for those already infected. From 2000 to 2005, the prevalence of HIV stabilized in Uganda while other Sub-Saharan countries experienced increases. There is some debate, however, about whether the decrease in the number of citizens living with HIV was due to the effectiveness of the ABC model or to the fact that many people had already died of HIV. The most recent statistics show a slight increase in cases of HIV in Uganda since 2006. Interestingly, it was about 2006 that the United States introduced free AIDS medications and shifted the focus from a complete sex education message to "abstinence only" approaches. Some claim that risky behaviors are on the rise as a result of the lack of condom promotion. Some have even suggested that the wide availability of AIDS medications has changed the perception of HIV—from a death sentence to a manageable condition, reducing fear and increasing high-risk behaviors (AVERT, 2010).

Regardless of how one interprets the history of HIV/AIDS in Uganda, most would agree that the story of AIDS in that country shows that strong leadership, commitment, and early response are crucial to turning the tide on the rapid and deadly spread of the virus. Translated to Black churches in the United States and the soaring rates of HIV infection in Black communities, the message is that more vocal leadership is urgently needed from the group who historically has led the fight for social justice for African Americans.

Conclusion

> ### Box 15.8. Lazarus, the Beggar
>
> If [each church is willing to light one small candle], Lazarus will no longer be overlooked by church folk who are so busy dressing themselves in purple and eating sumptuously every day that they give no thought, devote no time, and direct no resources to a major problem that sits right outside their door. If churches in communities all across America light one small candle, it will be said instead that Lazarus is now being looked after and loved by the people of God, who are concerned about and caring for their neighbors and friends who are infected and affected by HIV/AIDS.
>
> —McMickle (2008, p. 136, based on Luke 16:19–31)

An interview with a former leader of a large Episcopal church in Harlem (Harris, 2010, p. 29) found that the hard work of the Black churches there has had an impact in the region. "Today, right now as we speak, in Harlem, there is not one major church, not one, that does not have some kind of AIDS program. . . . We've just turned the circle completely from night to day."

Case Example

The following composite case illustrates the challenges faced by many local ASOs, as well as by the leadership in Black churches.

Mary McKinley walks into her office at Healthy Living Center and opens the blinds to allow the warmth of the sun to come in. Her assistant gives her the morning messages and she settles in to start her day. Healthy Living Center, a nonprofit agency, provides outreach and education to the community around areas of reproductive health. The Center also has a clinic that provides low-cost reproductive health screenings, free HIV testing, brochures about safe sex, and female and male condoms. Healthy Living Center is located on the northeast side of Simon, Georgia, surrounded by a major university and many up-and-coming businesses, and it is close to a major highway. Mary, a Caucasian social worker with a bachelor's degree, has worked at this agency for eight years and serves as the agency's faith-based outreach director. She provides health education and prevention services to houses of worship in the surrounding community of Simon. This quiet and picturesque town boasts a population of 35,000 and is located fifteen miles from the large metropolitan area of Rose, Georgia. She attends a large nondenominational Christian church in Rose, and enjoys the works she does at the agency. Her agency recently received a grant for a program to target the African-American community, a segment of the population that Healthy Living Center has not targeted in the past.

Mary sifts through her messages and is disappointed that she does not see one from the church she has been trying to reach for the past three weeks, Greater Mount Ethel Baptist Church. This church has deep roots in the community and served as a hub for community organizing during the civil rights movement. Church members were very active in sit-ins and protests, and the church building served as a central meeting location for organizing efforts. This small congregation was able to confront discrimination practices by community leaders and push for change in local laws.

According to his secretary, Pastor Adolphus R. Gates of Greater Mount Ethel Baptist Church has been in meeting after meeting and has not had a chance to get back to Mary. Pastor Gates grew up and still resides in the small town of Simon, where his church is located. He has been married for twenty-one years to Thelma; they have two children together. He adores his small congregation of approximately 250 members. Though small in numbers, the church is heavily rooted in the local African-American community: most members have lived all their lives in this small town and are committed to seeing it thrive through, "the love of the Lord."

Greater Mount Ethel has five main ministries: a very active youth ministry offering a place for youth to hang out rather than being pulled into negative behavior; a missionary circle whose purpose is to visit the sick, feed the hungry, and look out for the needs of the downtrodden; a health ministry that asserts that a healthy life is a life in line with God's vision for his people; a music ministry that delivers the word of God through Christ-centered music; and a Christian education arm to foster members' growth in their faith and knowledge of God.

Pastor Gates reads through the messages his secretary left for him and notices that once again, Mary, from Healthy Living Center, has called. "Why won't she just leave me alone?" he thinks. He stares at the message sheet and the four other messages she has left that are lying on his desk. He doesn't understand the pressure she is putting on him to incorporate an AIDS outreach ministry in his church. They already have a health ministry that has an information station in the vestibule and the church holds an annual "Sunday of Health and Wellness," which he thinks should be enough. They are a small church in a community that is suffering financially and the church is experiencing the same economic crunch. There is barely enough money to print worship service programs every Sunday, let alone brochures and pamphlets for an AIDS program. Besides, his parishioners, many of whom have been with his church for years, are not experiencing HIV/AIDS in proportionate rates to the larger population of the United States, or even the neighboring urban center of Rose. Pastor Gates agrees that HIV/AIDS is a pandemic reaching far and wide, but he thinks "HIV/AIDS is a big city issue" and things like that don't happen in his backyard. He believes firmly that the spread of HIV is due to homosexuality and that particular sinful behavior is not present in his congregation. He knows this because he preaches against it from the pulpit from time to time. He prays for the souls of those infected with HIV, but he has no idea of the number of people in his congregation or his community who are living with this virus. What Pastor Gates doesn't know is that five members of his congregation are living with HIV and two have been diagnosed with AIDS. Also, the county health department just released data that show there has been a significant spike in new HIV cases, with thirty new infections found last year. There are also two same-sex couples who attend his church, though both have made concerted efforts to keep this information private, because they are fearful of the repercussions. Pastor Gates has again rationalized his decision to do nothing, and he places the phone message in the stack with the others and hopes this lady will get the hint and not call again. HIV/AIDS is not an issue his church will tackle because the need is not great enough and the resources aren't available.

When Mary comes back from lunch she finds a voice mail message from Yolonda Craig. Yolonda identifies herself as the leader of the Health and Wellness Ministry at Greater Mount Ethel Baptist Church. She has heard through the grapevine that Mary has been trying to get in contact with the church, seeking a potential collaboration to address HIV-prevention education and testing. She leaves her phone number and asks for a return call at Mary's earliest convenience. Mary is elated that she has finally heard from this pivotal church in the community and is excited about a possible collaboration. However, after speaking in person with Yolonda, she learns that the church leadership is "not on board." Pastor Gates vehemently opposes the idea of "mentioning AIDS and condoms" from the pulpit and would like her to stop calling. Her spirits are crushed—until Yolonda tells her that although the pastor is not interested, she is. She would like to meet with Mary to formulate a plan to get him on board. Mary understands the importance of having insiders in the church who can open doors that otherwise would remain closed and potentially locked. They agree to meet later in the week to devise a plan.

After two weeks of planning, Mary suggests to Yolonda that she get the church's first lady, Thelma Gates, involved because, as the pastor's wife, she may be able to soften the blow when the information about HIV/AIDS is presented. They also believe that if they present the information to Thelma first, she will be able to help them gauge questions, comments, and concerns that the pastor may raise. This turns out to be an excellent idea. Thelma agrees to come to their meeting, listen to ways they can incorporate HIV/AIDS education into the church, and tour Mary's facility. They don't know that Thelma lost a close childhood friend to AIDS years ago. Thelma doesn't mention this, even to her husband, because she fears her friend contracted the virus by doing things that are an abomination to God. This loss motivates Thelma to help get the safe sex message out not just to the people in the community, but also and especially to her congregation.

Thelma is impressed by the agency. She has heard of Healthy Living Center, but never had a reason to visit. She is shocked when she sees clients in the lobby who to her don't "look sick." She checks in with the secretary, who escorts her to the conference room where Mary and Yolonda are waiting. The door closes behind her and the meeting begins. After two hours, their mission is accomplished. Thelma is on board and has agreed to speak with her husband on behalf of Mary and Yolonda. She also has agreed to take the initiative to coordinate a meeting with all the parties. She tells the women that this may take a while because her husband is very stubborn and set in his ways and knows this will be a struggle for him as it relates to his faith. "After twenty-one years of marriage I know the man's first answer is always 'No'. Then, after some time, I make him think it was his idea and we move to a 'Yes,'" she says with a smile. On the way out, she takes a tour of the facility, noting the high-tech equipment, welcoming employees, and atmosphere of under-standing and support. She is intrigued and begins to ask questions specific to HIV. As they talk about prevalence rates in their community and the impor-tance of getting tested, Thelma's curiosity gets the best of her. She asks Mary to show her how an HIV test is administered and volunteers to get one her-self. After the realization that the process is effortless, she is further motivated to share this information with her husband and help Mary and Yolonda with their mission.

Two weeks and several meetings later, the Sunday of Health and Wellness service has arrived. Yolonda prepares to speak with the congregation about a variety of health topics relevant to African Americans. She will staff the booth in the vestibule at the end of service to hand out literature about high blood pressure, diabetes, obesity, heart disease, and the new health topic this year, HIV/AIDS. Pastor Gates has agreed to allow Healthy Living Center to distribute their materials to his congregation. He does not agree, however, to speak specifically about the disease from the pulpit nor to actively encourage his congregation to get tested and use condoms. He also specifically prohibits Yolonda from pushing the HIV/AIDS information onto her fellow members and requests that this disease receive no more attention than the rest. As he begins his morning announcements, he takes a hard swallow and says, "Today is the start of Health and Wellness week. I want you to know that Yolonda has been working feverishly to make sure you all are educated on issues related to your health. On your way out this afternoon, please stop by the table in the vestibule to pick up pamphlets, brochures, and literature on a host of health topics."

They were not successful in incorporating an intense HIV/AIDS initiative in the church, but the dialogue has begun. Although he has allowed the infor-mation to be distributed, the pastor keeps the burden of responsibility on individuals regarding what they will do with the information, rather than placing the burden on the church as advocates and educators about this dis-ease. Although their ultimate goal had not been reached, all parties, including Thelma, are optimistic about the potential for change in the church commu-nity. Often change happens incrementally, and this is a positive first step.

The next day, Mary asks for a face-to-face meeting with Thelma at Healthy Living Center. She says she has important news to share and would like to speak with her as soon as possible. Thelma is still riding on the excitement of yesterday and is ecstatic to meet with Mary again. She plans to discuss how things went and brainstorm about ways that she can further help the faith community. Thelma arrives and walks into Mary's office. She is greeted with a big hug and Mary closes the door. As Mary begins to speak, Thelma Gates drops her head as she hears the unimaginable news. She clutches her heart, holds on to the arm of her chair, and lets out a loud shriek before the tears falls down her face. The test results for her HIV test are in: she is HIV positive.

Questions for Reflection

1. Do you identify yourself as a spiritual person? A religious person? If you attend organized services or events at a faith-based organization or place of worship, such as a church, consider whether you have ever heard any mention of HIV or AIDS in that location. Was it welcomed? If you have not heard a reference to HIV/AIDS, how might you present a prevention message at your place of worship?

2. Imagine that you have a client who attends an African-American church. Not only does he have AIDS, but he is also secretly gay. After someone sees him leaving your ASO, they "out" his status to the pastor. The pastor confronts him with hostility for his secrecy and says, "How did this happen? I hope you haven't been defiling yourself by being with a man!" How can you assist your client? Brainstorm and list various interventions you might discuss with him.

3. What is your racial or ethnic identity? Imagine that you are developing a training session on how to effectively work with members of your racial or ethnic group. What do you think should be taught? Name at least five tips for practicing with people of your population group. Are these tips valid for all members? Most members? Do any of these tips relate to religious or spiritual competence?

4. Review the list of possible approaches to involvement for churches. Identify whether each is a micro-level, mezzo-level, or macro-level intervention. Which ones do you think would have the greatest positive impact on the community? Why? Brainstorm about other ways that a local church might engage in the fight against AIDS.

5. The case example illustrates numerous themes identified throughout the chapter. Identify as many as you can. In your opinion, what could have been added or changed about the case example to make it more realistic? Why? At the end of the case example, the church's first lady, Thelma, discovers she is HIV positive. How do you think she might have gotten the virus?

References

AVERT. (2010). *HIV and AIDS in Uganda.* Retrieved from http://www.avert.org/aids-uganda.htm

Baker, S. (1999). HIV/AIDS, nurses, and the Black church: A case study. *Journal of the Association of Nurses in AIDS Care, 10*(5), 71–79.

Balm in Gilead, The, Inc. (2010). *The Balm in Gilead: Programs overview.* Retrieved from http://www.balmingilead.org/index.php/about/mission.html

Berkley-Patton, J., Bowe-Thompson, C., Bradley-Ewing, A., Hawes, S., Moore, E., Williams, E., . . . , Goggin, K. (2010). Taking it to the pews: A CBPR-guided HIV awareness and screening project with Black churches. *AIDS Education and Prevention, 22*(3), 218–237.

Centers for Disease Control and Prevention (CDC). (2010). *HIV among African Americans.* Retrieved from http://www.cdc.gov/hiv/topics/aa/

Conrad, P., & Schneider, J.W. (1992). *Deviance and medicalization: From badness to sickness.* Philadelphia: Temple University Press.

Douglas, K. (2003). *Sexuality and the Black Church: A womanist perspective.* Maryknoll: Orbis Books.

Douglas, K., & Hopson, R. (2001). Understanding the Black church: Dynamics of change. *Journal of Religious Thought, 56/57*(2-1), 95–113.

Francis, S., Lam, W., Cance, J., & Hogan, V. (2009). What's the 411? Assessing the feasibility of providing African American adolescents with HIV/AIDS prevention education in a faith-based setting. *Journal of Religion and Health, 48*, 164–177.

Francis, S., & Liverpool, J. (2009). A review of faith-based HIV prevention programs. *Journal of Religion and Health, 48*, 6–15.

Gant, L. M. (in review). And so *why* is gospel against AIDS so effective in faith communities? *Journal of National Medical Association.*

GlobeNewswire. (2010, February 5). *Clergy takes fight for HIV/AIDS legislation to Capitol Hill to mark Black AIDS Day: Policies that address AIDS' disproportionate toll on Blacks long overdue.* Retrieved from http://www.globe newswire.com/newsroom/news.html?d=183742

Gospel Against AIDS. (2003). *Gospel against AIDS: A program of hope for—and from—our community.* Retrieved from http://www.gospelaa.org/index.php

Griffin, H. (2006). *Their own received them not: African American lesbians and gays in Black churches.* Cleveland: Pilgrim Press.

Griffith, D., Campbell, B., Ober Allen, J., Robinson, K., & Kretman Stewart, S. (2010). YOUR Blessed Health: An HIV-prevention program bridging faith and public health communities. *Public Health Reports, 125,* 4–11.

Harris, A. (2010). Sex, stigma, and the Holy Ghost: The Black church and the construction of AIDS in New York City. *Journal of African American Studies, 14*(1), 21–43.

Hatcher, S., Burley, J., & Lee-Ouga, W. (2008). HIV prevention programs in the Black church: A viable health promotion resource for African American women? *Journal of Human Behavior in the Social Environment, 17*(3–4), 309–324.

Hicks, K., Allen, J., & Wright, E. (2005). Building holistic HIV/AIDS responses in African American urban faith communities: A qualitative, multiple case study analysis. *Family and Community Health, 28*(2) 184–205.

Lindley, L., Coleman, J., Gaddist, B., & White, J. (2010). Informing faith-based HIV/AIDS interventions: HIV-related knowledge and stigmatizing attitudes at Project F.A.I.T.H. churches in South Carolina. *Public Health Reports, 125,* 12–20.

Lorber, J. (1997). *Gender and the social construction of illness.* Oxford: Rowman & Littlefield.

Metropolitan Community Church of San Francisco. (2012). *History of MCC San Francisco: From a nomadic tribe to our Castro home.* Retrieved from http://www.mccsf.org/history.html

McKnight, E. (2005, June). Restoring our faith: HIV/AIDS and Black faith communities, An interview with Pernessa Seele. *Harvard Journal of African American Public Policy*, 71–77.

McMickle, M. (2008). *A time to speak: How Black pastors can respond to the HIV/AIDS pandemic.* Cleveland: Pilgrim Press.

Runnels, R. (2011). *Answered prayers: Using the Church to promote HIV/AIDS awareness, prevention, and treatment.* Texas Department of State Health Services. Retrieved from http://www.dshs.state.tx.us/hivstd/conference/2004/trackd.shtm

Sagle, D. (2007, March 28). Religious leaders think Black Church can do more to fight AIDS. *Jet, 111*(12), 16–18.

Smith, J., Simmons, E., & Mayer, K. (2005). HIV/AIDS and the Black church: What are the barriers to prevention services? *Journal of the National Medical Association, 97*(12), 1682–1685.

Swartz, A. (2002, Sept–Oct). Breaking the silence: The Black church addresses HIV. *HIV impact*: A newsletter of the Office of Minority Health, U.S. Department of Health and Human Services (DHHS), 3–4.

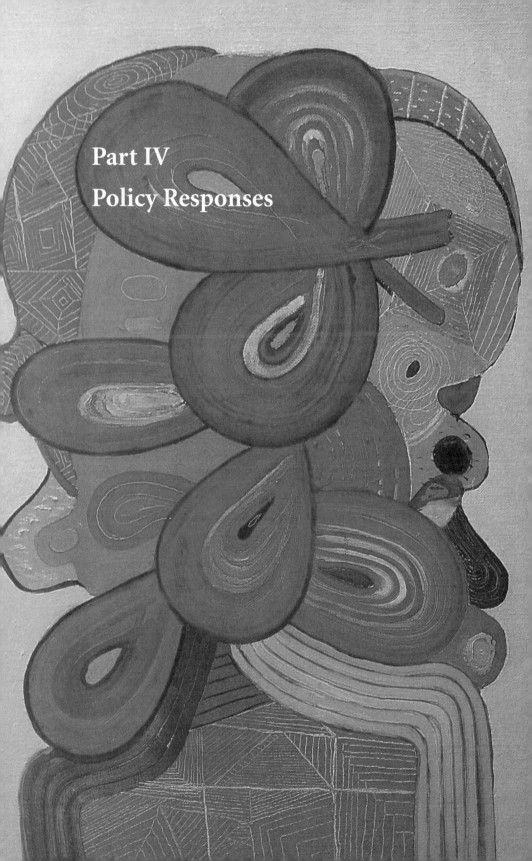

Part IV
Policy Responses

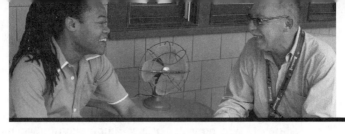

16

Housing for People Living with HIV and AIDS

Russell L. Bennett and Terry W. Ellington

> The primary and essential function of housing, to provide a safe and sheltered space, is absolutely fundamental to the people's health and well being.
>
> **—Dearbhal Murphy**

Introduction

This chapter will address why and how housing is an HIV/AIDS (human immunodeficiency virus and acquired immune deficiency syndrome) issue and the role that social workers play in ensuring that housing continues to be a critical component of care. Topics discussed in this chapter include:

- Why housing is an important HIV/AIDS issue

- A brief history of HIV/AIDS housing

- Housing needs of persons living with HIV/AIDS (PLWHA)

- Housing plus services

- Structural impacts of housing on both the micro- and macro-levels

- Current issues facing HIV/AIDS housing provision

This chapter presents two case studies to guide thinking on housing-related challenges faced by persons living with HIV/AIDS.

Why Housing?

When considering HIV/AIDS, many individuals first think of medical care. Although critical to the overall health and well-being of persons living with HIV/

AIDS, the provision of safe, decent, and affordable housing is intrinsically linked to HIV care. The question of "Why housing?" is a common question when considering the set-aside of funding specifically for HIV care. The allocation of specific resources or creation of systems solely for the care and treatment of persons living with HIV/AIDS has been termed HIV "exceptionalism." Practitioners and policy advocates alike have questioned and debated such set-asides related to HIV/AIDS specific housing. The question, however, of "Why housing for persons living with HIV/AIDS?" can be countered through the consideration of three basic housing fundamentals.

The first of these basic housing fundamentals is the supposition that housing is a basic human need. In his paper, "A Theory of Human Motivation," Abraham Maslow (1943) introduced the theory of the hierarchy of needs that posits that individuals have to fulfill basic physiological needs such food, housing, and clothing before they can address other social or individual needs. Maslow's hierarchy of needs provides a basic theoretical underpinning of social work practice and is even emphasized in the Preamble to the Code of Ethics of the National Association of Social Workers (NASW; 2008). It is important for social workers to understand that pursuing a job, getting health care, being active in the community, or conducting any other activity that one might believe is important to be engaged in society is dependent on an individual's ability to access, receive, and maintain these basic needs. Social workers must address housing as a basic condition when considering a person living with HIV/AIDS, to ensure the client will have access to care and other supports.

Based on the premise that housing meets a basic human need, the second housing fundamental is that housing is a right. In 1948, the General Assembly of the United Nations adopted the Universal Declaration of Human Rights and in it declared that "everyone has the right to a standard of living adequate for the health and well-being of himself and of his family, including food, clothing, housing and medical care and necessary social services" (United Nations [UN], 1948, Article 25). The UN declaration went beyond even the U.S. Constitution, as housing is not a protected right in the United States. Even before the federal government's increased role in housing during the Great Depression, social work pioneers were recognizing the need for safe, decent, affordable housing and its connection to health, stronger family life, and stronger communities. While these early U.S. housing policies promoted an increase in safe and decent housing for American families, the funding for the programs was not allocated. Although not addressed until later and through the development of new programs, a concern over housing affordability also began to shape U.S. housing policy during this time. Housing as a basic human right and the violations of such a right when safe, decent, and affordable housing is not available is evident when we examine the housing situations of persons living with HIV/AIDS. Furthermore, the critical connection of housing to improved health has spurred HIV/AIDS advocates to assert their own declaration on HIV/AIDS (National AIDS Housing Coalition [NAHC], 2008), which emphasizes the connection of unstable housing to an increase in HIV infection, HIV-risk behaviors, and poor health outcomes. More than sixty years after the passage of the UN declaration, many citizens in the United States, including persons living with HIV/AIDS, still are not guaranteed the right to safe, decent, and affordable housing.

> **Box 16.1. Quick Fact**
>
> The U.S. Department of Housing and Urban Development (HUD) is the federal agency designated to oversee housing policy in the United States (http://www.hud.gov).

Questions for Reflection

1. Consider the concept of "housing as a right." Do you believe all Americans have a right to a standard of living adequate to ensure safe, decent, and affordable housing? Why or why not?

2. How do your answers relate to the values of social work? To social work practice?

In considering persons living with HIV/AIDS, housing is health. This connection between housing and health represents the third housing fundamental. Housing and health have been connected in practice and research related to the effects of the type of housing, adequacy of housing, and stability of housing to health. This connection between housing and individual health speaks to a broader concept of housing, one in which housing represents a home. A home provides a safe and healthy environment for individuals to live, grow, and thrive. Over the past several years, the NAHC has conducted a series of research institutes to pull together practitioners, researchers, and policy makers to examine the linkage between housing and health (NAHC, 2010). HIV/AIDS researchers have connected stable housing to HIV prevention, access to care, maintenance of care, and improved health outcomes. Research has shown that housing is an effective intervention that improves the health and well-being of persons living with HIV/AIDS. The work of the NAHC and other policy advocates helped to spur the slogan, "Housing is health care," which speaks to the intrinsic connection between safe, decent, and affordable housing and individuals' health.

A History of HIV/AIDS Housing and the Federal Response

Box 16.2. Characteristics of Three Decades of HIV/AIDS Housing

1980s

- Local, grassroots responses
- Housing primarily emergency, intensive care, or hospice related
- No federal funding
- Lack of access to mainstream housing due to discrimination, lack of supports, or HIV-related poverty
- First antiretroviral (ARV) drug AZT released (1987)

1990s

- Passage of the Cranston-Gonzalez Housing Act includes Housing Opportunities for Persons with AIDS (HOPWA), the only federal HIV/AIDS housing program (1990).
- Passage of Ryan White Comprehensive AIDS Relief Emergency (CARE Act provides medical care to persons living with HIV/AIDS, 1990).
- HOPWA provides local and state governments first federal resources to develop community housing response (1992).
- HUD forms the Office of HIV/AIDS Housing to prioritize HIV/AIDS housing needs (1994).
- Creation of the National AIDS Housing Coalition (NAHC), first national advocacy organization dedicated to HIV/AIDS housing (1995).

- Housing programs begin to expand to include additional care and services.

- Advent of new HIV/AIDS drugs that allow for longer, healthier life change the face of HIV/AIDS housing.

- FDA approves protease inhibitors (1995–1996).

2000s

- Shifts in the epidemic bring about shifts in housing approaches, and greater desire for more independent and integrated housing.

- Individuals living with HIV/AIDS are living longer, living in poverty, and primarily minority.

- Congress reauthorizes the Ryan White CARE Act (2000).

- NAHC launches first of a series of research summits to link housing to health care (2003).

- Congress passes the Ryan White HIV/AIDS Treatment Modernization Act (2006).

- The journal *AIDS and Behavior* dedicates a whole issue to HIV/AIDS housing (2007).

- Congress passes the Ryan White HIV/AIDS Treatment Extension Act (2009).

- The White House creates the National AIDS Strategy under the Obama Administration, linking housing to HIV/AIDS care (2010).

With the advent of HIV/AIDS in the early 1980s, communities had to respond immediately to individual housing needs. Early approaches to meeting the housing needs included small housing programs supported through volunteers and local funding. The housing programs were often geared either toward short-term emergency housing or the provision of hospice care. Early programs were characterized as providing a safe place or home to live and die in dignity. The lack of knowledge about HIV/AIDS created an environment of fear and discrimination. During the early years of the epidemic, with the lack of new drug treatments, persons infected with HIV lost jobs and, with it, their homes. Often faced with discrimination due to their HIV status, persons living with HIV/AIDS had difficulty accessing health care and other social supports. Stories of individuals being denied housing due to long waiting lists for federally subsidized housing, discrimination due to HIV status, housing not connected to health care or other supports, and the lack of adequate resources or infrastructure to respond to the need began to create momentum for a federal response.

The 1990s brought many milestone moments for HIV/AIDS housing. In 1990, President George H.W. Bush signed into law the Cranston-Gonzalez Affordable Housing Act. The Act was the most significant housing legislation passed since the 1970s and created new housing resources for state and local governments, including programs to serve the disabled, elderly, homeless, and persons living with HIV/AIDS. The Act created the HOPWA program and provided resources "to devise long-term comprehensive strategies for meeting the housing needs" of persons living with HIV/AIDS (U.S. Code, 1992). The creation of the HOPWA program marked the prioritization of a federal program solely dedicated to the housing needs of persons living with HIV/AIDS. Congress first appropriated funding to the HOPWA program in 1992 and the program has grown to $335 million in 2010 (HUD, 2010a). The program provides an array of housing activities including emergency, transitional, and permanent housing linked to supportive services to ensure access to health care.

Box 16.3. Quick Fact

The HOPWA program is the only federal program designated to meet the housing needs of persons living with HIV/AIDS (HUD, n.d.a, n.d.b).

Questions for Reflection

1. Consider the history of the local and federal responses to the housing needs of persons living with HIV/AIDS. How do these two responses differ? How are they the same? What are the pros and cons of each response?

2. How is the federal response to the housing needs of persons living with HIV/AIDS similar to other federal responses to social problems (e.g., the elderly and children)?

In 1994, shortly after the implementation of the HOPWA program, HUD Secretary Henry Cisneros under the Clinton Administration, at the behest of HIV/AIDS housing advocates, established the Office of HIV/AIDS Housing in the Office of Community Planning and Development. The Office of HIV/AIDS Housing was charged with the administration of the HOPWA program, as well as implementation of HUD's HIV/AIDS initiatives. The creation of the office established a federal priority on HIV/AIDS housing issues. Recognizing the need for a national voice on HIV/AIDS housing issues, advocates again came together to establish the NAHC. NAHC was created in 1995 to generate a national advocacy voice around HIV/AIDS housing policy.

By the end of the 1990s, the face of HIV/AIDS was changing. Individuals living with HIV/AIDS were living longer and healthier lives with the continued development of ARV medications. With these changes in lifestyle came changes in housing needs. Persons living with HIV/AIDS desired housing options that promoted independent living and integration into communities rather than HIV-specific housing. They preferred rent subsidies that allowed for individual choice in the selection of a housing unit over congregate living facilities. Community-based housing arrangements also meant the development of new case management and care models that engaged clients within their homes versus a service facility. Accessing mainstream housing resources such as public housing or housing vouchers demonstrates not only that persons living with HIV/AIDS were willing to live integrated within a community, but also that low-income persons living with HIV/AIDS had the greatest need for housing. Although it is a critical component to ensuring housing for persons living with HIV/AIDS, the HOPWA program does not provide enough resources to fully meet the needs of low-income persons living with HIV/AIDS that have housing needs. To expand access among persons living with HIV/AIDS to available housing resources, it is essential for policy-makers and social workers to create the connection to other affordable housing programs or mainstream housing.

Nearly three decades since the beginning of the HIV/AIDS epidemic, the 2000s brought about a shift in overall HIV/AIDS care. Reauthorization of the Ryan White CARE Act in 2000, 2006, and 2009 has brought up old issues related to HIV/AIDS "exceptionalism" and considerations of mainstreaming HIV/AIDS into such medical systems as Medicaid. When the Act was reauthorized in 2006 as the Ryan White

HIV/AIDS Treatment Modernization Act, it changed how the funds were administered, through devolution of the distribution process from the federal government to more local levels (Health Resources and Services Administration [HRSA], 2007). The new distribution process made better attempts to allocate funds to new areas impacted by the disease, including the South and rural areas.

Throughout the 2000s, the HOPWA program received steady, yet small, increases in funding from Congress. Concern, however, that HIV/AIDS housing and its contribution to the care of persons living with HIV/AIDS may be lost to the mainstreaming rhetoric has prompted the NAHC to launch a series of research summits focused on the connection of housing to health outcomes among persons living with HIV/AIDS (NAHC, 2010). In 2007, the journal *AIDS and Behavior* dedicated an issue to HIV/AIDS housing research, which connects housing to health outcomes. Through these studies, researchers demonstrate the connection between housing and HIV prevention, access to care, maintenance of care, and positive health outcomes among persons living with HIV/AIDS. Further solidifying housing as a critical component of HIV/AIDS care was inclusion of housing as a necessary component of care in The White House National HIV/AIDS Strategy (NHAS), released in 2010.

Box 16.4. Exercise—Out of Reach

The Out of Reach report produced by the National Low Income Housing Coalition (Pelletiere, DeCrappeo, Crowley, & Teater, 2010) examines the differences in housing cost, the income required, and the hours of work necessary to live affordably. Go to the Out of Reach website and choose a state and an area (i.e., metropolitan area or county) in which you are interested. Consider the following questions:

• How much money does an individual need to earn to pay no more than 30 percent of his or her income on housing costs? How many hours would the individual need to work? How does this vary for different areas, for example, a city, county, or rural area?

• What is the maximum amount that an individual earning Supplemental Security Income (SSI) can pay for housing costs if the individual is responsible for paying no more than 30 percent of his or her income? Considering where you live, is housing available to an individual living on SSI in your neighborhood?

- In considering housing costs, it is often suggested that families should move to find affordable housing options when none are available where they live. For an individual earning SSI, where can this individual move in order to pay no more than 30 percent of his or her income on housing costs? What other considerations does an individual need to consider when looking for housing (such as accommodations for an individual with a disability)? How might these factors influence an individual's choice of where to live?

Understanding Housing Need

The NAHC estimates that more than 50 percent of persons living with HIV/AIDS will need some type of housing assistance in their lifetime (NAHC, 2011). Both individual and community conditions work together to create a need for housing among persons living with HIV/AIDS.

Box 16.5. Barriers to Housing

Individual Challenges

- Poor credit history
- Limited rental history
- Unemployment or sporadic employment
- Criminal history
- High service needs, such as health, mental health, substance use
- Poverty, no income

Community Challenges

- Lack of affordable units
- No or limited services
- Lack of transportation
- Unsafe or indecent housing
- Discrimination, stigma, or NIMBY-ism ("not in my backyard")

Questions for Reflection

1. What other barriers might impact a low-income persons living with HIV/AIDS accessing housing?

2. As a social worker, what would you do to help overcome these barriers?

Four Conditions of Housing

It is important for social workers to consider the community context or environment in which individuals live and how that environment both positively and negatively influences housing need. To frame this discussion of the individual and community conditions that influence housing need, we will now consider four conditions of housing:

- Affordable housing: Housing where households pay no more than 30 percent of their adjusted gross income toward rent and utility costs. This is the affordability marker used by HUD (2009).

- Accessible housing: Policies, procedures, and services that promote access to housing resources (e.g., legal services and fair housing services).

- Available housing: Units of housing (affordable and with services) ready for occupancy by persons living with HIV/AIDS.

- Adequate housing: Safe and decent housing, including the physical condition of the property, as well as its location.

Affordable Housing

Among HIV/AIDS housing providers and other community stakeholders, the affordability of housing is often prioritized as a major barrier to accessing housing. Affordable housing is defined as housing where households pay no more than 30 percent of their adjusted gross income toward their rent and utilities. In this definition, two things are considered: a household's income, and the household's costs for housing, including rent or mortgage costs, and utilities. There are two ways to assess housing affordability—housing burden and the affordability gap.

Housing Cost Burden. A household's housing cost burden is the household's housing cost considered in ratio to the household's income. Lower-income households tend to have higher housing cost burdens than households with higher incomes. Households with a housing cost burden, or households spending more than 30 percent of their income toward housing cost, can be divided into two groups:

1. Households paying costs 30–50 percent of income are considered moderately housing cost burdened.

2. Households paying costs higher than 50 percent are considered extremely housing cost burdened.

Take for example a single person living with HIV/AIDS earning an SSI of $674 per month. If he or she pays $400 per month in rent, this person would be paying more than 59 percent (674 ÷ 400 = .593 or 59 percent) of income toward housing costs. At this percentage, this person would be considered extremely housing cost burdened. Unfortunately, low-income persons living with HIV/AIDS often have housing burdens of 50 percent or higher.

Box 16.6. What Is Your Housing Cost Burden?

Enter the following amounts and divide.

Your Housing Costs   Your Income

Rent/Utilities $_____ / Monthly Income $_____ = _____%

What percentage do you pay in housing costs each month?

Is your housing affordable (30 percent or less)?

Affordability Gap. The affordability gap is another way to examine housing affordability. The affordability gap is the additional income required monthly to achieve housing affordability—paying no more than 30 percent of income toward housing costs. Again, take as an example a single person receiving SSI. This person would receive approximately $674 per month or $8,088 per year. To pay no more than 30 percent of income toward housing costs, this person would have to pay $202 or less per month for rent. If a rental unit was available for $600 a month, the difference between the affordable rent ($202) and the actual rental amount ($600) is the affordability gap—in this case $398 ($600 – $202 = $398). The affordability gap of $398 is the amount that this person would need per month to live affordably. According to the NLIHC's Out of Reach (Pelletiere et al., 2010) report, nowhere in the United States can someone on SSI or earning minimum wage afford a one-bedroom at the national Fair Market Rent (see table 16.1). The Fair Market Rent is the average housing costs, including utilities, set annually by HUD (2010b). Considering that persons living with HIV/AIDS needing housing assistance are more likely to be extremely low income and often are on SSI, these households will need greater support to achieve housing stability.

Table 16.1. Affordability Gap for Low Income Households in the United States

	Household Income SSI ($674/month)	Household Income Minimum Wage ($7.25/hour)
Annual Income	$8,088	$15,080
Monthly Income	$674	$1,267
30% for Housing Costs	$202	$377
National Fair Market Rent (1-Bedroom Unit)	$959	$959
Affordability Gap	($757)	($582)

Source: Pelletiere, DeCrappeo, Crowley, & Teater (2010).

Accessible Housing

Housing accessibility can be defined in a variety of ways, but most definitions include having equal access to housing and services. Equal access includes policies, physical space, and services that promote access to housing.

> **Box 16.7. Accessibility to Housing**
>
> Accessibility to housing can be affected by the following:
>
> - Policies: Policies that do not ensure ease of access to promote housing stability including a lack of clear and fair eligibility and rental requirements; rigid credit, rental, or criminal history requirements; and housing discrimination.
>
> - Physical space: Structures that do not accommodate individuals with disabilities, including no stairs, doors wide enough for wheelchairs, and grab bars in bathrooms. Housing that lacks working kitchens and bathrooms.
>
> - Services: Housing that does not have easy access to health care, supportive services, transportation, and other community amenities.

Policies. Policies such as eligibility criteria, rental requirements, or screening requirements can limit access to available housing. For example, the requirements of strong credit, previous rental history, or no criminal history can limit some individuals from having access to available housing. In addition, discrimination based on race, sex, having children, birth country, religion, or disability (including HIV/AIDS) can limit access to housing. Such discrimination is prohibited under the federal Fair Housing Act and often under state or local housing laws (HUD, 2011). In some cases, a person with a disability may require a reasonable accommodation of a landlord's policies. For example, if a person with a disability requires a guide dog and the landlord does not permit pets, the landlord will need to make a reasonable accommodation or bend the rule to allow the person to have the dog.

Physical Space. Physical accessibility is important to persons living with HIV/ AIDS, especially persons who have physical disabilities. Physical modifications such as wheelchair ramps, grab bars in bathrooms, and doorways wide enough to accommodate wheelchairs are common, and can all be made to ensure a housing unit is accessible to someone with a disability, including persons living with HIV/ AIDS. Such reasonable modifications are allowable under the Fair Housing Act; the landlord may complete such modifications at a cost to the tenant.

Services. Access to health care, supportive services, transportation, and other community amenities, like a grocery store, are also important housing attributes to consider. Such access can often make a difference in housing stability for persons living with HIV/AIDS. In some cases, landlords may be unwilling to work with nonprofit organizations that provide necessary supportive services to help individuals stay stably housed. Persons living with HIV/AIDS often have other challenges that can affect their ability to pay rent or comply with lease requirements. Such challenges may include impaired mental health or substance use, poor health, health-related unemployment or sporadic employment, or a disability. If social workers ensure connection to supportive services, case management, and health care, they often can prevent housing eviction and homelessness.

Available Housing

The NAHC estimates that 50 percent of persons living with HIV/AIDS have a housing need (NAHC, 2011). It is important for the social worker to consider a variety of housing options that address a myriad of housing needs. Housing options should include assisted living, shared housing, and independent housing. As persons living with HIV/AIDS are living longer, and as HIV/AIDS care is increasingly being mainstreamed into regular health care, the need for certain housing types has changed. Shared housing arrangements (i.e., group homes) or hospice care facilities are less often the desired housing model. In most studies, persons living with HIV/AIDS most often desire to live in independent housing that is integrated into the community versus living in HIV/AIDS–only facilities. When examining the availability of housing, social workers should also consider subpopulations of persons living with HIV/AIDS. For example, among persons living with HIV/AIDS, persons with mental illness, substance use issues, or families may have different housing needs. Social workers should consider such needs when exploring the size, location, and type of housing available.

The HOPWA program, the federal program dedicated to the housing needs of persons living with HIV/AIDS, provides short- and long-term rental assistance, utility assistance, rent deposits, and construction funds to provide housing to persons living with HIV/AIDS. The HOPWA program alone, however, cannot meet the housing needs of all persons living with HIV/AIDS. Other federal programs such as Section 8 rental assistance, housing for persons with disabilities (Section 811), low-income tax credits, public housing, and homeless programs are other federal programs that can and do provide housing to persons living with HIV/AIDS. Even with these funding sources, there continues to be a shortage of affordable housing in many communities across the United States, especially for persons living with HIV/AIDS.

Adequate Housing

Adequate housing can be defined as housing that is both safe and decent. Safe and decent housing provides a healthy environment that promotes physical and mental health. Under most federal housing programs, all units must meet housing quality standards. Housing quality standards are the basic structural and safety requirements a unit must meet before a household may live in the unit. For example, standards may include having a working kitchen and bathroom, adequate space appropriate to the household size, no electrical hazards, a smoke detector, no lead-based paint, and walls, ceilings, and floors that are in good condition. For persons living with HIV/AIDS, a clean environment is important to the promotion of health. For such subpopulations of persons living with HIV/AIDS as women, children, and individuals with mental illness or substance use, issues of safety may also be a concern.

Housing Plus Services

For low-income persons living with HIV/AIDS access to health care, supportive services, and case management can often mean the difference between being housing stable and being homeless. This connection between housing and services has been termed Housing Plus Services. Housing Plus Services models link permanent affordable housing and supportive services designed to promote housing stability. The NLIHC has developed a guiding set of principles for Housing Plus Services programs (Pelletiere et al., 2010).

Box 16.8. Housing Plus Services Principles

- Housing is a basic human need, and all people have a right to safe, decent, and affordable permanent housing.

- All people are valuable and capable of being valuable residents and valuable community members.

- Housing and services should be integrated to enhance the social and economic well-being of residents and to build healthy communities.

- Residents, owners, and property managers and service providers should work as a team in integrated housing and services initiatives.

- Programs should be based on assessment of residents' and community strengths and needs, supported by ongoing monitoring and evaluation.

- Programs should strengthen and expand resident participation to improve the community's capacity to create change.

- Residents' participation in programs should be voluntary, with an emphasis on outreach to the most vulnerable.

- Community development activities should be extended to the neighboring area of residents.

- Assessment, intervention, and evaluation should be multilevel, focusing on individual residents, groups, and community.

- Services should maximize the use of existing resources, avoid duplication, and expand the economic, social, and political resources available to residents (Pelletiere, DeCrappeo, Crowley, & Teater, 2010).

Supportive services that are often used in conjunction with housing assistance include

• Case management, including access to benefits, advocacy, and referrals

• Mental health services

• Substance abuse services (alcohol and drugs)

• Transportation

• Nutritional services, including food

• Adult daycare and personal assistance

• Child care

• Education

• Employment assistance and job training

• Health care

• Legal services

• Life skills, including money management, social skills, and household management

• Peer support

Case Example I

Jackie was formerly a homeless, single mother who lives in Sunrise, a multi-family housing facility for families affected by HIV/AIDS. She and her two-year-old daughter lived at Sunrise with three other families; and during her years at Sunrise she developed a strong rapport with her case manager. Jackie also benefited from other services such as the on-site drug support group, childcare, and job training. During her time at Sunrise, Jackie found a job and had been approved for a housing voucher. The voucher gave Jackie the freedom to find her own apartment in the community where she grew up. Jackie worked with her housing case manager to locate an apartment close to the school that Jackie's daughter would attend. Jackie moved into her new apartment one month after receiving her voucher, and had her final visit with her housing case manager. The funding that provided the case management and other services were only provided to residents of the Sunrise, thus Jackie no longer had contact with her case manager.

About seven months later, the case manager from Sunrise was conducting intake and assessments at the local homeless shelter. She was surprised to find Jackie in the shelter. The case manager could tell Jackie had been drinking, and in conversation learned that Jackie's daughter had been placed in foster care. Slowly the case manager learned that Jackie got sick due to her HIV and has not been able to work. Because she had little income, she got behind on her rent and utility payments, resulting in the electric company turning off her power. Before long, Jackie was so far behind that she decided to leave the apartment before being evicted. She ended up depressed and turned to what she knew would provide comfort—alcohol.

At first, Jackie's story seemed like the perfect success story, but what happened? What factors contributed to Jackie becoming homeless again? What could have helped Jackie remain housed successfully?

Due to the various funding streams, typically, federal funding that supports housing activities comes through a separate program and department that is different from the program that supplies funds for supportive services. Agencies attempting to create Housing Plus Service models usually rely on a variety of funding sources to make their programs work (Greiff, Proscio, & Wilkins, 2003; Hannigan & Wagner, 2003). Federal housing programs serving the persons living with HIV/AIDS, elderly, persons with disabilities, or persons experiencing homelessness provide both the housing and supportive services funding. In recent years, due to shrinking funding, housing advocates have called for federal housing programs to focus more on housing and less on services. Although this does focus resources on the development of new housing units, the reduction of services can make it much more challenging to provide and coordinate the supportive services that are necessary to ensure that persons living with HIV/AIDS achieve and maintain housing stability.

Box 16.9. Elements of a Housing Plan

A housing plan is a strategy agreed upon by the tenant and social worker through which housing goals are developed and monitored. The plan outlines the actions to be taken or services that need to be connected to ensure that the tenant remains housing stable. A primary focus of a housing social worker is to empower the tenant to remain lease compliant, thus preventing homelessness. Worker roles may include the following:

• Completed intake sheet including income and expense form

- Determination of client's housing history (former places of residence and any incidences that could impact future housing, such as evictions, foreclosures, etc.)

- Determination of client's goals for housing (e.g., to live in his or her own apartment)

- Identification of barriers (past evictions, low income, lack of employment, poor credit, ongoing issues with substance abuse, criminal background, etc.)

- Exploration of possible housing options (public housing, section 8, HOPWA resources, key target program, homeownership, shared living, family, etc.)

- Referrals to community resources (housing, employment, substance abuse treatment, food stamps, etc.)

- Advocacy with property managers and other referral sources

- Creation of a workable budget

- Postoccupancy counseling (including money management, assessment, additional referrals, etc.)

The role of the social worker engaged in HIV/AIDS housing is multifaceted and involves both direct (micro-level) and community (macro-level) practice. Consider the broad roles that HIV/AIDS housing social workers may play:

- Case management: includes outreach, engagement, assessment, education, setting housing goals and creating a housing plan; referrals to housing and related supportive services and/or resources;

- Eligibility determination: includes assessment of persons living with HIV/AIDS for eligibility for housing programs;

- Housing resource specialist: includes educating persons living with HIV/AIDS on housing options and availability of housing, developing relationship with new landlords, developing new units of housing;

- Housing provider: includes providing direct housing assistance like rental or utility subsidies, managing a housing facility, or providing emergency housing;

- Client advocate: includes advocating for access or maintenance of housing, supportive services, or other resources;

- Employment or life skills trainer: includes providing or referring to programs that help persons living with HIV/AIDS to increase their incomes, teaching budgeting, money management, housing skills (paying rent, housing upkeep, abiding by the terms of a lease, etc.);

- Community planner: includes working with other government and nonprofit agencies to assess community need and develop housing strategies for persons living with HIV/AIDS, or seeking new housing resources; and

- A variety of other roles to ensure that persons living with HIV/AIDS have access to affordable housing options.

Considering all the roles that social workers can play related to housing for persons living with HIV/AIDS, it should be clear that housing alone may not always be sufficient for ensuring housing stability. Supportive services are often a necessary component of HIV/AIDS housing programs to ensure housing stability among persons living with HIV/AIDS.

Structural Impacts of Housing: Micro-Level and Macro-Level

Much of the current research related to HIV/AIDS and health outcomes has focused on housing as a structural issue, moving away from individual risk characteristics.

Box 16.10. Risk Factors for HIV

Examples of Individual Risk Factors for HIV

(Micro-Level)

Race, sex, gender, risky sex practices, mental illness, substance use, criminal history

Examples of Social or Environmental Risk Factors for HIV

(Macro-Level)

Housing affordability, accessibility, availability, adequacy; community poverty or unemployment; lack of services or health care; rural areas

Increasingly in the United States, HIV infection is concentrated among persons in poverty, racial minorities, and persons with mental illness, substance use, or criminal backgrounds. Researchers and practitioners have used such individual factors to better understand disparities in health outcomes. Social workers may approach these individual-level risk factors through micro-level—direct or clinical—social work theories and practice. One important aspect of social work practice is the worker's ability to consider the broad perspectives that affect the well-being of individual clients. The ability to go beyond individual health, social, or psychosocial factors and consider the broader environmental or community conditionals, policies, or structural factors makes social work practitioners unique. HIV/AIDS prevention research has suggested that micro-level interventions focused on changing individual risk factors may not be entirely successful. Increasingly, researchers are making the connection that housing and other social or environmental factors indirectly and directly affect HIV prevention, access to care, and maintenance of care. "Housing is health care" has become an adage that conveys the message that, without stable housing, persons living with HIV/AIDS have poorer access to health care and other supportive services and poorer health outcomes. Considering housing's role, housing is

- HIV prevention. Individuals with stable housing are less likely to be engaged in risky behaviors, such as unsafe sexual practices or drug use, which can lead to HIV infection (Coady et al., 2007; Des Jarlais, Braine, & Friedman, 2007; German, Davey, & Latkin, 2007; Weir, Bard, O'Brien, Casciato, & Stark, 2007).

- Access to health care. Individuals with stable housing are more likely to access health-care services, including primary health care (Aidala, Lee, Abramson, Messeri, & Siegler, 2007; Bennett, Pope, & Dantzler, 2007).

- Maintenance of health-care and supportive services. Individuals with stable housing are more likely to be engaged and to remain engaged in health care. Homeless or unstably housed individuals are less likely to receive and adhere to care (Aidala et al., 2007; Smith, 2000).

- Positive health outcomes. Individuals with stable housing are more likely to live healthier lives. Homeless or unstable housed individuals have higher HIV-viral loads, increased infections, and a higher mortality rate (Leaver, Bargh, Dunn, & Hwang, 2007).

This view that social and environmental factors affect HIV-care and treatment is raising awareness that housing is an effective component of health care (Aidala, 2007). Such social work theories as Person in Environment are particularly suited to these research findings (Payne, 1997). Social workers need to understand the context of where an individual lives: for example, living in an area with high rates of poverty or unemployment, or living in a rural area may affect the ability of a person living with HIV/AIDS to access or maintain care, access transportation, or obtain other community services. Furthermore, the housing needs of persons living with HIV/AIDS may be more intense due to the environmental conditions in which they live (Bennett, 2009). Such an understanding of the macro-level structural issues—mainly a lack of stable housing—that may affect an individual with HIV/AIDS, helps social work practitioners to examine policies and practices that may be hindering effective HIV treatment and care. The assessment of housing status of persons living with HIV/AIDS must be a component of overall health-care and supportive service delivery. Housing represents the nexus between the environmental and structural factors in a community and the individual factors of persons living with HIV/AIDS.

Current Issues

As one considers the future, the view of HIV/AIDS housing seems, at best, a continually shifting component of overall HIV/AIDS care. Some key programmatic and policy shifts will need to be considered and will shape future HIV/AIDS housing strategies. Some areas for consideration include the following:

- The face of the epidemic is changing. As individuals at risk for and living with HIV/AIDS change, so do housing and related supportive service needs. Social workers should remain current on shifts that help to ensure programs are relevant and responsive to the needs of individuals and the communities in which they live.

- Housing is a home. Housing is not only a place, it is a home. A home promotes safety, family, health, and connection to other necessary community and social supports. Social workers must recognize that individual, environmental, and social conditions all have an effect on ensuring that persons living with HIV/AIDS have affordable, adequate, and accessible places to live.

• Housing models should vary depending on the needs of persons living with HIV/AIDS and the communities in which they live. Housing models must shift with the needs of persons living with HIV/AIDS while considering the housing resources that exist within a community. Housing models can range from group to independent living, rental to homeownership, intensive supportive services to voluntary supportive services, and many other models. Social workers should work with persons living with HIV/AIDS to determine the best housing options that optimize the household's housing goals, with consideration of both transitional and permanent housing.

• Advocate to strengthen housing quality and availability, services, and health care. The passage of the Affordable Health Care Act in 2010, national and state budget deficits, and a national emphasis on less government involvement with social programs all contribute to a potential reduction, merger, or loss of current HIV/AIDS programs. In the next few years, it will be critical for social work professionals not only to understand the unique needs of PLWHA, but also to understand the policies that affect PLWHA. Advocating on behalf of PLWHA will ensure that the housing, health, and supportive service needs of persons living with HIV/AIDS continue to be met.

Box 16.11. Quick Fact

The National HIV/AIDS Housing Coalition has developed a policy toolkit to support national and local advocacy efforts related to HIV/AIDS housing. See http://nationalaidshousing.org/policy-toolkit/

Questions for Reflection

1. What HIV/AIDS housing policy challenges do you see on a local, state, or federal level that social workers should advocate to change on behalf of persons living with HIV/AIDS?

2. How could some of the principles behind the benefits of housing be used to create positive and effective advocacy messages? For example, "Housing is health care."

3. How do these messages change based on the target audience? For example, policy makers versus persons living with HIV/AIDS.

The NHAS, with its emphasis on housing as an important component of care, and the continued emphasis on HIV/AIDS housing research, help to solidify housing's role as an important component of both HIV/AIDS care and services. If affordable, adequate, accessible housing is to continue to be available for persons living with HIV/AIDS, it will be incumbent upon social workers to understand the housing needs of PLWHA, to advocate for policies and programs to meet these housing needs.

Case Example II

> Walter had a serious need for housing. As a forty-two-year-old gay man who had lived with HIV for ten years, he had long felt ostracized by most of his family. He was nervous because he would soon have no place of his own, with only a homeless shelter as an option. What added to his problems in finding housing included his low income, his rental history that included two evictions for nonpayment of rent, and his past use of cocaine, which had resulted in legal trouble. Walter was living with his partner but they were not getting along; his partner was abusing Walter emotionally and sometimes physically. In fact, he believed he would have to move out at any moment. The stress of his situation was beginning to impact his health: he was very depressed, he was not eating well, he was not feeling well, and he did not feel like going anywhere or doing anything about it.
>
> The situation had not always been grim for Walter. Two years after his initial diagnosis, Walter's health was declining, he was unable to work, and was living from place to place with different relatives, most of whom he did not trust enough to share his status. Walter found an HIV case manager who was able to get him his own apartment where his rent was calculated based on his income. Walter was finally able to take his medications on a regular basis and his health improved.
>
> Walter made the unfortunate decision to allow a friend to move in with him. He and the friend began using cocaine. The cocaine became the priority in his life and that led to an arrest, which led to him being on probation, which led to him using more and not paying his rent, finally resulting in an eviction. The snowball effect had definitely kicked in.
>
> Walter decided it was time to be honest with his case manager about his situation because he was desperate. His case manager contacted a local facility that provided residential substance abuse treatment. However, the facility did

not have an immediate opening. His case manager found that the place received special funding from the HOPWA program, which allowed Walter to immediately be admitted. He stayed in the facility for several weeks until he had completed the program. While in treatment, Walter complied with his HIV medical regimen and his overall health and mental status dramatically improved.

Walter's case manager contacted the HOPWA program housing coordinator to ask about Walter's housing options, as he would soon be released from the facility. The coordinator knew that the public housing office in their city was not taking applications and other housing options might be limited due to his prior arrest and eviction records. The HOPWA housing coordinator enrolled Walter into their three-year transitional HOPWA tenant-based rental voucher program.

The HOPWA housing coordinator worked with Walter and the case manager to establish a housing plan that included such goals as engagement in budget and credit counseling, peer support groups, and referrals to other community resources. The housing coordinator assisted Walter with applying for applications for other subsidized programs and personally advocated on his behalf by informing apartment managers that Walter had been clean and sober for several years, paid his portion of the rent in a timely manner, and complied with all the requirements of his housing plan.

After several denials for housing—some property owners had more stringent requirements than others—the housing coordinator was eventually able to negotiate on Walter's behalf: a property manager approved him for a unit where the rent would be based on his income. Walter continued to receive housing information services and remained stable in his housing unit. Now that Walter had his own home, he had a place to store his medications, which he was able to take on a regular basis. He was close to public transportation and able to get to his medical and other appointments. Walter was even thinking of starting a support group. He wanted to help others because he knew what it felt like to be isolated and to have no one who was like him to confide in. Walter felt like things were getting to be a lot better and he had a future. The snowball had stopped rolling.

Questions for Reflection

1. What are the differences between the need for housing of a person living with HIV/AIDS, a person with a visual disability, a person with a disability that requires the use of a wheelchair, or a person with congestive heart failure?

2. Why is the term "Housing is health care" particularly important to a person living with HIV/AIDS?

3. If Walter were to lose his housing again, what would be his options? Why would a homeless shelter or a rooming house not be a good option?

4. What are the basics for developing a housing plan? Consider both individual and environmental factors in the housing plan.

5. What role did Walter's sexual orientation play in his difficulties?

6. How is having stable housing connected with HIV prevention and care?

Key Words and Concepts

- Housing is a basic human need.
- Housing is a right.
- Housing is health care.
- Housing burden
- Housing plan
- Housing Plus Services
- Housing Quality Standards
- Fair market rent
- Reasonable modifications
- Reasonable accommodations

Questions for Reflection

1. Why is there an affordable housing crisis in the United States? What are possible solutions?

2. How does having stable housing improve a person living with HIV/AIDS' medical adherence?

3. How does having stable housing improve a person living with HIV/AIDS' access to health care?

4. How are stable housing and HIV prevention connected?

5. Why are Housing Quality Standards important?

6. How could a person living with HIV/AIDS, who has an ongoing substance abuse issue, secure housing? What if the person also had a mental illness issue?

7. What are the local housing and supportive services in your community?

Web Resources

U.S. Department of Housing and Urban Development (HUD): http://www.hud.gov

Housing Opportunities for Persons with AIDS (HOPWA) program, HUD: http://portal.hud.gov/hudportal/HUD?src=/program_offices/comm_planning/aidshousing

National AIDS Housing Coalition (NAHC): http://www.nationalaidshousing.org

Policy Toolkit, NAHC: http://nationalaidshousing.org/policy-toolkit/

International Declaration on Poverty, Housing Instability, and HIV/AIDS, NAHC: http://nationalaidshousing.org/2008/07/endorseconference/

Information on HIV and homelessness: http://www.nationalhomeless.org/factsheets/hiv.html

Information on HIV and hospice care: http://www.thebody.com/content/art30590.html

National Low Income Housing Coalition (NLIHC): http://www.nlihc.org

Out of Reach, NLIHC: http://www.nlihc.org/oor/oor2010/

Advocates Guide (2011), NLIHC: http://www.nlihc.org/doc/2011-Advocates-Guide.pdf

Code of Ethics, National Association of Social Workers (NASW): http://www.socialworkers.org/pubs/code/code.asp

Universal Declaration of Human Rights, United Nations: http://www.un.org/en/documents/udhr/

Extraordinary photos of housing for people with HIV/AIDS: http://www.renaldi.com/portfolio/housing1.html

References

Aidala, A. (2007). Why housing? *AIDS and Behavior, 11*(Supl.), S1–S6.

Aidala, A., Lee, G., Abramson, D. M., Messeri, P., & Siegler, A. (2007). Housing need, housing assistance, and connection to HIV medical care. *AIDS and Behavior, 11*(6), S101–S115.

Bennett, R. L. (2009). *Community and individual factors that influence housing need among low-income persons living with HIV/AIDS.* Social Work Dissertation, The University of Alabama Tuscaloosa.

Bennett, R. L., Pope, C., & Dantzler, J. (2007). *Tampa EMSA HIV/AIDS housing plan: Responding to the need for permanent supportive housing for low income individuals and families living with HIV/AIDS.* Birmingham, AL: Collaborative Solutions.

Coady, M. H., Latka, M. H., Thiede, H., Golub, E. T., Ouellet, L., Hudson, S. M., . . . , Garfein, R. S. (2007). Housing status and associated differences in HIV risk behaviors among young injection drug users (IDUs). *AIDS and Behavior, 11*, 854–863.

Des Jarlais, D. C., Braine, N., & Friedman, P. (2007). Unstable housing as a factor for increased injection risk behavior at US syringe exchange program. *AIDS and Behavior, 11*(Suppl.), S78–S84.

German, D., Davey, M. A., & Latkin, C. A. (2007). Residential transience and HIV risk behaviors among injection drug users. *AIDS and Behavior, 11*(Suppl.), S21–S30.

Greiff, D., Proscio, T., & Wilkins, C. (2003). *Laying a new foundation: Changing the systems that create and sustain supportive housing.* New York: Corporation for Supportive Housing.

Hannigan, T., & Wagner, S. (2003). *Developing the "support" in supportive housing: A guide to providing services in housing.* New York: Corporation for Supportive Housing.

Health Resources and Services Administration (HRSA). (2007). *The Ryan White HIV/AIDS Program: A Living History.* Retrieved from http://hab.hrsa.gov/livinghistory/index.htm

Leaver, C. A., Bargh, G., Dunn, J. R., & Hwang, S. W. (2007). The effects of housing status on health-related outcomes in people living with HIV: A systemic review of the literature. *AIDS and Behavior, 11*(6), S85–S100.

Maslow, A. H. (1943). A theory of human motivation. *Psychological Review, 50,* 370–396.

National AIDS Housing Coalition (NAHC). (2008). *International declaration on poverty, housing instability, and HIV/AIDS.* Retrieved from http://national aidshousing.org/2008/07/endorseconference/

National AIDS Housing Coalition (NAHC). (2010). *National housing and HIV/AIDS research summit series.* Retrieved from http://nationalaidshousing.org/national-housing-and-hivaids-research-summit-series/

National AIDS Housing Coalition (NAHC). (2011). *Breaking the link between homelessness and HIV.* Retrieved from http://www.nationalaidshousing.org/PDF/Factsheets-Homelessness.pdf

National Association of Social Workers (NASW). (2008). *Code of Ethics of the National Association of Social Workers.* Retrieved from http://www.social workers.org/pubs/code/code.asp

Payne, M. (1997). *Modern social work theory* (2nd ed.). Chicago: Lyceum Books.

Pelletiere, D., DeCrappeo, M., Crowley, S., & Teater, E. (2010). *Out of reach 2010.* Retrieved from http://www.nlihc.org/oor/oor2010/

Smith, M. Y. (2000). Housing status and health care service utilization among low-income persons with HIV/AIDS. *Journal of Internal General Medicine, 15,* 731–738.

U.S. Code. (1992). Housing opportunities for persons with AIDS, 131 C.F.R. § 12901. Retrieved from http://www.law.cornell.edu/uscode/html/uscode42/usc_sec_42_00012901——000-.html

U.S. Department of Housing and Urban Development (HUD). (2009, February 18). *Affordable housing.* Retrieved from http://www.hud.gov/offices/cpd/affordablehousing/index.cfm

U.S. Department of Housing and Urban Development (HUD). (2010a). *CPD appropriations budget.* Retrieved from http://www.hud.gov/offices/cpd/about/budget/

U.S. Department of Housing and Urban Development (HUD). (2010b). *Fair market rents.* Retrieved from http://www.huduser.org/portal/datasets/fmr.html

U.S. Department of Housing and Urban Development (HUD). (2011). *Fair Housing: It's your right.* Retrieved from http://portal.hud.gov/hudportal/HUD?src=/program_offices/fair_housing_equal_opp/FHLaws/yourrights

U.S. Department of Housing and Urban Development (HUD). n.d.a. *HIV/AIDS housing.* Retrieved from http://portal.hud.gov/hudportal/HUD?src=/program_offices/comm_planning/aidshousing

U.S. Department of Housing and Urban Development (HUD). n.d.b. *Homelessness Resource Exchange.* Retrieved from http://www.hudhre.info/index.cfm?do=viewHopwaHome

United Nations (UN). (1948). *The universal declaration of human rights.* Retrieved from http://www.un.org/en/documents/udhr/

Weir, B., Bard, R. S., O'Brien, K., Casciato, C. J., & Stark, M. J. (2007). Uncovering patterns of HIV risk through multiple housing measures. *AIDS and Behavior, 11*(Suppl.), S31–S44.

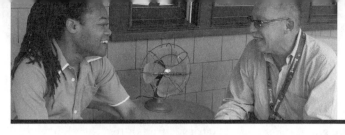

17

U.S. AIDS Policy: The Shifting Landscape

Randall H. Russell and Diana Rowan

AIDS has re-written the rules; to prevail, we must, too.
—Peter Piot, Executive Director,
Joint United Nations Programme on HIV/AIDS (UNAIDS, 2006)

Overview: HIV and AIDS in the Social Environment

Throughout the course of the AIDS (acquired immune deficiency syndrome) epidemic in the United States, policies have been shaped by those who responded to the immense human needs at a time of crisis. The frequency and duration of HIV (human immunodeficiency virus) coverage in the media is unparalleled in scope. When HIV was first introduced in the United States, there were no known treatments and the disease was greatly misunderstood. Consequently, those who had AIDS died painful deaths. Because of these circumstances, the AIDS epidemic and the disease itself became highly publicized. Gay men who came out and spoke about HIV and AIDS and the pain they caused, homophobia and the fear that erupted from those who openly stated their hatred of gay men, and the anger of AIDS survivors who found themselves being victimized, forever linked the gay rights movement and HIV/AIDS epidemic. The hatred at the time from the government, various faith-based communities, and societal leaders led gay men and women to create and sustain a national movement.

This chapter describes policy history that was influenced by a national movement in response to the AIDS epidemic similar to the public outcry in response to the Vietnam War. Indeed, more people have died from AIDS in the United States (more than 650,000 known deaths) (CDC, 2009) than in all modern wars including World War I, World War II, the Korean War, Vietnam, Iraq, and Afghanistan. The deaths associated with military combat occurred over one hundred years, while the deaths from AIDS occurred over thirty years. Furthermore, half of the deaths from the AIDS virus occurred within the first fifteen years of the epidemic.

The social conflicts of gay men, an incurable disease, and the messages portrayed by the media as "the war on AIDS" have contributed to the development of policies over the past three decades. The emergence of HIV/AIDS–related topics in mainstream discussions has forced our society to confront a variety of taboo topics. The following areas are only a few of the many public policy topics initiated by the introduction of HIV into the United States:

- Homosexuality and bisexuality

- Specific sexual behaviors

- Faith-based views of sexual behaviors, leading to conflicts with spiritual or religious beliefs

- Legal implications of poor treatment of individuals with a chronic communicable disease with regard to housing, health-care settings, employment, and basic human rights

- Research on the balance of public safety with access to treatment options

- Establishment of health-care systems that address complex, chronic conditions and show the efficacy and efficiency of treating the entire person

- Confrontation of disparities in access to information, diagnosis, care, and treatment for a variety of diseases due to the disproportionate share of infections in African Americans, Latinos, and men who have sex with men (MSM), and based on geographic differences

- Recognition that educating people about their health-care options empowers them to act with a better understanding of the consequences of their behavior.

In the United States, at least 1.1 million people are living with HIV and more than 650,000 have died from the impacts of HIV (CDC, 2009). These roughly 1.8 million people in the United States who have lived and died with HIV have friends, family, colleagues, caregivers, providers, and volunteers affected by HIV. When these groups who are affected by HIV are included, an estimated 20 million Americans have been personally touched by this epidemic. Some have said that the war on AIDS evolved from the guilt of a nation that betrayed its own citizens because of the stigmas associated with HIV and AIDS. Despite these setbacks, pure and passionate advocacy eventually arose to address the political issues that developed from the AIDS epidemic, in the hope of initiating domestic and global changes.

Policy and Advocacy

A policy is a course of action designed to outline an agreement by an organization, entity, group, governmental entity, or any other parties who agree to engage in using a policy to guide that interaction. Policies on HIV and AIDS have been developed in nearly every private, public, and faith-based setting, covering a wide spectrum of issues and systems. The policies addressed in this chapter are targeted at federal and state levels, but they are not intended to address the full spectrum of policy work influenced by the HIV/AIDS epidemic.

Advocacy, a cornerstone of social work practice, refers to organized education intended to influence policies and approaches taken by governmental and other entities, as they relate to people who are disadvantaged or at risk for marginalization. Successful HIV-specific advocacy templates have been created by multiple states and a wide variety of federal advocates focusing on a wide range of domestic and international efforts related to HIV. The case study at the end of this chapter illustrates the use of these tools to address specific issues related to HIV infection. Advocacy tools include the following:

- Messaging: Clearly stating the problem in simple terms and recommended solution(s) to the problem.

- Collaboration: Consumers (people living with HIV and AIDS), employees of HIV- and AIDS-related organizations, advocates, faith-based groups, allied disability or economic advocacy groups.

- Government partners: Those persons in federal, state, or municipal governmental positions who have information related to HIV, including surveillance data on the disease, current policies and procedures, information on how funds are spent and what outcomes were achieved from these spent funds, and a variety of other critical pieces of information.

- Organizing body: An agreed-upon entity to administer and organize advocacy efforts to centralize information and coordinate implementation of strategies.

- Strategies: Short- and long-term strategies involve both action and wisdom. Short-term gains at the cost of long-term and more-substantial accomplishments can be detrimental. To avoid these unintended consequences, a cohesive advocacy group is required, to develop plans that involve multiple actions aimed at multiple audiences.

- Cohesive advocacy group: A group of advocates representing an array of audiences typically includes
  - Multiple consumers
  - Staff members at nonprofit organizations that work on prevention, care, or treatment of HIV
  - Governmental partners who provide education, data, and the context of the larger situation
  - Allied organizations that share a common goal
  - Geographic representatives appropriate to the advocacy target
  - Health-care providers
  - Jail or prison representatives
  - Substance abuse or mental health representatives
  - Representatives by race, age, and gender that reflect the epidemic in the target area
  - Prevention and testing providers
  - Caseworkers and front-line staff

Importance of Social Policy to Social Workers

Social workers involved with the many facets of HIV and AIDS prevention, treatment, and care are directly impacted by social policy. Social workers intervene with clients who need education and linkage to resources. They also act as agency directors and program managers, researchers, and government workers. Governmental policies related to poverty, health insurance, health care, housing, substance abuse treatment, and mental health care directly affect people living with HIV and AIDS and their human service providers. How do people with no income access health care? How do they live and eat? What happens when someone has substance abuse addiction and is also mentally ill? What do the systems that could provide services offer to them? Which issues should be addressed first, given the resources available for various issues? What if the state cuts coverage for a service for an area that is currently funded, leaving a gap where no other resource is available? How does a social worker serve as an agency director when there is not ample funding to hire professionally trained people? It is clear that wherever social workers are employed, public policy drives their ability to meet the needs of clients and the community.

The Relationships between Policy, Practice, and Research

A policy is not a stagnant agreement—rather, it is dynamic. Research and organized input from practitioners should inform the policy-making process. Periodic surveys of case managers and consumers and reports of data on specific policies create an environment in which policies best serve the needs of consumers. Leadership to initiate this type of environment is often missing or unfunded, and therefore policies are not designed, developed, and assessed in timely ways. A lack of strong leadership can negatively affect the success of a policy in reaching its goals. Advocacy from the community is often the best way to enforce policies that affect people who have or are at risk for HIV infection. Data from policy evaluations can be leveraged to apply pressure toward positive change.

Historically, policy development in response to the AIDS epidemic in the United States has occurred primarily at the federal level. The following programs have direct impacts on people living with HIV or AIDS; discussion of these four programs follows:

- The Ryan White CARE Act

- Housing Opportunities for Persons with AIDS (HOPWA)—AIDS Housing Care Act

- Medicaid provides more than 30 percent of the insurance coverage for persons with HIV who are in treatment;

- Medicare provides multiple services and prescriptions for approximately 10 percent of persons with HIV who are in treatment; and

- The U.S. Department of Defense and the Veterans Affairs medical systems are the largest providers of HIV care and treatment in the United States.

- The Americans with Disabilities Act (ADA).

- The Patient Protection and Affordable Care Act (Health-care Reform).

- The AIDS Drug Assistance Program (ADAP).

- The U.S. Food and Drug Administration (FDA) and fast-track systems for drug approval.

- The Substance Abuse and Mental Health Services Administration (SAMHSA).

The Ryan White CARE Act
Brief History of the Reauthorization Process

The Ryan White CARE Act (often called the CARE Act) is the nation's largest HIV- and AIDS-specific federal grant program and is a critical source of care and treatment for people living with HIV or AIDS in the United States. Federal laws and programs typically have an authorization process that describes the ways in which the programs will be administered and funding distributed. The laws govern the way in which the funds will be used and the reports that will be required. Appropriation of funds for programs is a separate process. The CARE Act was first passed and authorized on August 18, 1990, with appropriations awarded in fiscal year 1991. It was reauthorized in May 1996 and October 2000; in December 2006 it was renamed the Ryan White HIV/AIDS Treatment Modernization Act. The CARE Act was reauthorized and renamed again in 2009, this time as the Ryan White HIV/AIDS Treatment Extension Act, though it is still referred to as the CARE Act. This extension will be active through September 2013, which is three months prior to the implementation of health-care reform.

Health Resources and Services Administration (HRSA), which is part of the U.S. Department of Health and Human Services (DHHS), oversees the CARE Act. Programs operated through DHHS and HRSA typically require reauthorization every five years. Therefore, the language that governs the Act is in place for five years and includes an expiration date. This does not preclude the U.S. Congress from continuing to appropriate funds after the expiration date, but it does make funding vulnerable to changes in the appropriation language.

The most challenging years of reauthorization of the CARE Act were in 1996 and 2006 and involved the formula for awarding funds throughout the United States. Until recently, the challenge has been that not every state required reporting names of HIV-positive individuals; many only required reporting names for AIDS diagnoses. Furthermore, for years funding was awarded based on cumulative AIDS cases, including those who had already died. Consequently, jurisdictions with only half of the AIDS population still living were receiving double the funding of similar regions with fewer AIDS deaths. Beginning in 2006, funding was awarded based on "estimated living HIV/AIDS cases"; essentially, the last ten years of diagnosed HIV/AIDS cases were used to develop algorithms to estimate cases in various jurisdictions. This change was made so that more of the funds would support those who were still alive. The introduction of highly active antiretroviral therapies (HAART) occurred in 1996, ten years before the implementation of this new approach to allocation of funds. The renewal of the 2006 reauthorization, with minor changes, was implemented for a three-year period through September 30, 2009. In 2009, the CARE Act was renewed for four more years, with a current expiration date of September 30, 2013.

The Ryan White Program, first conceptualized as an emergency measure, has grown to become a main part of the fabric of HIV care and services in the United States, and plays a critical role in the lives of low-income people with HIV who have no other source of care. Table 17.1 outlines the parts (formerly called titles) of the CARE Act (HRSA HIV/AIDS Bureau, 2011). It is essential for any human services professional working with people living with HIV or AIDS to be familiar with the terminology in this table.

Table 17.1. The Parts of the Ryan White Program

Section/Part	Description of Eligibility	Geographic Areas	Eligibility Criteria
Part A–subpart 1	EMAs—Emerging Metropolitan Areas	Major cities	50,000 or more population with disease burden of cumulative total of more than 2,000 AIDS cases during most recent five-year period.
Part A–subpart 2	TGAs—Transitional Grant Areas	Cities that are less major in size	50,000 or more population with disease burden of cumulative total of 1,000–1,999 cumulative AIDS cases in a five-year period.
Part B–Base and Supplemental	States and Territories	Fifty states, District of Columbia, Puerto Rico, Guam, the Virgin Islands, and five territories	States receive funding based on the state's share of living HIV (non-AIDS) and living AIDS cases, weighted to reflect the presence or absence of EMAs and TGAs, which are funded through Part A. Supplemental grants are available based on "demonstrated need."

Section/Part	Description of Eligibility	Geographic Areas	Eligibility Criteria
Part B–AIDS Drug Assistance Program (ADAP)	States and territories	Fifty states, District of Columbia, Puerto Rico, Guam, the Virgin Islands, and five territories	ADAP funds serve those with no insurance and below income levels established by every state; they cover ARV medications at a minimum. Supplemental grants are available for states with severe needs.
Part B–Emerging Communities (ECs)	Metropolitan areas	Areas that are not EMAs or TGAs	Metropolitan areas that have 500–999 cumulative reported AIDS cases over most recent five years, distributed via use of living HIV/AIDS cases from all eligible ECs.
Part C–Early Intervention Services	Competitive	Competitive	To reach people newly diagnosed with HIV, testing, case management, clinics (physicians, nurses), non-ADAP drugs.
Part C—Capacity Development and Planning	Competitive	Competitive	To support organizations in planning for service delivery and building capacity.
Part D–Services for Women, Infants, Children, Youth and Their Families	Competitive	Competitive	To provide family-centered and community-based services to children, youth, and women living with HIV and their families.
Part F–AIDS Education and Training Centers	Regional	Regional	National and regional centers that provide education and training for health-care providers who treat people with HIV.
Part F–Dental Programs	Competitive	Competitive	Reimburses dental schools and dental care providers to increase dental care for people with HIV and to educate providers.
Part F–Minority AIDS Initiative	Included in Ryan White and other HRSA programs	Competitive and through formula awards to Ryan White grantees	Provides funding to evaluate and address the disproportionate impact of HIV/AIDS on African Americans and other minorities.

Source: Kaiser Family Foundation (2009).

Strengths of the Ryan White CARE Act

Strengths of the Ryan White Program include these:

- A variety of approaches has been developed by different types of organizations across the United States. Because a variety of organizations has applied for funding, there is diversity in their approaches to care, and these approaches have further evolved over time.

- A high percentage (estimated at 50 percent) of those living with HIV in the United States are served through the various Ryan White Programs.

- The programs target those with the greatest needs.

- The establishment of medical home models for delivery of efficacious and efficient care is an advancement of the Ryan White Program.

- The development of strong care systems through the Ryan White Program can serve as a foundational model for health-care reform. This can be especially helpful as the United States moves toward providing health-care coverage for an estimated 50 million Americans currently without health-care access.

In 2010, nearly 2,200 providers throughout the fifty states, District of Columbia, Puerto Rico, U.S. Virgin Islands, Guam, and other territories delivered services funded through the Ryan White CARE Act (HRSA HIV/AIDS Bureau, 2011). These providers represented the following settings:

- Hospital or university-based clinics (17 percent)

- Publicly funded community health centers (11 percent)

- Publicly funded mental health centers (1 percent)

- Other community-based organizations (CBOs) (43 percent)

- Health departments (14 percent)

- Substance abuse treatment centers (3 percent)

- Other facilities (11 percent)

In 2010, there were more than 881,700 (duplicated) clients served, including 230,821 new (duplicated) clients. "Duplicated" clients refer to those who receive multiple services provided through Ryan White funds. Ninety percent of those served were living with HIV and 10 percent were affected by an HIV-positive individual.

The Ryan White Program was designed to serve those with the greatest need, and was to be used only as a funding resource of last resort. However, though the original CARE Act was designed to provide emergency care during the early times of crisis in AIDS care, the Act has transitioned to become the program that funds services for the majority of HIV and AIDS care in the United States, primarily for those with lower incomes. In 2008, 68 percent of those receiving services were at or below the federal poverty level (FPL) ($10,400 for one person in 2008, and $10,890 in 2012) and 22 percent were between 100 and 199 percent of the FPL. Of those served through 2010, at least 42 percent were HIV positive (non AIDS), 38 percent were HIV positive with AIDS as defined by the Centers for Disease Control and Prevention (CDC), and 15 percent were HIV positive with AIDS diagnosis unknown (HRSA, 2011).

The success of the Ryan White Program over the past twenty-one years appears to be directly correlated with the development of community-based systems of care across the United States. These systems are in communities ranging from very urban to very rural settings, and are designed to address the needs of the total person. For example, individuals who have a lower socioeconomic status are at higher risk for all sexually transmitted infections (STIs). Generally, this population also has less access to resources. The Ryan White Program ensures that this population has the best possible medical care and linkages to psychosocial, mental health, housing, substance abuse treatment, hepatitis treatment, and other highly used services. The evolution of community-based systems of care has led to establishment of the medical home model, which is now recommended for the broader health-care system. Currently, about 50 million people in the United States are without health-care insurance. The Ryan White CARE Act ensures high-quality care with the most efficient systems and thus can be used as a model for delivery of treatment to all individuals who have a chronic need for specialized care.

Weaknesses of the Ryan White CARE Act

Funding for the Ryan White CARE Act is discretionary, which means that it requires annual appropriations by Congress—a challenge in economically constrained environments. Furthermore, the discretionary funding process is subject to a range of factors that expose it to the current influences of the larger political and social context. The military, programs to provide relief for families affected by the economic downturn, other domestic social programs, and international relief efforts all compete for discretionary funds. The advancement of HIV and AIDS treatment has had substantial positive effects in lengthening and improving the lives of people living with HIV (PLWH). However, the development of life-extending treatments has increased the costs of care and lengthened the amount of time each client requires care. Therefore, AIDS care today requires more funding than AIDS care twenty years ago.

Currently, an estimated 1.1 million persons in the United States are living with HIV. Because of demands on the federal budget, the Ryan White CARE Act has been repeatedly flat funded. That is, Congress appropriates the same funding as in the previous year, even though each year the demand for services increases and costs for the same services rise. The flat-funding environment leads to the need for cost containment strategies in organizations providing the services. Recent strategies have included the following:

- Numerous states have made major changes to their ADAP. Many have lowered the income eligibility: now, in order to qualify for provision of life-saving medications, a person must now be "poorer" than before. Furthermore, some states have developed waiting lists, requiring new applicants to wait for a place to open up on the list.

- Psychosocial case management services have been curtailed.

- The flexibility of programs funded by Ryan White at local levels has been reduced. As a result, grantees cannot be as flexible to make sure the services needed in an area are covered. In the past, greater flexibility in the way funds were spent allowed localities to adapt their local systems of care to changing needs.

- A greater focus is placed on collecting client-level data to justify funding, even though some of the data do not accurately represent needs and the process provides an excessive administrative burden.

A further weakness of the current state of the Ryan White funding structure is that local governmental entities, through which funds are channeled, are often inflexible and not nimble enough to adapt to the changing needs of chronic communicable conditions.

Medical Case Management. Medical case management services through Ryan White include a range of client-centered services that link clients with health care, psychosocial care, and other services. The coordination of care and follow-up care are components of the case management. Services ensure timely and coordinated access to medically appropriate levels of health and support services. Services also provide continuity of care through ongoing assessments of the client, key family members, and personal support systems. This ensures that the goals and needs of the client and family members are met. HIV medical case management includes counseling to ensure readiness for complex HIV and AIDS treatment regimens and adherence to treatment. Key activities include

1. Initial assessment of service needs;

2. Development of a comprehensive, individualized service plan;

3. Coordination of services required to implement the plan;

4. Client monitoring to assess the efficacy of the plan; and

5. Periodic re-evaluation and adaption of the plan as necessary over the life of the client.

Case management can also include client-specific advocacy, through which the worker helps clients negotiate the best possible system of care for them. Case management includes review of the utilization of services and provides ongoing communication with clients, either face to face or by phone.

The Ryan White Program follows a medical model, and the case management function is delivered as medical case management. The 2006 reauthorization placed heightened emphasis on the medical aspects of care. Some say that as a result of this change the psychosocial aspects of holistic care, including transportation, housing assistance, substance abuse treatment, mental health care, and counseling, have fallen by the wayside (Rowan & Honeycutt, 2010).

With medical case management, local systems must refer from one case manager to another, rather than having a single case manager to serve as the central coordinator of care. Because case management through Ryan White funding is primarily concerned with medical adherence, there is often a need for an additional case manager for services provided by other organizations. This approach can actually limit access to needed psychosocial services, because case managers may not be sure what needs are being addressed by other case managers. The approach can undermine the core philosophy of case management to ensure continuity of care and unintentionally lead to reductions in access to mental health, substance abuse, housing, financial planning, and other psychosocial support services.

Current Ryan White policies require the grantees and subcontractors of grantees to deliver an increasing amount of client-level data. This extensive reporting may help to evaluate the effectiveness of various program elements. However, the time spent on data collection limits the ability of local jurisdictions to serve the growing and evolving needs of clients.

Implications for Macro Social Work. Macro-level social work with HIV and AIDS focuses on planning from a community perspective to maximize the impact of all funding. Jurisdictions differ in what local services are provided, what other systems may be in place (corrections, mental health, substance abuse treatment), how low-income housing solutions are reached by the community, and what HIV testing designs are used. These differences could be better accommodated if Ryan White funds were more flexible. All services provided must be discussed in detail in proposals for funding, and plans must be submitted to the city and state for approval. The reality is that the governmental entities that administer these funds are inflexible. When services are constrained at the federal level, for example, mandating medical case management provision, the ability of providers to meet local needs through Ryan White funds is reduced.

Ryan White funding is not equally distributed across the United States. Federal funds are not distributed directly to states, but instead are awarded to emerging metropolitan areas (EMAs) and transitional grant areas (TGAs). EMAs are political subdivisions, such as a large city or metropolitan area around a city, with a cumulative total of more than 2,000 AIDS cases during the most recent five-year period; TGAs have a cumulative total of 1,000 to 1,999 cases. Table 17.2 displays eligible EMAs and TGAs and the amount of Ryan White funds awarded in fiscal year 2011 (HRSA, 2011).

Table 17.2. Amount of Funding Awarded through Parts of Ryan White Program in 2011

Part A Emerging Metropolitan Area (EMA) or TGA	Total FY 2011 Part A Ryan White Award
Atlanta, GA	$ 21,577,871
Austin, TX	$ 4,400,041
Baltimore, MD	$ 21,097,384
Baton Rouge, LA	$ 4,004,606
Bergen–Passaic, NJ	$ 4,313,092
Boston, MA	$ 13,769,366
Charlotte–Gastonia, NC/SC	$ 5,748,542
Chicago, IL	$ 26,251,321
Cleveland, OH	$ 4,419,764
Dallas, TX	$ 14,625,082
Denver, CO	$ 7,826,960

Part A Emerging Metropolitan Area (EMA) or TGA	Total FY 2011 Part A Ryan White Award
Detroit, MI	$ 8,939,656
Ft. Lauderdale, FL	$ 15,006,261
Ft. Worth, TX	$ 3,864,274
Hartford, CT	$ 4,249,488
Houston, TX	$ 19,735,984
Indianapolis, IN	$ 3,913,252
Jacksonville, FL	$ 5,805,921
Jersey City, NJ	$ 5,078,282
Kansas City, MO	$ 4,308,949
Las Vegas, NV	$ 5,699,300
Los Angeles, CA	$ 40,064,159
Memphis, TN	$ 6,920,474
Miami, FL	$ 25,119,484
Middlesex-Somerset-Hunterdon, NJ	$ 2,757,588
Minneapolis–St. Paul, MN	$ 5,651,896
Nashville, TN	$ 4,720,797
Nassau–Suffolk, NY	$ 6,447,553
New Haven, CT	$ 7,042,480
New Orleans, LA	$ 7,370,711
New York, NY	$120,933,827
Newark, NJ	$ 14,054,011
Norfolk, VA	$ 6,044,862
Oakland, CA	$ 6,794,771
Orange County, CA	$ 5,975,990
Orlando, FL	$ 8,912,835
Philadelphia, PA	$ 24,102,413
Phoenix, AZ	$ 8,269,205
Ponce, Puerto Rico	$ 2,025,807
Portland, OR	$ 3,742,804
Riverside–San Bernardino, CA	$ 7,824,937
Sacramento, CA	$ 2,654,867
Saint Louis, MO	$ 6,528,396
San Antonio, TX	$ 4,413,444
San Diego, CA	$ 11,778,488
San Francisco, CA	$ 25,640,788
San Jose, CA	$ 2,844,809
San Juan, Puerto Rico	$ 15,411,549
Seattle, WA	$ 6,870,026
Tampa–St. Petersburg, FL	$ 9,411,546
Washington, DC (MD, VA, WV)	$ 31,386,544
West Palm Beach, FL	$ 8,781,650
Totals	$645,134,107

Source: HRSA (2011).

In addition to the funds allocated for each city, each community benefits from state Ryan White funds. Part C, Part D, and Part F funding may also operate within or support services in these areas. Several states receive no Part A funding.

While Chapter 2 provides a history of the young activist named Ryan White and the CARE Act named for him, the details of how appropriations are made are given here (Communities Advocating Emergency AIDS Relief Coalition, 2011). Figure 17.1 illustrates the distribution of the $2.3 billion in the CARE Act.

Figure 17.1. Ryan White FY 2011 Appropriations by Part

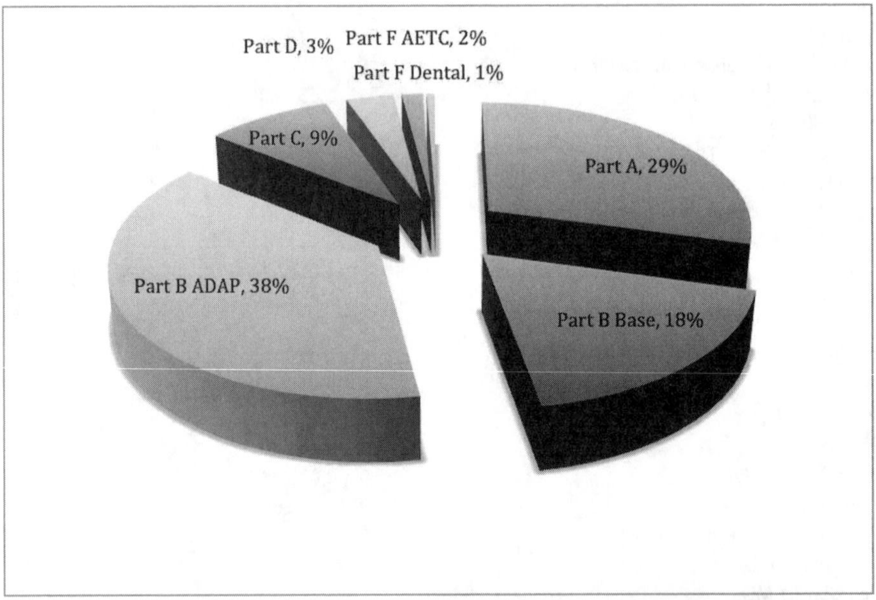

Program	FY 2011 Final
Part A	$677,700,000
Part B Base	$418,000,000
Part B ADAP	$885,000,000
Part C	205,600,000
Part D	$77,300,000
Part F AETC	$34,600,000
Part F Dental	$13,500,000
Total	**$2,311,700,000**

Source: Kaiser Family Foundation (2010).

AIDS Drug Assistance Program

Summary and History

ADAP is a carve out of the Ryan White CARE Act; in 2011 it provided $885 million for HIV medications for individuals with no health insurance. ADAP is funded through Part B of the Ryan White CARE Act and represented 38 percent of all Ryan White funding in 2011. In addition to federal Ryan White funding, several states and municipalities contribute portions of their awards to their ADAP to provide access to medications to more individuals living with HIV. The amounts contributed vary by area, but total more than $1 billion. Each state and territorial government administer their ADAP; in some cases, those entities opt to contract with a pharmacy benefits manager to run the program. They may also use their own state pharmacies or work with other distribution networks.

Project Inform

Several years ago, Project Inform, one of the nation's leading HIV/AIDS advocacy organizations, launched the ADAP Crisis Task Force to negotiate with pharmaceutical companies on the pricing for approved ARV therapeutic drugs, according to the DHHS Guidelines for the Use of Antiretroviral Agents in HIV-1-Infected Adults and Adolescents. Currently, the ADAP Crisis Task Force is operated by the National Alliance of State and Territorial AIDS Directors (NASTAD) and works with fourteen pharmaceutical manufacturers to obtain the lowest price for approved ARV medications. This is known as the "ADAP price," and it is by far the lowest price offered by manufacturers (NASTAD, 2011).

Disparities in Eligibility between States

Because each state government administers its own ADAP program, there are many state variations (Kaiser Family Foundation, 2010). These variations include the following:

- Eligibility criteria for program participation vary from 125 to 500 percent of the FPL.

- The types of drugs covered vary. Some states have formularies that cover ARV medications only, and others have an open formulary covering any medication required by someone who is eligible for ADAP, including medication therapies for high cholesterol, mental illness, hepatitis, and other treatments.

- States vary in whether or not they require co-pays for prescriptions.

- States differ in administration and distribution models, based on geography and demand for services. Cost-savings measures often lead to centralization of administrative processes, moving control away from localities.

Variations in how states administer programs have implications for clients' decisions on where to reside or relocate. A consumer may qualify in one state for ADAP coverage and receive full benefits, while the same consumer in another state would be denied the benefits because his or her income is more than $21,000 per year. This denial would occur even if the individual did not have health insurance coverage. These variations in access to care may or may not be addressed through health-care reform and Medicaid expansion. (Medicaid-related issues will be discussed further in the Medicaid expansion section of this chapter.)

State Waiting Lists. There are more than 7,000 persons on waiting lists for life-sustaining medications. The ADAP Advocacy Association, along with multiple other groups, continues to pressure the U.S. Congress to address this life-threatening concern (NASTAD, 2011). National, regional, local, and individual advocates have contributed to the dialogue at the Congressional level on how to approach the situation that has been created in the United States. The costs for each person who uses the ADAP program is approximately $10,000 annually. Therefore, each $1 million can serve one hundred people. To address the current ADAP access problem, Congress would need to appropriate an additional $70 million to retire the extensive waiting lists. Is it worth $70 million to prevent infections in untreated persons diagnosed with HIV? Is it worth $70 million to ensure that individuals have maximal quality and quantity of life? Recently, Texas had no ADAP waiting list and Florida had 3,398 persons on their waiting list as of October 13, 2011. Is it worth $70 million to flatten the difference between Texas and Florida? This approach to policy development has proven successful in the past. In today's context of broken economic systems and a depleted Wall Street, however, the answers are more complicated than ever.

Treatment Is Prevention. May 2011 brought exciting news to the HIV prevention and care community when the HIV Prevention Trials Network (HPTN) released the results of Clinical Trial 052. The HPTN trial had been designed to evaluate whether immediate versus delayed use of antiretroviral (ARV) medications would reduce transmission of HIV to uninfected partners (National Institutes of Health [NIH], 2011). HPTN Clinical Trial 052 showed a 96 percent reduction in HIV transmission in 877 sero-discordant couples that had used ARV medications immediately upon HIV diagnosis. (Sero-discordancy is when one person in a couple is HIV positive and the other is HIV negative.) Thus, the scientific research community has provided a powerful justification for providing all HIV-positive individuals who are suitable for ARV medications to have immediate access to them. It is clear through the release of HPTN Clinical Trial 052 that ARV therapy is an effective prevention strategy. This study provides powerful data to use as leverage with policy makers, to ensure unfettered access to ARV medications to everyone who needs them. This issue provides an excellent example of how research can affect policy change, which in turn can greatly impact social work practice, which then improves the quality of life of the individuals who receive life-saving medications, the individuals who are not infected through exposure to the virus by a partner with HIV, and society at large, which is interested in control of threats to public health.

Housing Opportunities for Persons with AIDS (HOPWA)
HOPWA Overview

As the Ryan White CARE Act was moving through Congress in 1990, the U.S. Department of Housing and Urban Development (HUD) also was addressing the HIV epidemic. The AIDS Housing Opportunity Act of 1992 (with the first appropriations coming in 1993) was the result of HUD's HIV/AIDS advocacy movement. HOPWA assists beneficiaries by providing stable housing as a basis for increased participation in appropriate health-care and other supportive services. Grantees measure program achievements and log those achievements as part of annual performance reports on housing. According to HUD (2010), the current national HOPWA outcome targets are as follows:

1. Maintain housing stability for at least 87 percent of HOPWA households in permanent housing (target to reach 90 percent by 2012).

2. Reduce risks of homelessness for at least 63 percent of clients in short-term or transitional housing (target to reach 70 percent by 2012).

(A more detailed discussion of the HOPWA program and the importance of housing for people living with HIV is found in chapter 16.)

Importance of Housing for Persons Living with AIDS

Housing Is Health Care. For individuals living with HIV/AIDS, stable housing, or the lack thereof, is one of the strongest predictors of access to treatment, health outcomes, and longevity. Before they can obtain and benefit from life-saving HIV treatments, people living with HIV must have safe and stable housing. Individuals who are homeless or who lack stable housing and are HIV positive are at a greater disadvantage than those who are housed. Housed individuals have lower CD4 counts and higher viral loads, and are less likely to enter early HIV care and receive and adhere to ARV therapy, and are more likely to be hospitalized, use emergency rooms, and experience higher rates of premature death. According to Wolitski and colleagues (2010), when a previously homeless person with HIV or AIDS is stably housed, there is a 57 percent reduction in hospitalizations, a 35 percent reduction in emergency room visits, and an 80 percent reduction in mortality.

Housing Is Prevention. HIV-prevention strategies will not succeed without attention to access to housing and other related factors. Based on current research, Wolitski and colleagues (2010) have identified several housing-related facts that impact HIV prevention and care:

- Living in an unstable housing situation is associated with increased risk behavior and higher HIV infection rates, controlling for substance use, mental health issues, access to services, and other factors that contribute to risk.

- Counseling, needle exchange, and other proven HIV-prevention interventions are less effective in reducing HIV risk among people who are homeless or unstably housed than among people who are housed.

- People living with HIV/AIDS who are homeless or unstably housed are two to six times more likely to have recently used hard drugs, shared needles, or engaged in high-risk sex.

- Homeless women are as much as five times more likely to report drug use and risky sexual behaviors, in part due to victimization through physical and sexual violence.

- At-risk youth who have stable housing are significantly more likely to use condoms and less likely to have multiple sex partners.

• When people living with HIV have their level of housing stability improved, their drug use is reduced and their risky sexual behaviors are reduced by as much as half. Those whose housing status worsens over time show increases in risky behaviors.

Box 17.1. Housing Is the Greatest Unmet Need of Americans Living with HIV/AIDS

• 1.1 million = The number of persons currently living with HIV/AIDS in the United States; 56,000 people are newly infected each year.

• Fewer than 60,000 = The number of households currently served by the federal Housing Opportunities for Persons with AIDS (HOPWA) program.

• 500,000 = The number of Americans living with HIV who will need some form of housing assistance during the course of their illness.

• More than 140,000 = The number of households with HIV in the United States that currently lack stable housing and have an unmet need for housing assistance.

The available research makes it readily apparent that access to adequate housing profoundly affects the health of Americans who are at-risk for or living with HIV.

Source: NAHC (2008).

Strengths and Weaknesses of HOPWA

The $350 million federal appropriation for the HOPWA program in 2011 greatly enhanced the quality of life and health care for the 60,000 people served. A study of housing needs across the United States in 2007, however, found that at least 50 percent of people living with HIV or AIDS are still in need of housing support. HUD's homeless programs, housing voucher programs (such as Section 8), public housing, U.S. Department of Veterans Affairs housing, and local housing solutions all address the housing needs of people with HIV. Nevertheless, the National AIDS Housing Coalition estimates that at any given moment there are 140,000 persons living with HIV who have partially or totally unmet housing needs (National AIDS Housing Coalition [NAHC], 2011).

Creative local plans that meet the housing needs of people with HIV have been developed in communities in many parts of the United States. These plans often result in funding for housing units, often called set-asides, that are restricted for use by individuals or families affected by HIV. Public housing authorities that lean toward a more progressive approach implement multiple programs to provide special needs housing, including units for those living with HIV. Other localities struggle to access any mainstream housing programs for those with HIV due to limited housing stock; lack of safe, low-cost housing; and conservative administrators who may be unwilling to consider special needs housing. Furthermore, the high poverty in both rural and urban communities results in increased pressure for safe and affordable housing, and housing resources are becoming less available for some at-risk populations.

Recent patterns show that housing advocacy approaches are more productive if they pursue development of more set-asides (HIV-dedicated units) rather than seeking funds to build new homes. Existing providers are often more interested in housing stable tenants who can pay rent in a timely manner than they are in contracting with organizations who are trying to build new housing developments. HIV housing advocates can capitalize on the situation in regions where the downturn in the housing market has created a large supply of foreclosed properties by developing a plan to house HIV-positive individuals or families with a reliable funding stream of governmental or nonprofit funding.

The Players in HIV/AIDS Policy Development

Successful development of HIV/AIDS policy involves many partners who consult with each other to develop effective programs to meet the needs of those living with HIV and AIDS (figure 17.2). Various entities have their own unique perspectives on the problems and proposed solutions. Policy development is typically based on a pre-identified area of need or area of study. For example, prevention and HIV testing could produce multiple national, regional, and local policies that influence whether funding is targeted toward traditional prevention messages or diagnostics.

Figure 17.2. State AIDS Director/Public Health Circle

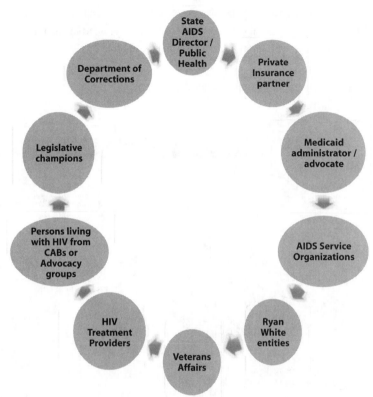

Perhaps the key element in determining who will be involved in decision making is identifying the issue or problem. For example, if the CDC's approach to funding prevention programs is not targeting women, but the incidence rates in a particular region indicate that women are greatly represented in new diagnoses of HIV disease, policy advocates can argue that the target population has been incorrectly identified. The need for equity should lead individuals and groups to research the topic and develop policies that directly impact previously unaddressed populations. After research has identified unmet needs, advocacy groups should seek out partners to collaborate on a resolution. Partnerships should be built with consideration of the stakeholders in the issue. Consumers, in this case newly diagnosed women, should be brought to the table and given a voice on the issue. Often lawmakers are most affected by the stories of members of the target population.

Three types of partners are critical for development of policies. The composition of groups differs based on the specific issue to be addressed. The groups included in Box 17.2 illustrate a typical combination of players present at the table to address issues; this box shows the partners to consider in an HIV/AIDS advocacy effort at the national level. The level of target advocacy efforts, whether local, state, or national, will determine which stakeholders and decision makers need to be brought on board.

Box 17.2. Partners to Consider in a National HIV/AIDS Advocacy Effort
Federal Government
• U.S. Department of Health & Human Services (includes HRSA, SAMHSA, CDC, NIH)
• U.S. Department of Housing and Urban Development
• U.S. Department of Justice
• U.S. Department of Education
• U.S. Department of Labor
• U.S. Department of Homeland Security
Private Sector Entities
• Kaiser Family Foundation
• Pharmaceutical industry lobbying consultants
• Ford Foundation
• Multiple other foundations depending upon specific issues involved
Community Based
• AIDS United (AIDS Action Council merged with National AIDS Fund)
• Federal AIDS Policy Partnership (more than 120 national, regional, and local organizations)

- National Minority AIDS Council

- Treatment Access Expansion Project

- Harvard Law and Policy Center

- HIV Medical Association

- American Academy of HIV Medical Care

- HIV Health

- National Alliance of State and Territorial AIDS Directors (NAS-TAD)

- National Association of Social Worker's HIV Spectrum Project

- AIDS Education Training Centers

- Cities Advocating for Emergency AIDS Relief (CAEAR)

- National Low Income Housing Coalition (NLIHC)

- National Alliance to End Homelessness

- National Association of Persons with AIDS

- Latino AIDS Commission

- National Council of La Raza

- Southern AIDS Coalition

- Professional Association of Social Workers in HIV and AIDS (PASWHA)

Case Example

Macro social work is part of systematic change. Policies at federal, state, and local levels all influence those living with or at risk of HIV infection. The following case example illustrates policy-level social work in HIV/AIDS care.

In 2004, the pharmaceutical company Pfizer was interested in expanding resources to states that had waiting lists for their ADAP. The Access Advocates program was designed to recruit leaders from various states that had ADAP waiting lists. The program oriented these leaders to national policies affecting local resources, and challenged advocates to develop statewide advocacy efforts on behalf of persons living with HIV.

There were 14 persons ultimately recruited for Access Advocates. Two individuals from seven states were chosen to participate in two in-person meetings and multiple conference calls. The seven states represented were Florida, Georgia, Louisiana, Mississippi, North Carolina, South Carolina, and Tennessee. The kick-off meeting, referred to as Access Academy I, lasted two and a half days and included national speakers who addressed the upcoming 2006 reauthorization of the Ryan White CARE Act, information regarding the CDC's new HIV testing guidelines, and an orientation on several federal programs including the Ryan White Program, HOPWA, substance abuse initiatives, and Medicare/Medicaid. The participants were then given multiple examples of how state advocacy design works. The orientation included a suggested framework for a successful HIV advocacy effort (figure 17.3). The board consisted of Dr. Gene Copello from the AIDS Institute, Anne Donnelly of Project Inform, and Dr. Marsha Martin from the AIDS Action Council.

The faculty outlined fundamental principles of state level advocacy and campaign design. The group worked through several practice scenarios and before the end of the last day of training they were asked to present their statewide advocacy model. Phase two, called Access Academy II, consisted of three conference calls over six months. Advocates all gave presentations on the implementation of their campaigns and the results of their efforts. The outcomes were as follows:

- Six statewide campaigns that translated into increases in state contributions to their ADAPs of $25 million over two years

- Support to establish the State Pharmacy Access Program for HIV-positive persons in the state of Texas

- Continued advocacy efforts in five of the original seven states

Recent Developments Affecting AIDS Policy

Several recent events are shaping how HIV and AIDS care and prevention interventions are being funded and delivered. Before looking at these changes, however, it is useful to look back at early perspectives on the rights of people living with AIDS. In 1983, a group of AIDS advocates came together in Denver, Colorado, and crafted what became known as the Denver Principles. These statements are as relevant

Figure 17.3. Keys to Effective Advocacy

1. Find a legislative leader or champion.
2. Recruit members to the table.
3. Gain buy-in from key stakeholders.
4. Key global objective: 100% access 0% disparity.
5. Communication: internal and external.
6. Enthusiasm and passion are key ingredients to build and maintain a strong network.

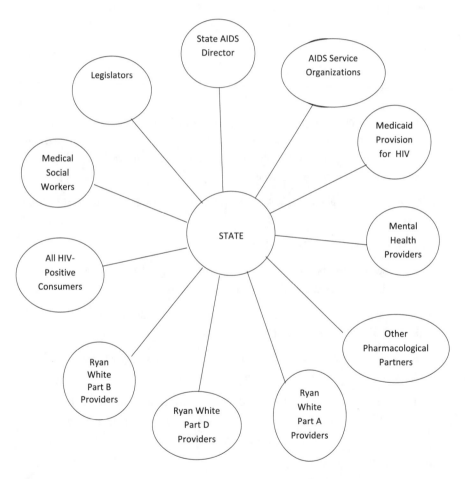

today as they were then, laying out an approach to guide all program design, language, funding criteria, and inclusion of those living with HIV. These fundamental principles have shaped how the nation has been committed to, or not committed to, HIV/AIDS awareness and prevention.

The Denver Principles

There is no better way to cite the history of the PWA (people with AIDS) self-empowerment movement than to quote the principles articulated in Denver in 1983 (Denver Principles, 1983). They are as relevant and powerful today as they were then.

The Denver Principles

(Statement from the advisory committee of the People with AIDS)

We condemn attempts to label us as "victims," a term which implies defeat, and we are only occasionally "patients," a term which implies passivity, helplessness, and dependence upon the care of others. We are "People With AIDS."

RECOMMENDATIONS FOR ALL PEOPLE

1. Support us in our struggle against those who would fire us from our jobs, evict us from our homes, refuse to touch us or separate us from our loved ones, our community or our peers, since available evidence does not support the view that AIDS can be spread by casual, social contact.

2. Not scapegoat people with AIDS, blame us for the epidemic or generalize about our lifestyles.

RECOMMENDATIONS FOR PEOPLE WITH AIDS

1. Form caucuses to choose their own representatives, to deal with the media, to choose their own agenda and to plan their own strategies.

2. Be involved at every level of decision-making and specifically serve on the boards of directors of provider organizations.

3. Be included in all AIDS forums with equal credibility as other participants, to share their own experiences and knowledge.

4. Substitute low-risk sexual behaviors for those which could endanger themselves or their partners; we feel people with AIDS have an ethical responsibility to inform their potential sexual partners of their health status.

RIGHTS OF PEOPLE WITH AIDS

1. To as full and satisfying sexual and emotional lives as anyone else.

2. To quality medical treatment and quality social service provision without discrimination of any form including sexual orientation, gender, diagnosis, economic status or race.

3. To full explanations of all medical procedures and risks, to choose or refuse their treatment modalities, to refuse to participate in research without jeopardizing their treatment and to make informed decisions about their lives.

4. To privacy, to confidentiality of medical records, to human respect and to choose who their significant others are.

5. To die—and to LIVE—in dignity.

As a result of the lack of proper education about HIV transmission, societal stigma and discrimination against individuals with HIV and AIDS remain realities in the United States. The war on AIDS continues, with transmission rates in marginalized communities on the rise and people who need care not receiving it. Several recent developments in the AIDS policy landscape are likely to have a great impact on AIDS policies in the future. They are discussed below.

The National HIV/AIDS Strategy

The White House released the National HIV/AIDS Strategy (NHAS) in July 2010. President Barack Obama delegated the responsibility for development of an NHAS for the United States to his Domestic Policy Council, which includes the director of the Office of National AIDS Policy. For decades, several organized groups and a large number of individuals had been advocating for a national approach to the HIV epidemic. The following key events helped to establish the NHAS:

- Through The U.S. President's Emergency Plan for AIDS Relief (PEPFAR), the United States became the global leader in provision of HIV treatment and prevention in developing areas of the world, which the pandemic disproportionately affects.

- The United States issued a declaration that HIV/AIDS had become a threat to national security.

- The CDC reported increased levels of HIV incidence in 2006, 2008, and 2009, demonstrating higher than previously expected annual new case counts.

One might wonder how AIDS can be a threat to national security. President Bill Clinton's administration was the first to declare HIV/AIDS as a national security threat. At the time, the high number of people dying from AIDS in other countries increased those countries' susceptibility to being overrun by groups who "intended to destroy the seeds of democracy" (Gellman, 2000). Internationally, the U.S. declaration, based on fear of upsets in global power, helped to increase HIV/AIDS awareness of the detrimental effects of this disease around the world. Still, the United States did not have a unified national plan for combating the HIV virus.

President George W. Bush called for the inclusion of an NHAS as part of health-care provision, and PEPFAR would be used to fund this initiative. PEPFAR was designed to distribute approximately $15 billion to HIV/AIDS high-risk nations around the world to increase life-saving treatment options from 2003 to 2008. Each participating nation was required to submit a national plan for the HIV/AIDS response. Internationally, the results increased the number of individuals receiving treatment from 50,000 to nearly 1.4 million in 2008, proving PEPFAR to be successful in advancing the fight on AIDS in other parts of the world. However, the United States did not move forward as planned on development and approval of the country's own national AIDS strategy. In 2010, the Obama administration developed and released the nation's first comprehensive and coordinated plan to fight HIV and AIDS in the United States, the National HIV/AIDS Strategy (NHAS).

The White House designed NHAS with input from multiple sources including the following (Office of National AIDS Policy, 2011):

• Online portals for individual comments

• Ten town hall meetings and listening sessions across the United States

• Multiple listening sessions from a variety of national, state, and regional advocacy groups

• Input from fourteen federal departments involving community input

• Consumer voices directly, through organizations, and from testimony

• Clinics and HIV/AIDS service organizations (ASOs) across the country

The National HIV/AIDS Strategy
Vision

The United States will become a place where new HIV infections are rare and when they do occur, every person, regardless of age, gender, race/ethnicity, sexual orientation, gender identity or socio-economic circumstance, will have unfettered access to high quality, life-extending care, free from stigma and discrimination.

—Office of National AIDS Policy (2011).

Goals

Reducing New Infections

- By 2015, lower the annual number of new infections by 25 percent (from 56,300 to 42,225)

- Reduce the HIV transmission rate, which is a measure of annual transmissions in relation to the number of people living with HIV, by 30 percent (from 5 persons infected per 100 people with HIV to 3.5 persons infected per 100 people with HIV)

- By 2015, increase from 79 percent to 90 percent the percentage of people living with HIV who know their status (from 948,000 to 1,080,000 people)

Increasing Access to Care and Improving Health Outcomes for People Living with HIV

- By 2015, increase the proportion of newly diagnosed patients linked to clinical care within three months of their HIV diagnosis, from 65 percent to 85 percent (from 26,824 to 35,078 people).

- By 2015, increase the proportion of Ryan White Program clients who are in continuous care (at least two visits for routine HIV medical care in twelve months at least three months apart) from 73 percent to 80 percent (from 237,924 people in continuous care to 260,739 people in continuous care).

- By 2015, increase the number of Ryan White clients with permanent housing from 82 percent to 86 percent (from 434,000 to 455,800 people). This goal serves as a measurable proxy of our efforts to expand access to HUD and other housing supports to all people living with HIV and AIDS.

Reducing HIV-Related Disparities and Health Inequities

While working to improve access to prevention and care services for all Americans, the following goals with regard to reduction of inequities are important:

- By 2015, increase the proportion of HIV-diagnosed Blacks with undetectable viral load by 20 percent.

- By 2015, increase the proportion of HIV-diagnosed Latinos with undetectable viral load by 20 percent.

(Note: All numbers in above list are based on current estimates, July 2010 [Office of National AIDS Policy, 2011]).

The implementation summary for the NHAS illustrates the outcome-oriented approach. Each goal includes specific objectives for fourteen different federal departments. The objectives focus on the outcomes outlined by funders, individuals in the community, and multiple facets of the health-care system. Each group and individual involved with the strategy must be fully engaged in the process to achieve the intended results. According to the U.S. Department of Health and Human Services (DHHS; AIDS.gov, 2011), establishment of the NHAS has led to the following outcomes:

- The twelve cities project, launched in September 2010 just after the announcement of the NHAS, identifies twelve cities where it is estimated that 44 percent of those with AIDS in the United States live (table 17.3). The twelve cities receive support from multiple federally funded initiatives aimed at prevention of new cases.

- State-level plans that tie into the NHAS are now required as part of Ryan White Program funding. The NHAS recommends that activities at state and local levels line up with the goals of the national plan.

Table 17.3. Twelve Cities Project

Metropolitan Area	Estimated AIDS Cases in 2007
New York City, NY	66,426
Los Angeles	24,727
Washington, DC	15,696
Chicago, IL	14,175
Atlanta, GA	13,105
Miami, FL	12,732
Philadelphia, PA	12,469
Houston, TX	11,227
San Francisco, CA	11,026
Baltimore, MD	10,301
Dallas, TX	7,993
San Juan, PR	7,858
Percent of U.S. total	44%

Source: Office of AIDS Policy (2011).

- Federal departments have specific implementation plans related to the NHAS available for the public, via download. The following departments have plans in place to support implementation of the strategy:
  - U.S. Department of Health and Human Services
  - U.S. Department of Housing and Urban Development
  - U.S. Department of Labor
  - U.S. Department of Justice
  - U.S. Department of Veterans Affairs
  - Social Security Administration.
- The following key entities within the federal government also have developed reports and documents:
  - U.S. Department of Defense
  - U.S. Department of State
  - Equal Employment Opportunity Commission
  - Appendix to the U.S. Department of Health and Human Services (DHHS) Operational Plan
- The Obama Administration lifted a twenty-two-year-old ban on HIV-infected persons entering the United States, effective January 4, 2010 (Preston, 2009).
- Multiple federal programs focusing on the NHAS have been funded through a competitive process. Furthermore, there has been an increased focus on ensuring that existing programs align with the NHAS goals.

Recently, perhaps because of the release of the NHAS and the focus of President Obama's administration on domestic and global HIV/AIDS awareness and prevention, there has been an increase in interest in HIV and AIDS across public sectors. The introduction of the social determinants of health (SDH) framework and the Patient Protection and Affordable Care Act—both of which are further explained below—are two fundamental changes at the federal level. The SDH framework helps to narrow the focus of the NHAS and determine the effectiveness of the approach.

Social Determinants of Health

In the summer of 2010, coinciding with the introduction of the NHAS, special editions of *Public Health Reports* included articles by Dr. Kevin Fenton and Dr. Hazel Dean. The articles described a framework for including environmental factors in reducing transmissions of chronic communicable diseases, called the social determinants of health, and included an authoritative report titled "Establishing a Holistic Framework to Reduce Inequities in HIV, Viral Hepatitis, STDs and Tuberculosis in the United States" (CDC, 2010). Based on international research, the articles identified a variety of factors (e.g., education, poverty, housing, and social environment) that influence behaviors related to disease transmission. Dr. Fenton and Dr. Dean identified these factors and examined each through four lenses:

1. Disease prevalence

2. Effectiveness of interventions

3. Illness and wellness responses

4. Attention to structural factors

Figure 17.4 clarifies the CDC's suggested approach to addressing the social determinants of health. Implementation of this model is intended to intervene across the life span and eventually lead to more effective and efficient ways to spend dollars for health care.

The Patient Protection and Affordable Care Act

The NHAS targets specific goals, and the social determinants of health framework seeks to advise policy makers on effective approaches to meeting those goals. These approaches are related to implementation of the recently passed Patient Protection and Affordable Care Act (PPACA). The PPACA, often referred to as ACA (Affordable Care Act) or health-care reform, provides opportunities for each state to maximize responses to prevention, care, and treatment that could dramatically affect the HIV/AIDS community. However, the methods chosen for implementation of the PPACA will ultimately be decided by the states.

Figure 17.4. Impacts on Social Determinants of Health

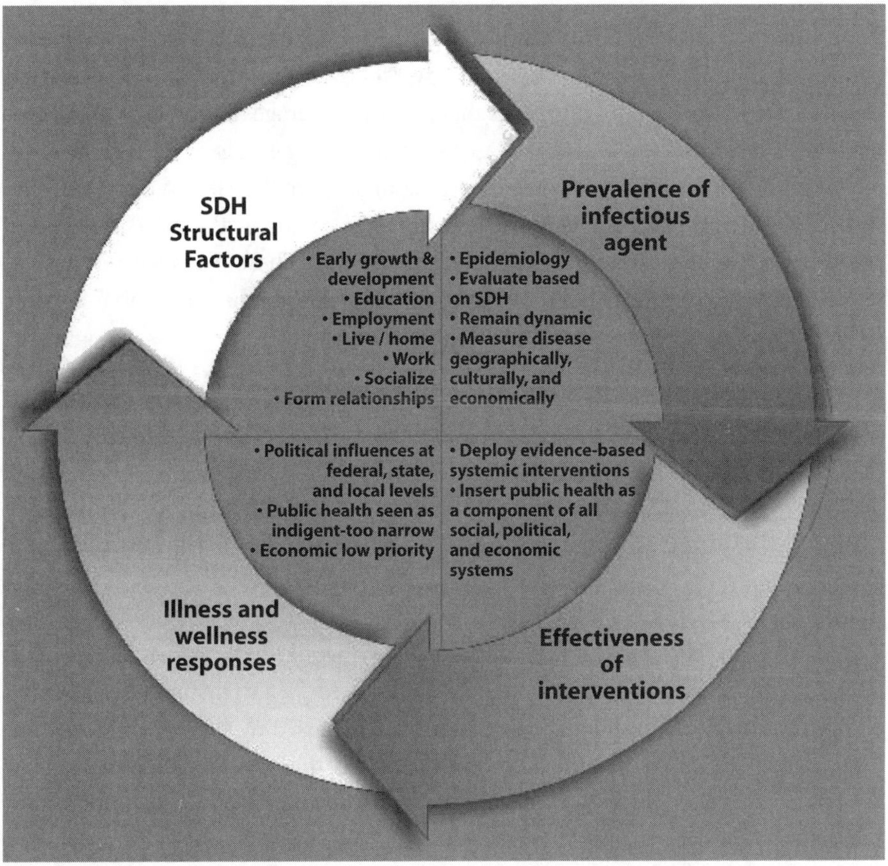

What Is Health-care Reform?

In brief, the ACA is designed to cover the currently 50 million Americans who cannot afford insurance, or are not eligible under current systems. The ACA plans to accomplish this goal through expansion of the dollars allocated to Medicaid. The amount of the expansion is roughly $28 million annually. Additionally, the ACA will require health-care coverage of all Americans through individual and employer-based plans that are affordable, with tax breaks and other approaches to ensure coverage through the private market. The ACA will be phased in over time, with lower amounts of state funding required initially, then larger amounts of state funding required later.

Health Insurance Exchanges

Public and private health insurance is regulated and controlled at the state level. While some U.S. citizens are directly covered by Medicare, most are covered through state-approved private plans that provide coverage on behalf of Medicare-managed care. Medicaid and all private plans, including employer-based plans, are approved by each state's insurance commission and are licensed to operate in the respective state. With the adaptations of managed care over the past fifteen years some states now have more than one hundred plans. These plans vary in nature, allowing insurance companies to maximize their profit margins through their ability to charge different premiums to different groups.

For example, if a person is currently covered through a Medicare Part D prescription plan, there may be fifteen private companies operating Part D plans in the specific state. There is one rate for this plan, which differs from Medicare Part A (for hospitalization insurance, including short-term skilled nursing care and hospice care) and Part B (for medical insurance, including outpatient visits and other services and supplies not covered by Part A). Insurance companies charge different premiums depending on the types of benefits provided. The ACA calls for every state to create a health insurance exchange, which would be a new entity intended to create a more organized and competitive market for health insurance by offering a choice of plans and establishing common rules regarding pricing of insurance. The intent is to help consumers better understand the options available to them while still providing private market choices. However, the governance of health insurance exchanges has yet to be agreed upon.

Medicaid Expansion

For Medicaid expansion, a similar approach will be used to determine at the state level what Medicaid will cover. Additionally, as part of the Medicaid expansion, the PPACA will include provisions for the development of a medical home. Beginning January 1, 2014, Medicaid will cover all persons whose income is up to 133 percent of the FPL, regardless of disability status. Today's Medicaid coverage varies by state. In some states, the eligibility threshold is as low as 24 percent of the FPL, and the states require that single adults also be disabled to receive benefits. The new changes will mean that 28 to 30 million people who otherwise would not receive health-care coverage will become eligible for Medicaid in 2014. The states will determine what they will cover based on federal minimum standards, and decide what disease states will be addressed under the medical home concept.

The Medical Home

A key concept of the Medicaid expansion is the creation of medical homes, or health homes. This approach to health-care delivery will allow for better identification and management of patients with certain diseases. Rather than providing only primary care, medical homes are designed to reduce the overall costs accrued by individuals who have been diagnosed with a chronic condition. Chronic illnesses have been identified as those that are most costly to the health-care system. It is likely that the medical home approach will be beneficial to management of HIV and other communicable diseases such as TB, hepatitis, and STIs. Studies are needed, however, to measure the effectiveness of the approach.

Implementation of Health-Care Reform

Currently, the PPACA lacks clarity; there has been a great deal of confusion regarding how to implement the program. While some states have nearly completed full implementation, including the installment of data collection systems, methods of enrollment, and other logistical challenges, other states have not yet begun the process. Presently, there is an active lawsuit representing twenty-six states and the National Federation of Independent Businesses, claiming the following infringements by the federal law:

- It is unconstitutional to require all citizens and legal residents to have qualifying health-care coverage or pay a tax penalty: By imposing such a mandate, the law exceeds the powers of the United States under Article I of the Constitution. Additionally, the tax penalty required under the law constitutes an unlawful direct tax in violation of Article I, Sections 2 and 9 of the Constitution.

- The health-care reform law infringes upon the sovereignty of the states and the Tenth Amendment to the Constitution. The law imposes onerous new operating rules that states must follow, and requires the states to spend billions of additional dollars without providing funds or resources to meet the states' cost of implementing the law. This burden comes at a time when states face severe budget cuts to offset shortfalls in already strained budgets.

A federal judge in Florida ruled that it is not unconstitutional to require all citizens and legal residents to have health-care coverage. However, the ruling on the requirement of states to pay any additional funding to meet the federal mandate is still pending, and will go to the U.S. Supreme Court in 2012 for a final decision (Office of the Attorney General of Florida, 2010).

National health-care coverage is closer to occurring in the United States than at any other time in the nation's history. The United States is one of the wealthiest nations in the world but does not provide for full national health-care coverage of its residents. Significant steps were made in 1965 with the introduction of the Medicaid and Medicare programs. Both Medicaid and Medicare, part of President Lyndon B. Johnson's set of Great Society domestic programs, remain as cornerstones in our nation's patchwork of health-care programs. The Clinton Administration's efforts to pursue national health-care legislation failed. The Obama Administration was able to pass health-care reform by a narrow margin in 2010. Implementation efforts have begun. This is a pivotal point in the nation's history, and social workers have an opportunity to lead the HIV and AIDS community through one of the most important reforms of this generation.

What About the Future of Ryan White Funding?

Utilization of the social determinants of health framework for care, political pursuit of the goals set forth in the NHAS and changes in coverage mandated by health-care reform will undoubtedly change the landscape of HIV and AIDS prevention, care, and treatment services. The Ryan White CARE Act expires on September 30, 2013, and the PPACA is slated to take full effect on January 1, 2014. While health-care reform is being implemented, many organizations and individuals have focused on sustaining the Ryan White CARE Act. The loss of funding for disease-specific conditions could mean that the growing demands on the HIV-specific care system will be merged with the larger health-care system. Yet, there will still be a need for a program such as Ryan White to provide emergency care to people who fall outside of other systems provided for by health-care reform. An example are undocumented residents with HIV, who will still not qualify for Medicaid benefits. Furthermore, many other supportive services needed by people living with HIV and AIDS are not delivered through the health-care system. Social workers in HIV and AIDS treatment and care roles will be very much interested to see if and how the CARE Act is reauthorized in 2013. Ideally, social workers should have a strong voice at the decision-making table.

Professional Association of Social Workers in HIV and AIDS

Over the past thirty years, social workers have played vital roles in HIV and AIDS prevention and care at micro, mezzo, and macro levels of intervention. Social workers are involved in policy, advocacy, program design, quality assurance, case management, medical case management, chemical dependency, mental health, housing, and many other issues. In 1988, Boston College organized a conference that merged the HIV/AIDS community with social workers. This conference has been held every year since in various cities across the United States, and there are typically 300 to 600 attendees each year.

Over the years, conference attendees and leaders have had discussions about the development of a professional association for social work in HIV and AIDS care. Two physician-related organizations focusing on HIV/AIDS support—the American Academy of HIV Medicine and the HIV Medical Association—have been in place for a number of years. The Association of Nurses in AIDS Care is another organization, though it was not established until May 2010. Dr. Vincent Lynch, the organizer of the annual national conference, approached key colleagues regarding the formation of a professional organization. Dr. Lynch asked them to facilitate a discussion with consistent conference attendees and other key players in order to determine the level of interest in launching a national association for social workers in HIV/AIDS care. The group decided to organize a committee to investigate the formation of what would be referred to as the Professional Association of Social Workers in HIV and AIDS (PASWHA).

In 2010, a national web-based survey collected 1,100 responses regarding the formation of an association of this group of professionals. More than 80 percent of the respondents indicated that they would join if such an organization existed. With the overwhelming positive support, a small group submitted an application for a 501(c) status and PASWHA was established. There are now more than three hundred PASWHA members involved in national advocacy. The board of directors of PASWHA undertake a multitude of other activities, on behalf of its members. (Visit www.paswha.us for more information on the professional organization.)

The formation of a national nonprofit professional organization in difficult economic times seems counterintuitive. However, social workers will be instrumental in determining the outcomes of health-care reform and the implementation of the NHAS. The formation of a national organization to support social workers who serve those with HIV and AIDS will ensure focused advocacy and care for people who confront stigma, poverty, discrimination, and a disproportionate exposure to chronic communicable diseases. Many social workers already play a vital role in HIV and AIDS prevention, treatment, and care, and they need the support of a larger group to continue to improve their interventions and advance advocacy efforts.

Questions for Reflection

1. Is it appropriate to allocate 70 percent of funding to twelve cities representing 44 percent of the nation's AIDS cases?

    a. Take into account HIV infections.

    b. Consider the loss to areas not in the twelve cities.

    c. Include the view that an increase in resources could mean reduced infections.

    d. Consider whether this number reflects a moral decision.

2. If you were to design a state response to HIV, where would the area of focus be?

    a. Expansion of Ryan White Program.

    b. Medicaid expansion.

    c. Multiple private plans in the health insurance exchange.

    d. State funding.

    e. The use of federal funds that flow to states.

3. How would you ensure that consumers (people living with HIV or AIDS) were involved in all policy decisions? How would this differ at federal, state, and local levels?

4. Is HIV exceptionalism over?

    a. If it is, should it be? Will the end of exceptionalism be better long term for individuals with HIV?

    b. If it isn't, why not?

    c. Imagine that your career does not involve work on policy development or implementation. How would you engage those working in the policy sector? What might you contribute to the process? Is any social work professional truly disengaged from policy work?

5. Peter Piot, the former executive director of Joint United Nations Programme on HIV/AIDS (UNAIDS), stated the following: "It does not make good sense to merge AIDS completely into the broader health or development agendas to the

point where it comes just one target or element of those agendas. . . . The fundamental drivers of the epidemic would not be tackled with any sense of emergency, making a sustained response an illusion. . . . If we agree to surrender the exceptionality of AIDS, we will come to regret our decision" (Piot, 2006, p. 530).

a. Imagine you met Dr. Piot at an AIDS conference. How would you respond to his assertion to work to maintain HIV and AIDS exceptionalism?

b. Do you think that AIDS exceptionalism is viewed as more or less important globally, as opposed to domestically?

c. How important do you think global policies on AIDS are in shaping policies in the United States?

References

AIDS.gov. (2011). *National HIV/AIDS Strategy.* U.S. Department of Health and Human Services (DHHS). Retrieved from http://www.aids.gov/federal-resources/policies/national-hiv-aids-strategy/

Centers for Disease Control and Prevention (CDC). (2009). *HIV/AIDS statistics and surveillance: Basic Statistics.* Retrieved from http://www.cdc.gov/hiv/topics/surveillance/basic.htm#ddaids

Centers for Disease Control and Prevention. (2010). *Establishing a holistic framework to reduce inequities in HIV, viral hepatitis, STDs, and tuberculosis in the United States: An NCHHSTP White Paper on social determinants of health.* Retrieved from http://www.cdc.gov/socialdeterminants/docs/SDH-White-Paper-2010.pdf

Communities Advocating Emergency AIDS Relief Coalition. (2011). *FY 2011 Ryan White Program Appropriations.* Retrieved from http://www.caear.org/about/appropriations.cfm

Denver Principles. (1983). *The Denver Principles of 1983.* Retrieved from http://data.unaids.org/pub/ExternalDocument/2007/gipa1983denverprinciples_en.pdf

Gellman, B. (2000, April 30). AIDS is declared threat to security. *The Washington Post.*

Health Resources and Services Administration (HRSA). (2011). *Ryan White HIV/AIDS Program Part A, Part B and ADAP Emergency Relief FY 2011 Awards.* U.S. Department of Health and Human Services (DHHS), Health Resources and Services Administration (HRSA). Retrieved from http://www.hrsa.gov/about/news/2011tables/110926hivaids.html#FinalPartA

Health Resources and Services Administration (HRSA) HIV/AIDS Bureau. (2011). *About the Ryan White HIV/AIDS Program.* U.S. Department of Health and Human Services (DHHS), Health Resources and Services Administration (HRSA). Retrieved from http://hab.hrsa.gov/abouthab/aboutprogram.html

Kaiser Family Foundation. (2009). *HIV/AIDS policy: Fact sheet. The Ryan White Program.* Retrieved from http://www.kff.org/hivaids/upload/7582_05.pdf

Kaiser Family Foundation. (2010). *AIDS Drug Assistance Programs (ADAP) formularies, number of medications by drug class, as of December 31, 2009.* Retrieved from http://www.statehealthfacts.org/comparetable.jsp?ind=551&cat=11

National AIDS Housing Coalition (NAHC). (2008). *HIV/AIDS Housing: Improving health outcomes.* Retrieved from http://www.hivhousing summit.org/BriefingBook/NAHCOneSheets_final_health_rev-2.pdf

National AIDS Housing Coalition (NAHC). (2011). *National AIDS Housing Policy.* Retrieved from http://nationalaidshousing.org/policy-toolkit/the-tools/

National Alliance of State and Territorial AIDS Directors (NASTAD). (2011). *ADAP Crisis Task Force.* Retrieved from http://www.nastad.org/Docs/022152_ADAP%20Crisis%20Task%20Force%20Fact%20Sheet%20-%20April%202011.pdf

National Institutes of Health (NIH). (2011, May 12). Treating HIV-infected people with antiretrovirals protects partners from infection: Findings result from NIH-funded international study. *NIH News.* Retrieved from http://www.niaid.nih.gov/news/newsreleases/2011/pages/hptn052.aspx

Office of AIDS Policy. (2011). *Implementing the National HIV/AIDS Strategy: Overview of agency operational plans.* Retrieved from http://www.aids.gov/federal-resources/policies/national-hiv-aids-strategy/nhas-operational-plan-overview.pdf

Office of National AIDS Policy. (2011). *The National HIV/AIDS Strategy.* The White House, President Barack Obama. Retrieved from http://www.white house.gov/administration/eop/onap/nhas

Office of the Attorney General of Florida. (2010). *The states' lawsuit challenging the constitutionality of the health care reform law.* Retrieved from http://www.healthcarelawsuit.us

Piot, P. (2006). AIDS: From crisis management to sustained strategic response. *Lancet, 368,* 526–530.

Preston, J. (2009, October 30). *Obama lifts a ban on entry into the U.S. by HIV-positive people. The New York Times.* Retrieved from http://www.nytimes .com/2009/10/31/us/politics/31travel.html

Rowan, D., & Honeycutt, J. (2010). The impact of the Ryan White Treatment Modernization Act on social work within the field of HIV/AIDS service provision. *Health & Social Work, 35*(1), 71–74.

U.S. Department of Housing and Urban Development (HUD). (2010). *Housing Opportunities for Persons with AIDS (HOPWA).* Retrieved from http://www.azhousing.gov/azcms/uploads/SPECIAL%20NEEDS/HOPWA FactSheet2011.pdf

Wolitski, R.J., Kidder, D.P., Pals, S.L., Royal, S., Aidala, A., Stall, R., . . . , and for the Housing and Health Study Team. (2010). Randomized trial of the effects of housing assistance on the health and risk behaviors of homeless and unstably housed people living with HIV. *AIDS and Behavior, 14*(3), 493–503.

Timeline: HIV, AIDS, and Social Work

1930s
: Scientists determined the virus that causes AIDS probably transferred to humans in the Congo region of Africa during the 1930s.

1945–1955
: The polio epidemic in the United States kills 20,000 people.

1970s
: HIV, which was an unknown virus at the time, was probably being transmitted among the first people with HIV in the United States.

December 1980
: First cases of "new pneumonia" reported.

June 5, 1981
: CDC (Centers for Disease Control) publish in *Morbidity and Mortality Weekly Report* the first reports of a rare pneumonia affecting five gay men in Los Angeles, followed by the first cases of Kaposi's sarcoma in New York.

July 3, 1981
: *New York Times* reports on forty-one cases of Kaposi's sarcoma affecting gay men in New York and California.

Fall 1981
: The term "gay cancer" emerges; there are 108 cases of the "homosexual disorder" reported nationwide.

November 1981
: The term GRID appears, standing for Gay-related Immune Deficiency: there are two hundred cases of GRID reported by year's end. The CDC warn it is reaching "epidemic proportions."

December 1981
: There are 12 cases of PCP (pneumocystis carinii pneumonia) in San Francisco, and 108 cases nationwide.

: Nine people have died of PCP by year's end.

March 1982
: The first transfusion-related case of GRID is identified, and concerns about the safety of the blood supply begin.

Mid 1982
: San Francisco budgets $180,000 to combat new disease.

: The syndrome is named AIDS (acquired immune deficiency syndrome).

: San Francisco AIDS Foundation is established.

July 1982   The CDC says the syndrome is an epidemic because cases are doubling every six months.

December 1982   First hemophiliac cases are reported, with a connection to the U.S. blood supply suspected.

                 First AIDS hotline opens in New York City.

                 First AIDS cases are reported in Africa.

Early 1983   Total number of people living with AIDS (PLWA) nationally is 1,112; total number of people living with AIDS in San Francisco is 176.

                 The term ARC (AIDS-related complex) emerges.

May 1983   Scientists in France and the United States conclude that the cause of AIDS is a retrovirus.

                 President Ronald Reagan says the word "AIDS."

Summer 1983   CDC establishes first AIDS case definition.

October 1983   The city of San Francisco closes all gay bathhouses.

Late 1983   People with AIDS Bill of Rights created in Denver by first national gathering of people living with AIDS (called The Denver Principles).

                 Federal AIDS budget climbs to $4.3 million.

                 First San Franciscan woman is diagnosed with AIDS.

                 There have been a total of 826 AIDS cases reported in San Francisco; of those, 369 have already died.

April 1984   Dr. Robert Gallo isolates a retrovirus his team calls HTLV-III, later to be called HIV (human immunodeficiency virus). They argue with a team in France, headed by Dr. Luc Montagnier, who separately identifies the same virus his team called LAV.

July 1984   *Time* magazine marks first major coverage of AIDS in a mainstream periodical.

February 1985	Blood banks begin testing donated blood as the Food and Drug Administration (FDA) approves the first test.
March 1985	ELISA, the first HIV antibody test kit, is licensed for public use.
May 1985	AZT (azidothymidine), an early antiretroviral medication, is approved for use by the FDA.
	In the United States, $106.5 million is spent on AIDS research.
June 1985	First International AIDS Conference is held in Atlanta, GA.
October 1985	Rock Hudson dies of AIDS.
November 1985	First TV movie about AIDS airs, *An Early Frost.*
Late 1985	There are 13,000 people living with AIDS in the United States.
	AIDS has been reported in fifty-one countries, including China.
1986	Ninety-one percent of all U.S. insurance companies deny coverage to HIV-positive individuals.
April 1986	Every fourteen hours, a San Franciscan dies of AIDS.
June 1986	Ryan White, a ten-year-old boy with hemophilia and with HIV, appears in the media.
Late 1986	The CDC announces that universal precautions are required in all hospitals and blood-related environments.
January 1987	Statistics suggest 50 percent of all HIV-positive cases will progress to AIDS.
June 1987	ACT-UP (AIDS Coalition to Unleash Power) is founded in New York City by playwright and activist Larry Kramer to end the AIDS crisis by direct action. The slogan SILENCE = DEATH is born.
	The Pope hugs a person with AIDS.
	Pianist Valentino Liberace dies of AIDS.
July 1987	After four years in office, President Ronald Reagan publicly addresses AIDS for the first time.

August 1987	The AIDS Quilt, a product of The Names Project, founded by AIDS activist Cleve Jones, goes to Washington, DC.
January 1988	The average life span for a White person with AIDS is two years; for a Black person with AIDS it is nineteen weeks.
April 1988	Greg Louganis, who secretly knew he was HIV positive, hits his head on a diving board during the Olympics, requiring stitches.
August 1988	Studies say AZT delays onset of AIDS.
	ACT-UP successfully pressures the FDA to speed up the drug approval process.
December 1988	The World Health Organization (WHO) institutes World AIDS Day to be held every December 1.
January 1989	Dr. Lorraine Day, San Francisco surgeon, claims AIDS is airborne.
May 1989	ACT-UP New York disrupts services at St. Patrick's Cathedral in New York, making international headlines.
June 1990	Ryan White dies at age eighteen.
July 1990	The Americans with Disabilities Act includes people with HIV/AIDS.
	Ryan White CARE Act is inaugurated.
Late 1990	There are 154,917 people with AIDS in the United States; 95,774 others have died.
Early 1991	The CDC estimate 1 million U.S. HIV infections; the World Health Organization (WHO) estimates 10 million worldwide.
Mid 1991	Musician Freddy Mercury of the rock band Queen dies of AIDS.
Late 1991	NBA player Magic Johnson announces he is HIV positive. Karl Malone speaks out against having to play basketball with him.
	Kimberley Bergalis, one of several patients who claimed to have been infected with HIV after visiting a dentist who tested HIV

	positive, dies. Mandatory testing for all health-care workers is debated as a result of her accusations.
	The red ribbon introduced as the international symbol of AIDS awareness at the Tony Awards in New York City.
June 1992	Tennis professional Arthur Ashe confirms he has AIDS.
Late 1992	Robert Reed, the actor who played the father on *The Brady Bunch*, dies of AIDS.
November 1992	President Bill Clinton is elected, stating that the first order of business is AIDS, and recommends sizable increases in Ryan White CARE Act funding.
October 1993	The 9th International AIDS Conference in Berlin reports that a vaccine or cure may never be found.
February 1994	Prophylactic treatment with AZT becomes the standard of care to avoid perinatal HIV transmission.
March 1994	First issue of *POZ Magazine* is published.
	Actor Tom Hanks wins an Oscar for portraying a gay man with AIDS in the film *Philadelphia*.
Early 1995	Olympian Greg Louganis discloses he has HIV.
	Joint United Nations Programme on AIDS (UNAIDS) is established.
April 1995	Total number of panels in the AIDS Quilt: 30,704. Size of the Quilt: 13 acres.
	The CDC announce that AIDS has become the leading cause of death among Americans aged twenty-five to forty-four years old.
August 1995	The first protease inhibitor anti-retroviral medication is approved by the FDA (Saquinavir).
	Rapper Easy-E dies of AIDS.
March 1996	The FDA approves the first viral load test, the p-24 antigen assay.

May 1996	Triple combination therapy becomes the standard of care for anti-retroviral use.
	Scientists discover that HIV hides in reservoirs in the body, making a total elimination of the virus much more elusive than thought.
June 1996	Dr. David Ho reports on "Hit hard, hit early" at the Eleventh International AIDS Conference.
	Oral collection (OraSure) for HIV antibody test is approved by the FDA.
October 1996	The AIDS Quilt is displayed in its entirety for the last time. The Clintons come to see it, a presidential first. Cleve Jones advocates to President Clinton for more funding.
November 1996	Worldwide death toll is 6.4 million. Worldwide number of people living with HIV is estimated to be 22.6 million.
	Congress passes a law to discharge all military personnel living with HIV, currently more than 1,000 individuals. The provision is later repealed.
Mid 1997	Unexpected side effects seen with new protease inhibitor AIDS drugs: the protease paunch, buffalo hump, and other forms of lipodystrophy.
Early 1998	AIDS deaths in the United States drop by 47 percent.
August 1998	*Bay Area Reporter* headlines, "No Obituaries," which was the first time since 1982.
December 1998	AIDS is the leading cause of death in Africa and kills more people worldwide than any other infectious disease.
November 1999	The federal government tells states they must track HIV infection, by name or code.
November 2000	Needle Stick Safety and Prevention Act is signed by President Clinton, a law requiring all medical facilities to use safe syringes and blood drawing devices.

June 2001	There are 320,282 people with AIDS in the United States; 438,795 others have died. The CDC estimate that one-third of all Americans who have HIV don't know it. The CDC estimate that 31 million have HIV worldwide, with the majority in Africa.
	Fuzeon, the first entry inhibitor ARV, is released amid great optimism.
February 2002	Dr. Anthony Fauci of the CDC reports HIV rates ten times higher in the African-American community compared to other ethnic groups.
June 2002	One in four new infections in the United States is estimated to occur among people under the age of twenty.
	UNAIDS reports that about half of all adults living with HIV/ AIDS worldwide are women.
April 2003	The OraQuick Rapid HIV Antibody Test becomes available in California. Clients can now receive their HIV test results in twenty minutes instead of one to two weeks.
2004	Kofi Annan, secretary general of the United Nations, compares the war on terror with the war on AIDS.
	President George W. Bush launches a major initiative, PEPFAR (President's Emergency Program for AIDS Relief) to combat AIDS worldwide.
2005	The WHO, UNAIDS, the U.S. government, and the Global Fund to Fight AIDS announce results of joint efforts to increase anti-retroviral drugs in developing countries. An estimated 700,000 people have been reached by the end of 2004.
	Failed research shows that an HIV vaccine is still years away. Medication advances continue but long-term side effects of ARV are becoming more evident.
2006	Circumcision is shown to reduce HIV infection among hetero-sexual men.
	Experts conclude HIV had its origins in the rainforest of the Congo in Africa in wild chimpanzees. Evidence suggests the

simian form of HIV (SIV) entered the human species through ape bites or through people eating chimpanzee meat or brains.

2007   WHO and UNAIDS recommend that male circumcision should always be considered as part of a comprehensive HIV-prevention package.

2008   Controversial Swiss study claims people adhering to their HIV medications have a small risk of transmitting HIV through unprotected sex.

Dr. Luc Montagnier of France is awarded the Nobel Prize for discovering HIV in 1984, much to the dismay of Dr. Robert Gallo of the United States.

2009   Newly elected U.S. President Barack Obama calls for the first-ever National HIV/AIDS Strategy (NHAS). The White House releases the strategy in July 2010.

On December 18, 2009, the U.S. Congress eliminates long-standing ban on the use of federal funding for needle exchange in the United States.

2010   January 4, 2010, United States lifts its travel ban for people with HIV. South Korea, China, and Namibia do the same.

On March 23, 2010, President Obama signs the Patient Protection and Affordable Care Act (PPACA) into law, signaling the most significant health-care reform in the United States since the 1960s. Medicaid expansion is expected to provide health coverage to many people living with HIV and AIDS that are not covered under current rules.

The Centre for the AIDS Programme of Research in South Africa (CAPRISA) 004 microbicide trial is hailed a success after results show the gel reduces the risk of HIV infection by 40 percent.

Results from the iPrEx trial (Preexposure prophylaxis initiative) show a reduction in HIV acquisition among men who have sex with men taking PrEP (preexposure prophylaxis). The study is named Scientific Breakthrough of the Year by *Time* magazine.

The CDC release reports that they advocate for an approach to reduction of communicable diseases (such as HIV) that considers environmental factors, called social determinants of health. This approach is directly in line with the social work perspective of the person-in-environment, which has been embraced and followed by the profession since the 1980s.

2010   Professional Association of Social Workers in HIV and AIDS (PASWHA) is formed.

2011   On December 1, World AIDS Day, President Obama announces intent to provide anti-retroviral medications to 6 million people around the world, an increase of over 2 million people. He reports a commitment to ending the AIDS pandemic "once and for all."

On May 12, 2011, the HIV Prevention Trial Network releases results of Clinical Trial 052, which found that immediate use of anti-retroviral medication following HIV diagnosis reduced the transmission of HIV in sero-discordant couples by 96 percent. The study provides scientific evidence that "treatment is prevention."

2012   The CDC release a report that shows that poorer men, men who were recently released from prison, and young Black men have higher rates of high-risk sexual behaviors than other populations.

2013   The last reauthorization of the legislation for the Ryan White HIV/AIDS Program (called the Ryan White Treatment Extension Act of 2009) is due to sunset in 2013. It is not an entitlement program and therefore its budget line is subject to Congressional discretionary spending decisions.

Sources: This timeline is assembled from content presented in the following sources, combined with original content.

About.com. (2009). The history of HIV/AIDS. Retrieved from http://aids.about.com/od/newly diagnosed/a/hivtimeline_2.htm

AIDS.gov. (2012). A timeline of AIDS. Retrieved from http://aids.gov/hiv-aids-basics/hiv-aids-101/overview/aids-timeline/

AVERT. (2011). AIDS timeline. Retrieved from http://www.avert.org/aids-timeline.htm

Black AIDS Institute. (2006). *AIDS in blackface*. Los Angeles: Author.

Contributors

Meredith Bagwell, MSW

Meredith Bagwell graduated from University of Texas at Austin School of Social Work in May 2009. She joined Michele Rountree's research team because of her passion for addressing the HIV/AIDS crisis. One particular area of research interest is the correlation between risk for HIV infection and women's experiences of intimate partner abuse. Bagwell intends to continue using her talents for research and writing to increase knowledge and prevention of HIV/AIDS.

Russell L. Bennett, PhD, LGSW

Rusty Bennett is founding executive director of Collaborative Solutions, Inc., a nonprofit consulting firm based in Birmingham, Alabama, delivering national technical assistance on housing and supportive services for populations with special needs. Bennett has more than fifteen years of experience in the federal government and nonprofit sectors on programs, policies, and research related to the housing and services for low-income persons living with HIV/AIDS. Bennett served as presidential management intern at the U.S. Department of Housing and Urban Development and holds a doctor of philosophy degree in social work, with an emphasis in housing and community development, from The University of Alabama.

Mary Boudreau, LMSW, RN

Mary Boudreau has worked with people with HIV for more than eighteen years, first as a social worker and now, after returning to school, as a nurse. She works as an infectious disease nurse in the health departments for two counties. Currently, Boudreau is studying at the University of Michigan at Flint to be a nurse practitioner. She has trained numerous social work students and is teaching nursing at Lansing Community College. She recently collaborated on a research project piloting an adolescent sex health history assessment instrument. Her other interests include vocal music, biking, and soccer.

Lisa E. Cox, PhD, LCSW, MSW

Lisa Cox is associate professor of social work and gerontology at The Richard Stockton College of New Jersey, and associate fellow with the University of Pennsylvania's Institute on Aging. She has worked in the field of HIV/AIDS for more than twenty-five years. Through the 1990s she was a pioneering AIDS clinical trial social worker with the Terry Beirn Community Programs for Clinical Research on AIDS (CPCRA) Richmond AIDS Consortium, a program funded by the National Institutes of Health (NIH). She has published numerous peer-reviewed and empirically based journal articles on HIV adherence, and has presented nationally and internationally. Cox regularly teaches a college-level HIV/AIDS seminar course, and serves on the National Advisory Board of National Association of Social Workers (NASW-DC) HIV/AIDS Spectrum Project.

Jeff Driskell, PhD, LICSW

Jeff Driskell is assistant professor at Salem State University in the School of Social Work, and holds a doctor of philosophy degree from Boston College. Driskell has worked in direct HIV-related services for more than ten years. During this time, he has provided both care and prevention services to individuals living with HIV/AIDS. Driskell spent more than five years as a member of a research team at The Fenway Institute, the largest provider of care and prevention needs related to lesbian, gay, bisexual, and transgender (LGBT) individuals in the United States. While at Fenway, he helped develop and implement a five-year study targeting HIV-infected gay and bisexual men. His research focused on prevention tailored to the needs of HIV-infected gay and bisexual men. More specifically, his research addresses the challenges of HIV disclosure and sexual risk behavior. More recently, his service and research efforts have been centered on the needs of gay and lesbian elders. In collaboration with Boston College Graduate School of Social Work, Driskell has been co-planner for the Annual National Social Work Conference on HIV/AIDS for the past nine years.

Kevin Edwards, MSW

Kevin Edwards holds a master of social work (MSW) degree from the University of North Carolina at Charlotte. He currently works as an HIV case manager for the Mecklenburg County Health Department in Charlotte, North Carolina. He is also adjunct instructor in the human services program at Mitchell Community College. Edwards has worked in the field of HIV and AIDS for twenty-five years. He has provided direct services to persons living with HIV and AIDS and worked as director of client services for an AIDS service organization (ASO). His social work experiences involve HIV, mental health, and the homeless population. He has co-authored a professional article on social work with Latinos who are living with

HIV/AIDS. He enjoys spending time with his life partner, Jeffery, and their two dogs, Shadow and Makiah.

Terry W. Ellington, BA

Terry Ellington is executive director of Carolinas CARE Partnership, a nonprofit AIDS service organization (ASO) that administers housing programs for people living with HIV/AIDS, HIV prevention and counseling and testing programs, and coordinates community action efforts. Ellington has more than thirty years of experience in working on affordable housing issues that includes supervision at a housing counseling agency approved by the U.S. Department of Housing and Urban Development (HUD). In addition, Ellington has served on national, local, and state boards and committees that address homelessness issues. Ellington has conducted numerous presentations around the country on implementing best practices for developing housing resources for people living with HIV/AIDS. Ellington has a bachelor of arts degree in English from the University of North Carolina at Charlotte and has received many training certificates from entities such as the Centers for Disease Control and Prevention (CDC) and HUD.

Maestro A. Evans, DCC, MSW, LCSW

Maestro Evans has a broad range of experience in working with HIV/AIDS direct service and prevention programs. Evans' work tenure includes working eight years for the Centers for Disease Control and Prevention (CDC) as a health education specialist, where he works as a leader in the development of national trainings and HIV-prevention interventions as well as project officer for capacity building assistance providers. He has worked for eight years at AID Atlanta, Inc., the Southeast's largest AIDS service organization (ASO) where he was responsible for the development, implementation, evaluation, and management of all services provided to persons who are living with and affected by HIV/AIDS in the Atlanta area. Evans has also served as a clinician at Anchor Hospital, CHRIS Homes, Georgia Department of Pardons and Parole, and North DeKalb Mental Health Center. He is the CEO of Spiritus Counseling Consultants, Inc. In addition to his noted professional achievements, he received a doctor of Christian counseling degree from Pillsbury College and Seminary, a master of social work degree from Clark Atlanta University, and a bachelor of arts degree in speech communication from the University of Georgia. He is a licensed clinical social worker in the state of Georgia, and licensed as a clinical Christian counselor by the National Christian Counselors Association.

Kimi Fey-Powers, PA-C, MSW

Kimi Fey-Powers started her work in the HIV/AIDS field as an AmeriCorps member at an AIDS service organization (ASO) in Charlotte, North Carolina. She helped newly diagnosed clients navigate services including Medicaid, Medicare Part D, and AIDS Drug Assistance Program (ADAP) as well as support groups and food pantries. While earning her master of social work degree, she performed HIV testing and counseling as a community health educator. Inspired by the caring in the HIV/AIDS medical community, Fey-Powers decided to become a physician assistant. She now practices in a neighborhood clinic in Portland, Oregon.

Susan E. Grettenberger, PhD, LMSW, MPA

Susan Grettenberger is currently social work program director and associate professor at Central Michigan University in Mt. Pleasant, Michigan. She has served as an HIV program evaluator for the state of Michigan, conducted program evaluation with HIV programs, and volunteered with HIV-affected individuals. She presents regularly about spirituality in social work and researches the role of faith-based organizations in social services. Grettenberger's work with HIV and AIDS is an integral part of her understanding that social work is a community-based, social justice–focused profession.

Lamont C. Holley

Lamont C. Holley was born in the mountains of Staunton, Virginia. After graduating from Johnson C. Smith University, a historically Black college/university (HBCU) in Charlotte, North Carolina, he worked in banking for more than a decade before deciding to change careers to pursue his passion for social work. Holley has worked with people living with HIV and AIDS and done HIV and AIDS prevention work since 1999. Currently, he works with the Mecklenburg County Health Department in Charlotte as an access coordinator, connecting people living with HIV and AIDS to care and doing psychosocial support. He is currently a master of social work student at the University of North Carolina at Charlotte. Holley enjoys spending time outdoors, cooking, doing artistic crafts, exercising, and spending time with the love of his life, Panda Jane, his Boston Terrier.

Vincent J. Lynch, PhD, MSW

Vincent Lynch is director of continuing education at Boston College Graduate School of Social Work in Chestnut Hill, Massachusetts. He has served in that position since December 1986. He holds a master of social work degree from Boston University and a doctor of philosophy degree from Boston College. He has expertise in developing and delivering workshops on varied clinical social work topics such as empathy in psychotherapeutic relationships, psychopharmacology, motivational interviewing, case management, trauma, services to older adults, and therapy for couples and families. Lynch also founded (and continues to chair) the Annual National Conference on Social Work and HIV/AIDS, now in its twenty-fourth year. This four-day conference on HIV/AIDS psychosocial issues is held in a different city across the country each year and draws more than 500 HIV/AIDS social workers annually. Since 1988, he has obtained more than $1 million in grants, contracts, and gifts from governmental and corporate sources to support the ongoing work of this conference. Awards presented to Lynch in recognition of his HIV/AIDS educational work include the Distinguished Recent Contributions Award of the Council on Social Work Education (1998), The Harlem Life Award (1998), and the National Association of Social Workers Massachusetts Chapter's Greatest Contribution to Social Work Education Award (2001). He has edited (and coedited) four books that address HIV/AIDS social work issues.

Alan Rice, MSW, LCSW

Alan Rice has been co-director of social work and case management for the Center for Comprehensive Care at St. Luke's–Roosevelt Hospital in New York City since July 2005. Rice has been providing social work service to the HIV and AIDS population since 1983. He was selected as one of the first dedicated HIV hospital social workers while at Beth Israel Medical Center and helped establish early HIV and AIDS policies for the hospital, New York City, and the nation. Rice is adjunct professor at the Wurzweiler School of Social Work at Yeshiva University where he teaches courses on substance abuse and HIV and AIDS. He continues to remain involved on the national scene of HIV and AIDS and is president of the Professional Association for Social Workers in HIV and AIDS (PASWHA).

Michele A. Rountree, PhD, MSW

Michele A. Rountree is associate professor with University of Texas at Austin School of Social Work. Her scholarship focuses on the areas of health promotion, disease prevention, and health disparities as they relate to meeting the needs of marginalized populations. Much of her research has involved the examination of HIV/AIDS risk reduction interventions for women who have experienced intimate partner abuse. In addition, her scholarship efforts include the development and evaluation of evidence-based HIV/AIDS interventions and prevention strategies tailored to populations with alarming incidence rates, such as African-American and Latina women.

Diana Rowan, PhD, MSW, LCSW

Diana Rowan is assistant professor of social work at the University of North Carolina at Charlotte. Her doctor of philosophy degree in social work is from the University of Texas at Arlington. She has a master of social work degree from Our Lady of the Lake University of San Antonio and a bachelor of science degree in recombinant gene technology from the State University of New York at Fredonia. Rowan is currently a Centers for Disease Control and Prevention (CDC) Minority AIDS Research Initiative (MARI) principal investigator for a four-year CDC-funded study on the use of social media as a mechanism for accessing young Black men who have sex with men (YBMSM) for HIV prevention. She has published on numerous topics related to HIV prevention and care with at-risk communities, including the house/ball community. She has direct social work practice experience as a psychotherapist working with multiple areas of focus including HIV and AIDS, substance abuse, anxiety and depression, sexual therapy, Christian counseling, and supervision for social work clinical licensure. Rowan's teaching focuses on advanced practice with individuals and groups, and she has taught an elective course on social work with HIV and AIDS numerous times. Rowan has traveled and worked extensively in numerous countries of southeastern Africa, conducted funded cross-cultural research in Sub-Saharan Africa on HIV stigma, and taught a service-learning-oriented social work study abroad course in Malawi. She is president of Mu Chapter of Phi Beta Delta Honor Society for International Scholars and coauthor of *An Experiential Approach to Group Work*.

Randall H. Russell, MSW, LASW

Randall Russell has served in the HIV community for thirty years as a volunteer, leader of AIDS service organizations (ASOs), advocate, and technical assistance provider for the Centers for Disease Control and Prevention (CDC), the Health Resources and Services Administration's (HRSA) Ryan White Program, and the U.S. Department of Housing and Urban Development's (HUD) special needs housing program. He has also served as founder of the Professional Association of Social Work in HIV and AIDS (PASWHA), the Southern AIDS Coalition, and Collaborative Solutions. He has also served as president of the National AIDS Housing Coalition. In 2011, Russell became the CEO of Lifelong AIDS Alliance in Seattle, Washington, where he strives to develop practical solutions for persons with HIV after the implementation of the Affordable Care Act in Washington state. Russell has been a successful grantee of HUD, HRSA, and the CDC at various times throughout his career. He is an avid social worker and hiker, and is a proud gay Eagle Scout.

Ayana Simon, MSW, P-LCSW

Ayana Simon is a social worker at Wake Forest Baptist Medical Center in Winston Salem, North Carolina. She earned a bachelor of science degree in Public Health Education from the University of North Carolina at Greensboro and a master of social work degree from the University of North Carolina at Charlotte. She is a certified health education specialist as well as a provisionally licensed clinical social worker in North Carolina. Simon is a member of the Phi Alpha National Social Work Honor Society and is of Baptist faith.

Rebecca Stamler, MA

Rebecca Stamler graduated from the University of North Carolina at Charlotte with a master of arts degree in counseling and a graduate certificate in substance abuse. She is a member of the Charlotte Transgender Healthcare Group. Her primary focus includes working with people with chemical dependency, people who identify as sexual minorities, and people with HIV and AIDS. Stamler has served as a volunteer with AIDS service organizations (ASOs) in Provincetown, Massachusetts, and Charlotte, North Carolina. She has volunteered at Time Out Youth in Charlotte, which serves lesbian, gay, bisexual, transgender, and questioning (LGBTQ) youth. Stamler has presented education sessions at several professional conferences, including the National Meeting of the American Counseling Association (ACA) and the TransFaith in Color Conference.

Marsha Zibalese-Crawford, DSW, MSW

Marsha Zibalese-Crawford is associate professor with a dual appointment in the School of Social Work, and the Geography and Urban Studies Department at Temple University. Zibalese-Crawford combines a focus on the needs of families and youth with a rich array of experience developing organizational partnerships in the community, both public and private. She has earned a national and international reputation on program evaluation, youth violence, at-risk youth, and substance abuse in community research, through the dissemination of research and applied research results at workshops at the local level, as well as at international, national, and regional conferences.

Index